Polysomnography

Guest Editors

LAWRENCE J. EPSTEIN, MD
DOUGLAS B. KIRSCH, MD

SLEEP MEDICINE CLINICS

www.sleep.theclinics.com

September 2009 • Volume 4 • Number 3

SAUNDERS an imprint of ELSEVIER, Inc.

W.B. SAUNDERS COMPANY
A Division of Elsevier Inc.

1600 John F. Kennedy Boulevard • Suite 1800 • Philadelphia, PA 19103-2899

http://www.sleep.theclinics.com

SLEEP MEDICINE CLINICS Volume 4, Number 3
September 2009, ISSN 1556-407X, ISBN-13: 978-1-4377-1273-5, ISBN-10: 1-4377-1273-8

Editor: Sarah E. Barth
Developmental Editor: Donald Mumford

Sleep Medicine Clinics (ISSN 1556-407X) is published quarterly by Elsevier, 360 Park Avenue South, New York, NY 10010. Months of issue are March, June, September and December. Application to mail at periodicals postage rates is pending at New York, NY and at additional mailing offices. Subscription prices are $150.00 per year (US individuals), $76.00 (US students), $339.00 (US institutions), $149.00 (Canadian individuals), $106.00 (Canadian students), $373.00 (Canadian institutions), $185.00 (foreign individuals), $106.00 (foreign students), and $373.00 (foreign institutions). Foreign air speed delivery is included in all *Clinics* subscription prices. All prices are subject to change without notice. **POSTMASTER:** Send change of address to *Sleep Medicine Clinics*, Elsevier Health Sciences Division, Subscription Customer Service, 3251 Riverport Lane, Maryland Heights, MO 63043 Customer Service (orders, claims, online, change of address): **Elsevier Health Sciences Division, Subscription Customer Service, 3251 Riverport Lane Maryland Heights, MO 63043 Tel: 1-800-654-2452 (U.S. and Canada); 314-447-8871 (outside U.S. and Canada). Fax: 314-447-8029. E-mail: journalscustomerservice-usa@elsevier.com (for print support); journalsonlinesupport-usa@elsevier.com (for online support).**

Reprints. For copies of 100 or more of articles in this publication, please contact the Commercial Reprints Department, Elsevier Inc., 360 Park Avenue South, New York, NY 10010-1710. Tel.: 212-633-3812; Fax: 212-462-1935; E-mail: reprints@elsevier.com.

Printed and bound in the United Kingdom
Transferred to Digital Print 2011

GOAL STATEMENT

The goal of *Sleep Clinics of North America* is to keep practicing physicians up to date with current clinical practice by providing timely articles reviewing the state of the art in patient care.

ACCREDITATION

The *Sleep Clinics of North America* is planned and implemented in accordance with the Essential Areas and Policies of the Accreditation Council for Continuing Medical Education (ACCME) through the joint sponsorship of the University of Virginia School of Medicine and Elsevier. The University of Virginia School of Medicine is accredited by the ACCME to provide continuing medical education for physicians.

The University of Virginia School of Medicine designates this educational activity for a maximum of 15 *AMA PRA Category 1 Credits*™ for each issue, 60 credits per year. Physicians should only claim credit commensurate with the extent of their participation in the activity.

The American Medical Association has determined that physicians not licensed in the US who participate in this CME activity are eligible for a maximum of 15 *AMA PRA Category 1 Credits*™ for each issue, 60 credits per year.

Credit can be earned by reading the text material, taking the CME examination online at: http://www.theclinics.com/home/cme, and completing the evaluation. After taking the test, you will be required to review any and all incorrect answers. Following completion of the test and evaluation, your credit will be awarded and you may print your certificate.

FACULTY DISCLOSURE/CONFLICT OF INTEREST

The University of Virginia School of Medicine, as an ACCME accredited provider, endorses and strives to comply with the Accreditation Council for Continuing Medical Education (ACCME) Standards of Commercial Support, Commonwealth of Virginia statutes, University of Virginia policies and procedures, and associated federal and private regulations and guidelines on the need for disclosure and monitoring of proprietary and financial interests that may affect the scientific integrity and balance of content delivered in continuing medical education activities under our auspices.

The University of Virginia School of Medicine requires that all CME activities accredited through this institution be developed independently and be scientifically rigorous, balanced and objective in the presentation/discussion of its content, theories and practices.

All authors/editors participating in an accredited CME activity are expected to disclose to the readers relevant financial relationships with commercial entities occurring within the past 12 months (such as grants or research support, employee, consultant, stock holder, member of speakers bureau, etc.). The University of Virginia School of Medicine will employ appropriate mechanisms to resolve potential conflicts of interest to maintain the standards of fair and balanced education to the reader. Questions about specific strategies can be directed to the Office of Continuing Medical Education, University of Virginia School of Medicine, Charlottesville, Virginia.

The faculty and staff of the University of Virginia Office of Continuing Medical Education have no financial affiliations to disclose.

The authors/editors listed below have identified no professional or financial affiliations for themselves or their spouse/partner:
Josna Adusumilli, MD; Sarah Barth (Acquisitions Editor); Suzanne E. Beck, MD; Cynthia Brown, MD (Test Author); Kelly A. Carden, MD, MBA; Alejandro Chediak, MD, FAASM, FACP, FACCP; Nancy A. Collop, MD; Maryann Deak, MD; Conrad Iber, MD; Douglas B. Kirsch, MD; Elise Maher, MA, RPSGT; Carole L. Marcus, MBBCh; Jahan Naghshin, MD; Michael H. Silber, MBChB; Kyuhyun Wang, MD; and, Rajive Zachariah, BA.

The authors/editors listed below identified the following professional or financial affiliations for themselves or their spouse/partner:
Lawrence J. Epstein, MD (Guest Editor) is employed by Sleep Health Centers.
Clete A. Kushida, MD, PhD is an industry funded research/investigator for XenoPort.
Teofilo Lee-Chiong, Jr., MD (Consulting Editor) is an independent contractor for NIH, Restore, Respironics, Schwarz Pharma, and Takeda, and is a consultant for Elsevier.
David T. Plante, MD's spouse owns stock in Pfizer.
Anil Natesan Rama, MD, MPH serves on the Speakers Bureau for Jazz Pharmaceutical and Cephalon.
Patrick Sorenson, MA is an industry funded research/investigator for Sleep Foundations.
Patrick J. Strollo, Jr., MD is an industry funded research/investigator for Respironics and ResMed.
David P. White, MD is employed by Respironics, Inc., and is a consultant for Itamar Medical, Aspire Medical, and PAVAD.
John W. Winkelman, MD, PhD serves on the Speaker's Bureau for Boehringer-Ingelheim, GlaxoSmithKline, Sanofi-Aventis, Sepracor, and Takeda, serves on the Advisory Board for Pfizer, GlaxoSmithKline, Schwarz-Pharma, Takeda, Boehringer-Ingelheim, and Novartis, and has received research support from GlaxoSmithKline, Boehringer-Ingelheim, Schwarz-Pharma, and Sepracor.

Disclosure of Discussion of Non-FDA Approved Uses for Pharmaceutical Products and/or Medical Devices.
The University of Virginia School of Medicine, as an ACCME provider, requires that all faculty presenters identify and disclose any off-label uses for pharmaceutical and medical device products. The University of Virginia School of Medicine recommends that each physician fully review all the available data on new products or procedures prior to clinical use.

TO ENROLL

To enroll in the Sleep Clinics of North America Continuing Medical Education program, call customer service at 1-800-654-2452 or visit us online at: www.theclinics.com/home/cme. The CME program is available to subscribers for an additional fee of $99.95.

Sleep Medicine Clinics

FORTHCOMING ISSUES

December 2009

Behavioral Sleep Medicine
Kenneth L. Lichstein, MD,
Guest Editor

March 2010

Dental Sleep Medicine
Dennis R. Bailey, MD,
Guest Editor

June 2010

Dreaming
James F. Pagel, MD,
Guest Editor

RECENT ISSUES

June 2009

Circadian Rhythm Sleep Disorders
Kenneth P. Wright, Jr., PhD,
Guest Editor

March 2009

Epidemiology of Sleep Disorders: Clinical Implications
Edward O. Bixler, PhD,
Guest Editor

December 2008

Respiratory Disorders and Sleep
Ulysses J. Magalang, MD,
Guest Editor

RELATED INTEREST

Child and Adolescent Psychiatric Clinics of North America, October 2009,
Vol. 18, No. 4
Child and Adolescent Sleep
Jess P. Shatkin, MD, MPH and Anna Ivanenko, MD, PhD, *Guest Editors*
www.medical.theclinics.com

THE CLINICS ARE NOW AVAILABLE ONLINE!

Access your subscription at:
www.theclinics.com

Contributors

CONSULTING EDITOR

TEOFILO LEE-CHIONG, Jr., MD
Head, Division of Sleep Medicine, National Jewish
Health; and Associate Professor of Medicine,
University of Colorado Denver School of Medicine,
Denver, Colorado

GUEST EDITORS

LAWRENCE J. EPSTEIN, MD
Instructor in Medicine, Division of Sleep Medicine,
Brigham and Women's Hospital, Harvard Medical
School, Boston, Massachusetts; Medical Director,
Sleep Health*Centers*, Brighton, Massachusetts

DOUGLAS KIRSCH, MD
Regional Medical Director, Sleep Health*Centers*,
Brighton, MA; Instructor in Medicine, Harvard
Medical School, Boston, Massachusetts

AUTHORS

JOSNA ADUSUMILLI, MD
Sleep Disorders Fellow, Brigham and Women's
Hospital, Boston, Massachusetts

SUZANNE E. BECK, MD
Associate Professor of Clinical Pediatrics,
Sleep Center, Division of Pulmonary Medicine,
Department of Pediatrics, The Children's
Hospital of Philadelphia, University of
Pennsylvania School of Medicine,
Philadelphia, Pennsylvania

KELLY A. CARDEN, MD, MBA
Medical Director, Sleep Centers of Middle
Tennessee, Sleep Center at StoneCrest,
Smyrna, Tennessee

NANCY A. COLLOP, MD
Associate Professor, Division of Pulmonary
and Critical Care Medicine, Department of
Medicine, Johns Hopkins University,
Baltimore, Maryland

**ALEJANDRO D. CHEDIAK, MD, FAASM,
FACP, FACCP**
Associate Professor of Medicine, University
of Miami at Mount Sinai Medical Center, Miami
Beach, Florida; Medical Director, Miami Sleep
Disorders Center, South Miami, Florida

MARYANN DEAK, MD
Clinical Fellow in Sleep Medicine, Division of Sleep
Medicine, Brigham and Women's Hospital,
Harvard Medical School, Boston, Massachusetts

LAWRENCE J. EPSTEIN, MD
Instructor in Medicine, Division of Sleep Medicine,
Brigham and Women's Hospital, Harvard Medical
School, Boston, Massachusetts; Medical Director,
Sleep Health*Centers*, Brighton, Massachusetts

CONRAD IBER, MD
Professor of Medicine, University
of Minnesota; Director of Pulmonary
and Critical Care Division, Department
of Medicine, Hennepin County Medical Center,
Minneapolis, Minnesota

DOUGLAS KIRSCH, MD
Regional Medical Director, Sleep Health*Centers*,
Brighton, MA; Instructor in Medicine,
Harvard Medical School, Boston,
Massachusetts

CLETE A. KUSHIDA, MD, PhD, RPSGT
Acting Medical Director, Stanford Sleep Disorders
Clinic, Standford, California; Director, Stanford
Center for Human Sleep Research, Palo Alto,
California; Associate Professor, Stanford
University Medical Center, Stanford Sleep
Medicine Center, Stanford, California

ELISE MAHER, MA, RPSGT
Sleep Health*Centers*, Medford,
Massachusetts

CAROLE L. MARCUS, MBBCh
Professor of Pediatrics; and Director, Sleep
Center, Division of Pulmonary Medicine,
Department of Pediatrics, The Children's
Hospital of Philadelphia, University of
Pennsylvania School of Medicine, Philadelphia,
Pennsylvania

JAHAN NAGHSHIN, MD
Sleep Fellow, University of Pittsburgh,
Pennsylvania

DAVID T. PLANTE, MD
Clinical Fellow in Sleep Medicine, Department
of Medicine, Brigham and Women's Hospital,
Harvard Medical School, Boston,
Massachusetts

ANIL NATESAN RAMA, MD, MPH
Medical Director, Division of Sleep Medicine,
The Permanente Medical Group, San Jose,
California

MICHAEL H. SILBER, MBChB
Professor of Neurology, Department of Neurology;
Co-director, Center for Sleep Medicine, Mayo
Clinic, Rochester, Minnesota

PATRICK SORENSON, MA
Technical Education Specialist, Division of Sleep
Medicine, Department of Neurology,
Massachusetts General Hospital, Boston,
Massachusetts; Adjunct Professor in
Polysomnographic Technology, Northern Essex
Community College, Lawrence, Massachusetts

PATRICK J. STROLLO, Jr., MD, FCCP, FAASM
Associate Professor of Medicine, Department of
Medicine; and Clinical and Translational Science;
and Medical Director, UPMC Sleep Medicine
Center, University of Pittsburgh, UPMC
Montefiore, Pittsburgh, Pennsylvania

KYUHYUN WANG, MD
Clinical Professor, Division of Cardiology,
Department of Medicine, University of Minnesota,
Minneapolis, Minnesota

DAVID P. WHITE, MD
Clinical Professor of Medicine, Division of Sleep
Medicine, Department of Medicine, Brigham and
Women's Hospital, Boston, Massachusetts;
Chief Medical Officer, Philips Respironics, Boston,
Massachusetts

JOHN W. WINKELMAN, MD, PhD
Assistant Professor of Psychiatry, Department
of Medicine, Divisions of Sleep Medicine and
Psychiatry, Brigham & Women's Hospital, Harvard
Medical School, Boston, Massachusetts; Medical
Director, Sleep Health Center®, Affiliated with
Brigham & Women's Hospital, Brighton,
Massachusetts

RAJIVE ZACHARIAH, BA
Tracy, California

Contents

Foreword   **xi**

Teofilo Lee-Chiong, Jr.

Preface   **xiii**

Lawrence J. Epstein and Douglas B. Kirsch

The History of Polysomnography   **313**

Maryann Deak and Lawrence J. Epstein

> Similar to the first anatomists or the first radiographers, sleep scientists and physicians used electroencephalography and later polysomnography as means of "peering in" to the workings of the human body with the hope of gaining understanding. The rapid advancement of sleep research, made possible by the development of polysomnography, permitted not only a deeper understanding of normal sleep, but a more complete picture of the pathologic processes that affect sleep. After 20 years, not only has polysomnography been fine-tuned as a research tool and vital diagnostic test, but it has also made possible the creation of a new medical specialty and a new allied health field.

Generating a Signal: Biopotentials, Amplifiers, and Filters   **323**

Patrick Sorenson

> Understanding the underlying science of the generation of electrophysiologic signals is necessary to monitor and interpret sleep studies accurately. There are many factors that can alter a signal observed on a polysomnogram. Armed with the knowledge of how an electrophysiologic signal is generated and recorded, those who study sleep and its disorders are expected to be able to separate true from artifactual signals, and know the difference between accurate signal data and unexpected alterations in these signals. At any step in the process the diagnostic accuracy of a polysomnogram may be altered or unreliable, which, if not detected and corrected, could adversely affect the care of the patient.

Recording Sleep: The Electrodes, 10/20 Recording System, and Sleep System Specifications   **333**

Kelly A. Carden

> The goal of this article is to review the current standards for monitoring and evaluating sleep and wake in clinical laboratory and research settings. The standard parameters used to record sleep and wake are electroencephalography, electrooculography, electromyography, airflow measurement, respiratory effort measurement, electrocardiography, oxygen saturation, snoring monitor, and sleep position evaluation. Each of these parameters is addressed in this article, including the application of the monitoring equipment, the derivations used, and the recommended specifications of the equipment.

Staging Sleep   **343**

Michael H. Silber

> Since the 1930s, various schemas have been suggested to describe the different electrophysiologic patterns of human sleep. This article reviews the historical

development of sleep staging. The development of the new American Academy of Sleep Medicine manual is reviewed, together with the scientific background underlying the choice of staging criteria. The rules for the different stages of wakefulness, non–rapid eye movement sleep, and rapid eye movement sleep are described, and variations recommended for scoring sleep in children.

Respiratory Monitoring Equipment and Detection of Respiratory Events   353

Jahan Naghshin and Patrick J. Strollo, Jr.

This article examines the current sleep laboratory tools available for diagnosing sleep disordered breathing. The authors discuss the advantages and disadvantages of each modality and the current state of monitoring in adults. It is important to consider that the use of more than one device may be required in identifying an sleep disordered breathing event. The precision of classifying a given event is dependent on the accuracy of the data generated by a given monitor and how those data are integrated by the scoring algorithm that is employed. The authors also provide a brief discussion of advanced signal processing in existing and emerging technology.

Differentiating Nocturnal Movements: Leg Movements, Parasomnias, and Seizures   361

Anil Natesan Rama, Rajive Zachariah, and Clete A. Kushida

The need to evaluate nocturnal movements is a common clinical problem in the practice of sleep medicine. Because reports of the movements occurring during sleep typically cannot be relayed by the patients themselves, the event descriptions often become second hand during evaluation by a sleep medicine clinician. Use of polysomnography, at times with use of specialized techniques, becomes an integral part of the diagnosis of these movements. This article describes the clinical steps involved in the diagnostic plan and reviews the most common sleep-related movements and their polysomnographic findings.

Cardiac Monitoring During Sleep   373

Conrad Iber and Kyuhyun Wang

Normal sleep is associated with slowing of the heart rate and occasional asymptomatic selflimited rhythm disturbances. Obstructive sleep apnea produces cyclical changes in heart rate and an increase in the occurrence of cardiac dysrhythmias. Sleep medicine practitioners should be familiar with routine methods, limitations, and scoring of cardiac events, including sinus tachycardia, sinus bradycardia, narrow and wide complex tachycardias, atrial fibrillation, and cardiac asystole. Other cardiac rhythms that are recognizable within the context of the sleep study should be reported. Changes in cardiac rhythm during polysomnography seldom result in adverse outcomes. Decisions regarding interventions for identified cardiac rhythms should be influenced by the nature of the dysrhythmia, risks identified by patient characteristics and comorbidities, and prevailing patient care strategies in managing heart disease.

Multiple Sleep Latency Test and Maintenance of Wakefulness Test   385

Douglas Kirsch and Josna Adusumilli

Degrees of excessive daytime sleepiness can be quantified by obtaining a comprehensive history in conjunction with various diagnostic studies, such as an overnight polysomnography, the multiple sleep latency test, and the maintenance of wakefulness test. Although the multiple sleep latency test and maintenance of wakefulness test are laboratory-based assessments of sleepiness and wakefulness, respectively, these findings on these tests may not always correlate with patient safety in the workplace or while driving. Further research is needed to improve the diagnostic accuracy of our assessments of excessive daytime sleepiness.

Pediatric Polysomnography 393

Suzanne E. Beck and Carole L. Marcus

Pediatric polysomnography is the diagnostic study of choice to evaluate for obstructive sleep apnea in children, and to evaluate cardiorespiratory function in infants and children with chronic lung disease, or neuromuscular disease when indicated. It is helpful to investigate atypical cases of parasomnias. It is important to understand that children are not just small adults when being studied in a sleep laboratory; they require a child friendly atmosphere and approach, need smaller and specialized equipment, and because of developmental and physiologic differences from adults, have age-adjusted rules for the scoring and interpretation of polysomnograms.

Polysomnographic Features of Medical and Psychiatric Disorders and Their Treatments 407

David T. Plante and John W. Winkelman

Psychiatric, neurologic, and medical illnesses, and their pharmacologic treatments affect the polysomnographic manifestations of sleep. Many patients undergoing sleep studies have multiple medical problems and often are taking many medications. Therefore, it is crucial that those interpreting sleep studies have an understanding of these effects. In this way, all the potential contributors to the polysomnographic findings can be addressed adequately. This article serves as a primer on changes in polysomnography (PSG) caused by commonly encountered disease states and their pharmacologic treatments.

Artifacts and Troubleshooting 421

Elise Maher and Lawrence J. Epstein

Recordings are made of the physiologic events during sleep to understand the mechanisms of sleep and wakefulness, identify sleep disorders, determine appropriate therapies, and monitor response to treatment. Correct interpretation depends on producing high-quality, artifact-free recordings. The objectives of this article are to illustrate common artifacts in polysomnographic recordings, to show how to differentiate between physiologic and nonphysiologic artifacts, to describe the known causes of artifacts, to learn to identify the source of artifacts, and to explain how to optimize the postrecording signals.

Portable Monitoring 435

Nancy A. Collop

The diagnosis of obstructive sleep apnea has been confirmed by polysomnography (PSG) for many years. PSG, however, often is considered inconvenient, expensive, and inefficient. The use of monitoring equipment that can be more portable and used in the home has been developed and frequently is used in countries outside the United States and by some federal agencies such as Veterans Administration hospitals in the United States. These portable monitors (PMs) often record fewer physiologic variables, are unattended, and can be performed in the home. It is anticipated that there will be more widespread use of portable monitors for diagnosing sleep apnea as sleep centers and insurance companies embrace this technology.

Manual Titration of Positive Airway Pressure in Patients with Obstructive Sleep Apnea   443

Alejandro D. Chediak

Positive airway pressure (PAP) devices are used to treat patients who have sleep-related breathing disorders including obstructive sleep apnea. After a patient is diagnosed with obstructive sleep apnea, the current standard of practice involves performing attended polysomnography, during which positive airway pressure is adjusted throughout the recording period to determine the optimal pressure for maintaining upper airway patency. Continuous positive airway pressure (CPAP) and bilevel positive airway pressure (BPAP) represent the two most common forms of PAP that are titrated manually during polysomnography to determine the single fixed pressure of CPAP, or the fixed inspiratory and expiratory PAPs of BPAP for subsequent nightly usage in the home. I recently cochaired the PAP Titration Task Force of the American Academy of Sleep Medicine, which reviewed the available literature on PAP titration protocols and strategies and, based on this analysis and expert consensus, developed recommendations for conducting CPAP and BPAP titrations. This article serves to review the task force recommendations and to provide a practical approach to using selected recommendations in the course of laboratory titration of PAP.

The Future of Sleep and Circadian Testing   455

David P. White

When one writes about the future, there is inherent and obvious speculation, as no one can predict with certainty what will come. That being said, this article reflects a combination of what would seem logical based on the evolving science and what, in the opinion of the author, is needed for the sleep field to grow and prosper. Whether any of this will turn out to be accurate, time will tell.

Index   465

Foreword

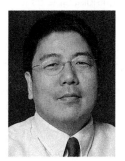

Teofilo Lee-Chiong, Jr., MD
Consulting Editor

The next time you go to a symphony, splurge on a good seat—let's say center aisle, third row. Go alone (preferably). Get to your seat at least a quarter of an hour before it starts, close your eyes, and listen to the orchestra go about the business of tuning their instruments and getting ready. Such a cacophony of sounds—much akin to the noise one might find on a busy street corner! Suddenly there is a hushed silence except for the footsteps of the conductor walking to the podium and the audience rushing to their seats. A cough here and there. Then, the music begins: perhaps a few violins to your left initially, followed almost imperceptibly by the cellos on your right, and finally, impatiently, by woodwinds and brass directly in front of you, and the percussion way out in the distance, its sound enveloping the violins as it thunders toward you. Suddenly, the entire place is transformed from solitary musicians and their isolated instruments into a symphony.

Such, too, is the nature of polysomnography, a word derived from the Greek roots, *poly* (many), *somnus* (sleep), and *graphein* (to write). Akin to an orchestra, polysomnography is the vocabulary with which we convey the complex, but unified, process of sleep. Early on, a single profound observation influenced the development of polysomnography: that sleep, although a function of the brain, affects other physiologic processes as well. Therefore, it was established early on that polysomnography, rather than simply measuring brain electrical activity alone, should include electroencephalography, electrooculography, and electromyography. This was eventually followed by the addition of respiratory sensors, oximetry, leg electromyogram, and other devices as technological advances allowed us to probe ever more comprehensively, and noninvasively, into the physiology as well as pathology of sleep.

It has been half a century since Nathaniel Kleitman, Eugene Aserinsky, and William Dement described rapid eye movement (REM) sleep, four decades after Allan Rechtschaffen and Anthony Kales standardized the method of scoring polysomnographic recordings in their classic paper, and two years since the American Academy of Sleep Medicine revised the sleep scoring guidelines. During this period, paper tracings had given way to the monitor screen and disc storage, and analog systems of recording sleep have been digitized and computerized.

The evolution of polysomnography continues even to this day. Recently, there has emerged a movement to simplify the process of monitoring sleep (ie, to measure only respiratory variables in persons suspected of having obstructive sleep apnea). We have, thus, both the capacity to expand the array of measuring devices during polysomnography, as well as increasingly more instruments that are more limited in scope—with avid proponents for each camp.

As musical compositions evolve into distinct styles, so too is polysomnography changing. Some patients and research subjects require the full components of the test and should get it; others may need only certain specific measures. The task that every clinician and researcher has to contend with is trying to distinguish the former

Sleep Med Clin 4 (2009) xi–xii
doi:10.1016/j.jsmc.2009.05.002

from the latter. No single technique is always the right one for every sleep disturbance and for every person. In 1907, Jean Sibelius and Gustav Mahler met for the first, and only, time in Helsinki. Both great composers by then, their conversation eventually turned to the topic of music. With characteristic austerity and economy that also marked his compositions, Sibelius stated that he writes, perhaps much like Beethoven, to capture a single concept. Mahler, Sibelius later recalled, had a different opinion, and said, "*Nein, die Symphonie müss sein wie die Welt. Sie müss alles umfassen.*" ("No, the symphony must be like the world; it must embrace everything.") Whether, we prefer Mahler or enjoy listening to Sibelius more, we have to agree that the two men are, implausible as it may seem, both correct, *but not always so.*

Teofilo Lee-Chiong, Jr., MD
Division of Sleep Medicine
National Jewish Health
University of Colorado Denver School of Medicine
1400 Jackson Street
Room J221
Denver, CO 60206, USA

E-mail address:
Lee-ChiongT@NJC.ORG (T. Lee-Chiong)

Preface

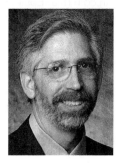 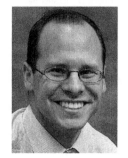

Lawrence J. Epstein, MD   Douglas B. Kirsch, MD
Guest Editors

For many sleep physicians, the polysomnogram has been the primary investigational and diagnostic tool of the specialty of sleep medicine for much of its lifespan. Studying sleep has always been a difficult process, but, before the polysomnogram, it was a less formalized and mostly visual examination. To quote Robert MacNish, a writer about sleep medicine in the mid 1800s, "The science is entirely one of observation: by that it must stand or fall, and by that alone it should be tested."[1] He refers, in that statement, to sleep and its relationship to phrenology, revealing not only that the study and understanding of sleep itself has changed significantly in the last two centuries but also that scientific observation of sleep has always been the basis of understanding sleep medicine. This issue of *Sleep Medicine Clinics* is devoted to understanding the development of sleep recording to its current form, describing the current use of the polysomnogram in clinical practice, and evaluating its potential for the future.

Recording the electrical activity of the brain, and the ability to assess change in activity over time, fundametally changed how sleep specialists now evaluate sleep. By combining electroencephalography with the observations of Drs. Kleitman, Aserinsky, and Dement, the basis of our current understanding of the structure of sleep was born. We begin with a review of the history of the polysomnogram, allowing better understanding of how early examination of sleep transformed into what we now see as routine.

The next couple of articles examine the mechanisms of signal generation, as well as the methods for detecting, recording, and displaying those signals. Once the electrophysiological signals are recorded, they must be scored and interpreted. Standardized scoring of the polysomnogram was, for many years, based on the work of Rechtshaffen and Kales.[2] However, within the last year, the work of a large group of physicians associated with the American Academy of Sleep Medicine (AASM) has produced The AASM Manual for the Scoring of Sleep and Associated Events in an attempt to update the rules for use of, terminology associated with, and the technical specifications for the polysomnogram.[3] The articles that comprise the majority of this issue review the new rules for scoring and interpreting the variety of signals obtained during a sleep study, including sleep staging, respiratory events, nocturnal body movements, cardiac monitoring, and other new information that is relevant from the AASM scoring manual. The articles that follow describe the many uses for the polysomnogram and the polysomnographic findings for many sleep and medical disorders.

While the polysomnogram has been a reasonably stable test for many years, some sleep specialists are already looking forward to introducing new aspects of testing based on currently ongoing research. Investigations into the next phase of sleep testing have, interestingly, gone in opposite directions. One line of investigation has explored how to get the same diagnostic information with less equipment and fewer signals, while another thread has looked at how to expand the amount and type of information obtained during a sleep study. The article on portable monitors explores the current understanding of how to use home sleep studies with fewer channels to diagnose obstructive sleep apnea. Then, using

Sleep Med Clin 4 (2009) xiii–xiv
doi:10.1016/j.jsmc.2009.05.003

sleep.theclinics.com

a forward-thinking approach, the final article of this issue attempts to predict not only what new evaluation techniques might be used but also how polysomnograms may aid in the diagnosis of medical disorders that lay beyond the current reach of sleep medicine.

We would like to thank the authors from across the country for all of their hard work involved in writing these articles, which we know take significant time and effort. Hopefully, their work will leave the reader with a better understanding of the past, present, and potential future of the polysomnogram.

Lawrence J. Epstein, MD

Douglas B. Kirsch, MD
Sleep Health*Centers*
1505 Commonwealth Avenue
Brighton, MA 02135, USA

E-mail addresses:
Lawrence_epstein@sleephealth.com (L.J. Epstein)
Doug_Kirsch@sleephealth.com (D.B. Kirsch)

REFERENCES

1. Macnish R. The philosophy of sleep. Glasgow: WR McPhun; 1836.
2. Rechtschaffen A, Kales A. A manual of standardized terminology, techniques and scoring system for sleep stages of human subjects. US Department of Health, Education and Welfare Public Health Service - NIH/NIND; 1968.
3. Iber C, Ancoli-Israel S, Chesson A, et al. The AASM manual for the scoring of sleep and associated events: rules, terminology and technical specifications. 1st edition. Westchester (IL): American Academy of Sleep Medicine; 2007.

The History of Polysomnography

Maryann Deak, MD[a],*, Lawrence J. Epstein, MD[a,b]

KEYWORDS

- Polysomnography • Sleep • Sleep stages
- Rapid eye movement • Sleep apnea • Narcolepsy

The state of sleep has fascinated people for a very long time. In his treatise on sleep and sleeplessness, Aristotle wrote that sleep is "a seizure of the primary sense-organ, rendering it unable to actualize its powers; arising of necessity... for the sake of its conservation." But, he wondered, "what are the processes in which the affection of waking and sleeping originates, and whence do they arise? We must also inquire what the dream is, and from what cause sleepers sometimes dream, and sometimes do not and whether it is possible or not to foresee the future (in dreams)."[1]

It should not be surprising to be curious about something that occupies a third of our lives. It was not until technology was developed that allowed one to peer inside the resting brain, however, that an understanding of sleep began. The development of sleep science and sleep medicine has been intertwined with the development of the polysomnogram, the method for recording the physiologic changes during sleep that has allowed the description of what happens during what one early writer called "the intermediate state between wakefulness and death."[2]

RECORDING SLEEP
Physiologic Recordings of Brain

Before the physiology of sleep could be explored, the scientific community needed a practical means of examining the natural oscillation of the brain from moment to moment. In 1875, Richard Caton (**Fig. 1**), a Scottish physiologist, was the first to record electrical rhythms originating from the brains of rabbits and monkeys.[3] In a brief

paragraph summary of a live presentation, Caton recounted his observation that every brain he tested had electrical currents as indicated by a galvanometer. He rightly conjectured that the activity he observed was related to brain function.

Years later, in 1929, German psychiatrist Hans Berger (**Fig. 2**) succeeded in recording electrical activity of the human brain.[4] Not only did this discovery grant scientists a window into the brain's activity; the ability now existed to measure it quantitatively. Berger coined the term "electroencephalogram (EEG)." Moreover, Berger was able to demonstrate pattern changes between wakefulness and sleep.

Physiologic Recording of Sleep

In the 1930s, several American investigators used the EEG to describe intricately the brain's electrical activity. Two main research groups generated prolific writings on the subject: Harvey, Hobart, Loomis, Davis, and others at Harvard University,[5,6] and Blake, Gerard, and Kleitman at the University of Chicago.[7,8] Loomis and coworkers[9] were the first to describe the characteristic features that now comprise non–rapid eye movement sleep. Loomis recorded overnight and daytime sleep in 30 individuals. He characterized sleep into five stages: A (alpha), B (low voltage), C (spindle), D (spindle and random), and E (random). Alpha was described as the normal waking rhythm. "Low voltage" occurred when alpha disappeared, which corresponds to today's stage 1 sleep. Stage C or "spindles" were 14-Hz waves, which were also accompanied by "random" or delta waves.

[a] Division of Sleep Medicine, Brigham and Women's Hospital, Harvard Medical School, 75 Francis Street, Boston, MA 02115, USA
[b] Sleep HealthCenters, 1505 commonwealth Avenue, Brighton, MA 02135, USA
* Corresponding author.
E-mail address: maryann_deak@sleephealth.com (M. Deak).

Sleep Med Clin 4 (2009) 313–321
doi:10.1016/j.jsmc.2009.04.001

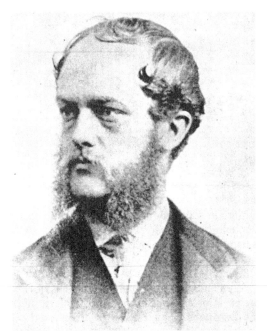

Fig. 1. Richard Caton. Pioneer who developed a method for recording electrical impulses from the surface of brains in animals.

Loomis described delta waves as becoming longer in stage D until they became predominant and spindles disappeared in stage E, similar to the current description of stage 3 sleep. Loomis

and colleagues[9] listed the stages in order of appearance and "in order of resistance to change by disturbances." Blake and Gerald[7] further explored sleep depth by studying the sleep of healthy adults, attempting to disturb sleep at each stage and measuring the amount and duration of a stimulus that was required to elicit a response from the research subject. They concluded that "deep sleep" is associated with large amplitude, slow waves at a frequency of 0.5 to 3 per second.

The series of articles that followed from the Harvard and the University of Chicago groups further described the stages initially proposed by Loomis. Not only did these experiments serve to explore and define the normal physiology of sleep, but the experimenters began to modify and improve the methods through which sleep was studied. Nathaniel Kleitman (**Fig. 3**) designed a means of measuring movement during sleep and used this technique during experimental sleep recordings.[8] Through the work of these scientists and others, EEG recording methods evolved, including use of amplifiers and high- and low-pass filters. Additionally, the experimenters learned that certain waveforms that characterize stages of sleep versus wakefulness were best recorded from specific regions of the brain.[8] The "14 per second rhythm"

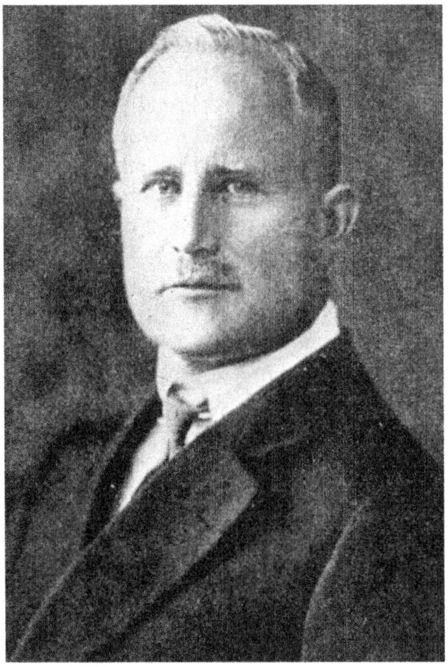

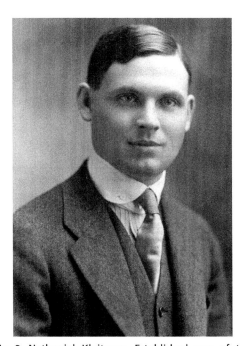

Fig. 3. Nathaniel Kleitman. Established one of the foremost laboratories for the study of sleep at the University of Chicago, where full-night sleep studies allowed the discovery of rapid eye movement sleep.

Fig. 2. Hans Berger. He made the first recording of electrical activity of the human brain.

that was termed a "spindle" was best seen at the vertex. The "10 per second" trains that were present in wakefulness with eyes closed were observed most frequently at the occiput. As a result, certain channels of the EEG gained importance in the recording of sleep. In addition to EEG and movement, sleep researchers experimented with channels that recorded new ancillary information, such as heart rate and respirations.[9]

In the 1950s, the discovery of rapid eye movement sleep (REM) by Kleitman's group advanced the field of sleep research. Kleitman had a particular interest in eye movement as a potential indicator of cortical activity in sleep. Aserinsky, a graduate student working with Kleitman at the University of Chicago, began directly observing eye movements in sleeping infants, noting distinct periods of eye motility and quiescence in sleep. He observed similar periods in sleeping adults. To avoid the necessity of direct observation, Kleitman and Aserinksy devised the electro-oculogram (EOG) as a means of conveniently and quantitatively measuring eye movements. This device distinguished between slow eye movements and REM. When used in conjunction with EEG and body movement channels, EOG extended the ability to evaluate the physiology of sleep.

During one experiment, Kleitman and Aserinksy observed the sleep of 20 healthy adults, awakening some of the subjects during periods of REM or quiescence for questioning on the content of their dreams.[10] They noted that patients were more likely to report vivid dreams, particularly involving visual imagery, during periods of REM than during periods when eye movements were not present. During periods without REM, the patients could not recall dreams or dreams were ill-defined. The EEG that accompanied REM periods consisted of a low voltage pattern that did not contain spindles or delta waves. Additionally, Aserinsky and Kleitman noted that respiration and heart rate increased during periods of REM. They concluded that the REMs and accompanying autonomic changes represented physiologic alterations associated with dreaming.

Although the discovery of Aserinsky and Kleitman brought the field closer to the notion that REMs represented a distinct stage of sleep, the periodicity and order of sleep stages was not understood. To conserve resources, experimenters had hitherto used short sleep recordings or intermittent sampling of sleep throughout the night to examine sleep. Kleitman and Dement wished to explore REM further to confirm the presence of characteristic concomitant EEG changes and determine the frequency of such periods. They realized that they needed to study full nights

of uninterrupted sleep intensively to achieve their goal. Kleitman and Dement (**Fig. 4**) used EEG, EOG, and movement channels to study 126 nights of sleep in 33 adults.[11] They discovered a recurring sequence of sleep stages, beginning with light (stage 1) sleep and progressing to deeper stages of sleep until reaching stage 4. After stage 4, sleep would lighten again. REM periods occurred every 90 to 100 minutes, and the periods lengthened as the night progressed. The EEG during REM periods consisted of a characteristic pattern that closely resembled light sleep or stage 1. They noted that stage 1, however, which occurred only at sleep onset, was never associated with REM; and patients responded to auditory stimuli more readily during stage 1 than during REM. Importantly, they observed that body movement dropped sharply at the onset of REM and rebounded at the conclusion of REM. This sequence was predictable among individuals and within one individual from night to night. From studying full nights of sleep, Kleitman and Dement were able to describe the human sleep cycle and created a new precedent for EEG recording.

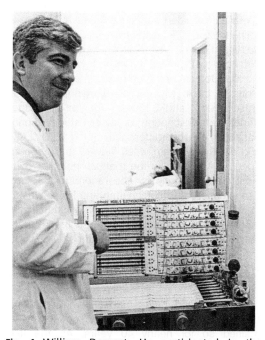

Fig. 4. William Dement. He participated in the discovery and description of the human sleep cycle and started the first sleep clinic at Stanford University. (*From* Dement WC, Kushida CA, Chang J. History of sleep deprivation. In: Kushida C, editor. Sleep deprivation: basic science, physiology, and behavior. New York: Taylor and Francis (previously Marcel Dekker); 2005. p. 38; with permission.)

FROM RECORDING TO SCORING SLEEP
The Rechtschaffen and Kales Manual

After Dement and Kleitman's article was published in 1957,[11] sleep researchers began to routinely use their description of clinical sleep stages. Over the subsequent 10 years, the sleep community expressed growing concern about the reproducibility and interrater reliability of sleep scoring. Moreover, researchers wanted to ensure that results of research studies could be reasonably compared, which would not be possible if laboratories used different methods of scoring sleep. Monroe[12] published an article in 1969 that showed that interrater reliability between laboratories was low, particularly for scoring of non-REM sleep.

A group of sleep researchers decided to meet to begin discussing the development of a standard scoring system for stages of sleep. The first meeting of the Association for the Psychophysiological Study of Sleep was held in 1960, but it was not until 1967 that a committee of investigators with considerable experience scoring sleep records, led by Allan Rechtschaffen and Anthony Kales, was tasked with developing a terminology and scoring system that might be universally used by sleep researchers.[13] The group devised a manual of sleep scoring entitled *A Manual of Standardized Terminology, Techniques and Scoring System for Sleep Stages of Human Subjects*, which was published in 1968.[13] The work of Dement and Kleitman formed the cornerstone of the newly published manual. The Rechtschaffen and Kales manual included a detailed description of sleep stage scoring based on the characteristics of the EEG, EOG, and electromyogram when viewed in 30-second epochs. Additionally, the manual included technical considerations for the recording of sleep. The intention of Rechtschaffen and Kales was for the publication to be "viewed as a working instrument rather than a statute," with the idea that the handbook required revision over time.

Limitations of Rechtschaffen and Kales

The sleep community widely accepted the Rechtschaffen and Kales manual, which became the gold standard for sleep stage scoring and remained so for nearly 40 years. As the field advanced, limitations of the sleep manual became apparent. Moreover, the manual was not revised to account for changes in the field, as intended by the original editors. Of concern was the use of the Rechtschaffen and Kales manual to study pathologic sleep when it had only been designed to study normal sleep.[14] The manual did not take into account important phenomenon including arousals; autonomic nervous system activity, such as cardiac rate and rhythm; respiratory abnormalities; body movement; or behavior in sleep. The manual was designed for paper recordings; many technical considerations in the original manual were no longer applicable with the widespread use of digital recordings. Additionally, some researchers disagreed with specific channel choices in the original manual, such as the use of only one EEG channel of central derivation.

Development of a New Scoring Manual

Although there were earlier attempts to revise the rules for sleep scoring, including a system for scoring arousals[15] and a manual for scoring the sleep of newborns,[16] a full-scale revision of the scoring manual was not accomplished until the American Academy of Sleep Medicine (AASM) commissioned the development of a new scoring manual. The effort was spearheaded by a steering committee of sleep experts. Between 2004 and 2006, several task forces were assigned to review the published evidence on specific topics and write a review article. The topics covered by the task forces included visual scoring, digital scoring, arousal, movement, respiratory issues, and cardiac issues.[17] Two additional task forces reviewed sleep scoring for pediatric and geriatric patient populations. The work of the task forces, in concert with the steering committee, culminated in a series of review articles published in the *Journal of Clinical Sleep Medicine*,[18–24] followed by publication of the *AASM Manual for the Scoring of Sleep and Associated Events: Rules, Terminology, and Technical Specifications* in 2007.[17]

ROLE OF POLYSOMNOGRAPHY IN THE DEVELOPMENT OF SLEEP MEDICINE

From the 1930s through the 1950s, scientists worked to reveal the properties of normal sleep. Concomitantly, the technology of recording sleep evolved. By the end of the 1950s, experimenters were performing full-night recordings of sleep. Beginning in the early 1960s and going forward, sleep researchers began to apply the new technology to study sleep pathology. The field of clinical sleep medicine began to develop beside a growing discipline of sleep research.

Narcolepsy

Although the clinical manifestations of narcolepsy had been described previously, narcolepsy as a clinical entity was poorly understood in the late

1950s and early 1960s. Narcolepsy was not substantiated as an epileptic phenomenon by EEG studies in narcolepsy patients.[25] Many scientists theorized that narcolepsy was a psychiatric disorder, and the clinical features of narcolepsy represented "repression of feelings" that are "unacceptable to consciousness."[26] By recording sleep in narcolepsy patients, however, physicians gained new insight into the disorder.

In 1959, Charles Fisher recorded a sleep-onset REM period in a patient with narcolepsy at Mount Sinai Hospital. The next year, Gerald Vogel published a case report of a patient with narcolepsy, which documented sleep-onset REM on EEG during a sleep attack. As the patient described dreams at sleep onset, Vogel[27] surmised that narcolepsy patients had an inherent need to dream "for the projection of fantasy." Finally, in 1963, Rechtschaffen and coworkers[28] observed full-night sleep recordings in nine narcolepsy patients. The patients were each studied for 18 nights, between one and three nights in succession, and the data were compared with control subject data. The most striking finding was the presence of sleep-onset REM periods in narcolepsy patients. The authors conjectured that cataplexy, sleep paralysis, and hypnagogic hallucinations represented features of REM occurring in wakefulness. They further speculated about the underlying cause of narcolepsy. Based on the contemporary understanding that REM sleep originated in the pontine reticular formation, the authors surmised that "precocious triggering" of this region of the brain led to narcolepsy. The concept that a specific neuroanatomic localization could be tied to narcolepsy was novel. Once again, full-night sleep recordings completely revolutionized the existing theories about sleep and sleep disorders.

The Stanford Narcolepsy Clinic

When Dement moved to Stanford University in the early 1960s, he hoped to continue to research the sleep of narcolepsy patients.[29] When recruitment of patients proved difficult, Dement placed an advertisement in the San Francisco Chronicle, which yielded a large number of responders. Half of the patients who responded to the advertisement were diagnosed with narcolepsy with cataplexy. Dement and Stephen Mitchel began to follow narcolepsy patients clinically at regular intervals. Working within the constraints of testing permitted by insurance companies, they performed daytime sleep recordings on all patients and full-night sleep recordings whenever possible. The Stanford clinic represented the first

specialized sleep clinic of its kind, growing out of the clinical research interests of its founders. As research interests grew, so did the number and diversity of patients in the clinic, including insomnia patients. By the 1970s, several sleep centers developed, which also grew from clinical research interests. There are now over 1500 sleep centers and laboratories accredited by the AASM, which likely represents about half of the existing centers and laboratories.

Sleep Apnea

In 1956, Bickelmann and colleagues[30] described a patient with obesity, hypoventilation, muscular twitching, and hypersomnolence. They named this constellation of symptoms the "pickwickian syndrome," based on the similarity to a character in Charles Dicken's The Posthumous Papers of the Pickwick Club. In the 1956 paper, which was based on observations of the patient during the day, the authors ascribed the patient's sleepiness to hypercapnia. This idea was perpetuated and accepted by the medical community until further clinical studies using overnight sleep recordings demonstrated the existence of sleep apnea.

EEG, EOG, and body movement channels were used in the first full-night recordings of sleep. As the sleep field advanced, researchers began to study other aspects of sleep, including respirations. In the early 1960s, two groups of researchers in Europe examined full-night sleep recordings in patients with the pickwickian syndrome. In Germany, Jung and Kuhlo recorded EEG, chest movements with an inflatable belt, carbon dioxide content of expired air, and heart rate in three patients. They observed that pickwickian patients experienced discontinuous sleep, interrupted by apneic periods. The apneic episodes were followed by a deep breath and acceleration of heart rate, which the authors interpreted as "an emergency reaction to severe hypercapnia and hypoxia." The patients rarely attained deep stages of sleep or significant periods of REM sleep. With regard to the underlying etiology of the phenomena they observed, the authors surmised that pickwickian patients had decreased sensitivity to carbon dioxide, causing not only the apneas observed in sleep but chronic hypoventilation in wakefulness. In all three patients, loss of 10 to 20 kg of weight resulted in remarkable improvement in daytime symptoms, although apneas persisted in two out of the three patients.

In France, Gastaut and coworkers[31] studied a similar patient population with all-night sleep recordings. An important change in technique permitted a markedly different interpretation of their findings, however, compared with Jung and Kuhlo. Rather than testing the carbon dioxide content of expired air, the French group analyzed airflow in the nostrils and mouth. Both the German and French experimenters measured movement of the thorax. Gastaut and colleagues[31] observed that despite a cessation of airflow at the mouth and nose during an apnea, movement of the thorax and respiratory muscle activity persisted. The authors concluded that a blockage in the airway triggered the episodes of apnea, rather than central nervous system dysfunction related to sensitivity to carbon dioxide, as previously suggested. The idea of airway obstruction was further supported by studies that observed polygraph recordings before and after tracheostomy.[32,33] Improvement in patient symptoms that accompanied resolution of obstruction revealed that daytime somnolence was more likely to be related to sleep disruption than to hypercapnia. Using similar techniques to perform additional overnight recordings, Gastaut and others were able further to characterize apnea as obstructive, central, or mixed. Once again, innovative techniques for recording sleep were necessary to advance sleep research.

Growth of Clinical Application of Polysomnography

Advancement in sleep research in concert with full-night sleep recordings permitted valuable insights into disease processes, sometimes in unexpected ways. Another example was restless leg syndrome. When patients with restless leg syndrome underwent sleep recordings, they demonstrated periodic involuntary leg movements.[34] EEG proved that these periodic limb movements were not a form of epilepsy; rather, restless leg syndrome could be counted among the sleep disorders.

As full-night sleep recordings gained importance, so did the specific techniques use by laboratories. Because many of the research studies that described sleep apnea occurred in Europe, researchers outside of the United States began routinely using cardiac and respiratory channels in their full-night sleep recordings before their American counterparts. When French neurologist and psychiatrist, Christian Guilleminault, joined the Stanford group in 1972, he introduced the routine monitoring of respiratory and cardiac parameters in sleep recordings at the Stanford clinic.[29] Although the Stanford clinic began by treating narcolepsy and, later, added insomnia patients, the clinic was now equipped to diagnose

and treat patients with sleep apnea. Jerome Holland first coined the term "polysomnogram" in 1974 to describe the measurement of multiple physiologic parameters during sleep.[35]

Barriers to Use of Polysomnography

Barriers to the use of polysomnography (PSG) surfaced as the number of sleep clinics and use of sleep testing grew.[29,36] The studies required clinicians to work through the night, which was unpopular especially for an outpatient test. Also, it was nearly impossible for clinicians to work in clinic during the day and conduct sleep studies in the laboratory through the night. The studies were very involved for the patients, and the idea of spending a night in the sleep laboratory took some adjustment. From a practical standpoint, the studies were expensive, and PSG was not established as a reimbursable test until 1975. The polygraphs were large, used ink pens, and required careful calibration before each study (**Fig. 5**). Also, the studies generated a tremendous amount of paper, which was difficult for laboratories to manage. The sleep field worked to alleviate some of these concerns by lobbying for reimbursement and developing computer polysomnograms that made recording sleep easier. Additionally, the medical community did not easily accept sleep medicine as a field. Only after years of research and clinical work did the importance of sleep disorders begin to gain recognition.

PARALLEL GROWTH OF THE FIELD OF SLEEP TECHNOLOGY

Against the backdrop of increasing demand for PSG and the growing clinical applicability of PSG, it became more impractical for sleep clinicians to perform PSG on a nightly basis. The growing sleep field required a new group of skilled professionals to ensure accurate and meticulous execution of this important diagnostic test. The first technologists originated from diverse backgrounds, including electroneurodiagnostics and respiratory therapy.[37] In 1978, a group of technologists met at an academic meeting and created the Association of Polysomnographic Technologists. The group's mission was to unite a cohesive group of professionals for the promotion of education and advancement of the new field.[38] The group appointed a committee, the American Board of Registered Polysomnographic Technologists, to create a certification examination. In 1979, the first examination was administered by the renamed Board of Registered Polysomnographic Technologists. The profession of sleep technology has grown in parallel to the field of

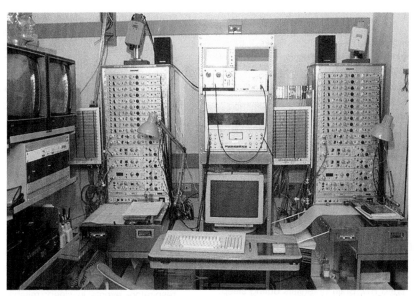

Fig. 5. Analog sleep system. Two-bed sleep laboratory at the University of Wisconsin, 1988. (*Courtesy of* S. Weber, Madison, WI.)

sleep medicine, experiencing an exponential increase in certified sleep technologists to over 13,000 technologists since the inception of the board examination.

Sleep medicine originated from other specialties. Once a sufficient body of knowledge requiring a unique skill set developed, an independent medical specialty evolved. A similar course has been followed by sleep technology. Training in electroneurodiagnostics, respiratory therapy, or cardiopulmonary technology is no longer sufficient to acquire all the skills required for sleep technology without additional training. Training in sleep technology was initially available only as on-the-job training. This localized training resulted in site-specific protocols and inconsistency in the practice of sleep technology. To address this issue the AASM launched a sleep technology initiative in 2005 in conjunction with the American Association of Sleep Technology (the successor to Association of Polysomnographic Technologists) and the Board of Registered Polysomnographic Technologists.[37] The goals of the initiative were to standardize training in sleep technology, raise the educational level of sleep technology training programs, and ensure proper credentialing of all technologists.

The AASM created the accredited sleep technologist education program (called ASTEP) to standardize on-the-job training training. Step 1 is a standardized didactic entry course. Step 2 is on-the-job training in a laboratory along with completion of computerized self-education modules. The last step is credentialing by the Board of Registered Polysomnographic Technologists

following 18 months of on-the-job training. At the same time, college-based sleep technology allied health programs are being developed. The programs are accredited by the Commission on Accreditation of Allied Health Education Programs, the accrediting body for allied health training programs. These programs can be in addition to respiratory therapy or electroneurodiagnostic training, or stand-alone sleep technology programs. Once there are sufficient college-based programs to supply the field adequately, the on-the-job training programs will be phased out. At that point, the field of sleep technology will have the same training pathways as other allied health fields. In addition, state legislatures have begun to establish licensing requirements for sleep technologists. The field of sleep technology has come of age.

SUMMARY

Similar to the first anatomists or the first radiographers, sleep scientists and physicians used EEG and later PSG as means of "peering in" to the workings of the human body with the hope of gaining understanding. The rapid advancement of sleep research, made possible by the development of the PSG, permitted not only a deeper understanding of normal sleep, but a more complete picture of the pathologic processes that affect sleep. The twentieth century not only fine-tuned the PSG as a research tool and vital diagnostic test, but also made possible the creation of a new medical specialty and a new allied health field.

REFERENCES

1. Aristotle. On sleep and sleeplessness. Beare JI, trans. Adelaide, Australia: eBooks@Adelaide, University of Adelaide; 2007
2. Macnish R. The philosophy of sleep. Glasgow: W.R. McPhun; 1836.
3. Caton R. The electric currents of the brain. Br Med J 1875;2:278.
4. Berger H. Uber das elektroenenkeephalogramm des menschen [On the human electroencephalogram]. Archiv f. Psychiatr Nervenkr 1929;87:527–70 [in German].
5. Davis H, Davis PA, Loomis AL, et al. Changes in human brain potentials during the onset of sleep. Science 1937;86(2237):448–50.
6. Davis H, Davis PA, Loomis AL, et al. Human brain potentials during the onset of sleep. J Neurophysiol 1938;1:24–38.
7. Blake H, Gerard RW. Brain potentials during sleep. Am J Physiol 1937;119:692–703.
8. Blake H, Gerard RW, Kleitman N. Factors influencing brain potentials during sleep. J Neurophysiol 1939; 2:48–60.
9. Loomis AL, Harvey EN, Hobart GA. Cerebral states during sleep as studied by human brain potentials. J Exp Psychol 1937;21:127–44.
10. Aserinsky E, Kleitman N. Regularly occurring periods of eye motility, and concomitant phenomena, during sleep. Science 1953;118(3062):273–4.
11. Dement W, Kleitman N. Cyclic variations in EEG during sleep and their relation to eye movements, body motility, and dreaming. Electroencephalogr Clin Neurophysiol 1957;9(4):673–90.
12. Monroe LJ. Inter-rater reliability and the role of experience in scoring EEG sleep records: Phase 1. Psychophysiology 1969;5(4):376–84.
13. Rechtschaffen A, Kales A. A manual of standardized terminology, techniques and scoring system for sleep stages of human subjects. Los Angeles: Brain Information Service/Brain Research Institute University of California; 1968.
14. Himanen SL, Hasan J. Limitations of Rechtschaffen and Kales. Sleep Med Rev 2000;4(2):149–67.
15. EEG arousals: scoring rules and examples: a preliminary report from the Sleep Disorders Atlas Task Force of the American Sleep Disorders Association. Sleep 1992;15(2):173–84.
16. Anders T, Emde R, Parmelee AH. A manual of standardized terminology, techniques and criteria for scoring of states of sleep and wakefulness in newborn infants. Los Angeles (CA): UCLA Brain Information Services, NINDS Neurological Information Network; 1971.
17. Iber C, Ancoli-Israel S, Chesson A, et al. The AASM Manual for the scoring of sleep and associated events: rules, terminology and technical specifications. 1st edition. Westchester (IL): American Academy of Sleep Medicine; 2007.
18. Penzel T, Hirshkowitz M, Harsh J, et al. Digital analysis and technical specifications. J Clin Sleep Med 2007;3(2):109–20.
19. Silber MH, Ancoli-Israel S, Bonnet MH, et al. The visual scoring of sleep in adults. J Clin Sleep Med 2007;3(2):121–31.
20. Bonnet MH, Doghramji K, Roehrs T, et al. The scoring of arousal in sleep: reliability, validity, and alternatives. J Clin Sleep Med 2007;3(2): 133–45.
21. Caples SM, Rosen CL, Shen WK, et al. The scoring of cardiac events during sleep. J Clin Sleep Med 2007;3(2):147–54.
22. Walters AS, Lavigne G, Hening W, et al. The scoring of movements in sleep. J Clin Sleep Med 2007;3(2): 155–67.
23. Redline S, Budhiraja R, Kapur V, et al. The scoring of respiratory events in sleep: reliability and validity. J Clin Sleep Med 2007;3(2):169–200.
24. Grigg-Damberger M, Gozal D, Marcus CL, et al. The visual scoring of sleep and arousal in infants and children. J Clin Sleep Med 2007;3(2):201–40.
25. Daly DD, Yoss RE. Electroencephalogram in narcolepsy. Electroencephalogr Clin Neurophysiol 1957; 9(1):109–20.
26. Switzer RE, Berman AD. Comments and observations on the nature of narcolepsy. Ann Intern Med 1956;44(5):938–57.
27. Vogel G. Studies in psychophysiology of dreams. III. The dream of narcolepsy. Arch Gen Psychiatry 1960;3:421–8.
28. Rechtschaffen A, Wolpert EA, Dement WC, et al. Nocturnal sleep of narcoleptics. Electroencephalogr Clin Neurophysiol 1963;15:599–609.
29. Dement WC. History of sleep physiology and medicine. In: Kryger MH, Roth T, Dement W, editors. Principles and practice of sleep medicine. 4th edition. Philadelphia: Elsevier; 2005. p. 1–12.
30. Bickelmann AG, Burwell CS, Robin ED, et al. Extreme obesity associated with alveolar hypoventilation; a pickwickian syndrome. Am J Med 1956; 21(5):811–8.
31. Gastaut H, Tassinari CA, Duron B. [Polygraphic study of diurnal and nocturnal (hypnic and respiratory) episodal manifestations of Pickwick syndrome]. Rev Neurol (Paris) 1965;112(6):568–79 [in French].
32. Kuhlo W, Doll E, Franck MC. [Successful management of pickwickian syndrome using long-term tracheostomy]. Dtsch Med Wochenschr 1969; 94(24):1286–90 [in German].
33. Lugaresi E, Coccagna G, Mantovani M, et al. [Effects of tracheotomy in hypersomnia with periodic respiration]. Rev Neurol (Paris) 1970;123(4):267–8 [in French].

34. Lugaresi E, Coccagna G, Tassinari CA, et al. [Polygraphic data on motor phenomena in the restless legs syndrome]. Riv Neurol 1965;35(6):550–61 [in Italian].

35. Atkinson JW. The evolution of polysomnographic technology. In: Butkov N, Lee-Chiong T, editors. Fundamentals of sleep technology. Philadelphia: Lippincott, Williams & Wilkins; 2007. p. 1–5.

36. Kuhl W. History of clinical research on the sleep apnea syndrome: the early days of polysomnography. Respiration 1997;64(Suppl 1):5–10.

37. Epstein LJ. Polysomnographic technologists: troubled waters ahead? J Clin Sleep Med 2005;1(1):14–5.

38. Shepard JW Jr, Buysse DJ, Chesson AL Jr, et al. History of the development of sleep medicine in the United States. J Clin Sleep Med 2005;1(1):61–82.

Generating a Signal: Biopotentials, Amplifiers, and Filters

Patrick Sorenson, MA[a,b],*

KEYWORDS

- Biopotential • Ion channels • Action potential
- Neurotransmitter molecules • Neuron • Synapse
- Amplification • Filters

The diagnosis of sleep disorders is directly dependent on the knowledge and the skills that determine how electrophysiologic signals are monitored and recorded. To understand the signals recorded and displayed on a sleep study evaluation, commonly referred to as a polysomnogram (PSG), it is necessary to describe how these electrophysiologic signals are generated at the cellular level and recorded through noninvasive means onto a polygraph. The manifestations of electrophysiologic activity allow one to monitor and interpret biopotential activity from the cerebral cortex, the eyes, and selective muscles. Biopotentials, by definition, are signals derived from an electric quantity (voltage or current or field strength) caused by chemical reactions of charged ions. Biopotentials permit those who study sleep and its disorders to record data for the evaluation of sleep stages, pathologic electroencephalographic (EEG) findings, cardiorespiratory function, and body movements. These data parameters are necessary to determine the presence or absence of sleep disorders diagnosed with a PSG, as discussed elsewhere in this issue.

Any discussion of the biopotentials monitored during a sleep study should include the morphologic manifestations of PSG-related electrophysiologic activity and how that information is appropriately recorded and displayed for interpretation. The quality of the electrophysiologic data on a PSG is directly dependent on the knowledge

and skills of the sleep technologist and the polysomnographers who evaluate and interpret these data. The knowledge and skills necessary to perform and interpret a PSG are confined to three main categories: (1) the knowledge of biopotentials and their appropriate and inappropriate manifestations, (2) the knowledge and skills necessary to apply electrodes and sensors to collect electrophysiologic data appropriately for a PSG, and (3) a thorough knowledge of amplification techniques and theory necessary to monitor and interpret the PSG data recorded. All three categories must be mastered and practiced. Lack of attention to, or mastery of, any of these categories may significantly impair the collection and subsequent interpretation of the PSG.

THE NEURON: PHYSICAL AND ELECTRICAL PROPERTIES

The primary function of neurons is to receive, modify, and transmit messages. This includes information exchanges between separate neurons and exchanges between different parts of the same neuron. Neurons, like other cells in the body, are structurally independent; there is no protoplasmic continuity between neurons. Neurons are negatively charged relative to the extracellular fluid that surrounds them. The plasma membrane of any cell provides a resistance to the flow of ions between the intracellular and

a Division of Sleep Medicine, Department of Neurology, Massachusetts General Hospital, 5 Blossom Street - 2nd Floor, Boston, MA 02114, USA
b Northern Essex Community College, Lawrence, MA, USA
* Division of Sleep Medicine, Department of Neurology, Massachusetts General Hospital, 5 Blossom Street - 2nd Floor, Boston, MA 02114.
E-mail address: psorenson@partners.org

Sleep Med Clin 4 (2009) 323–331
doi:10.1016/j.jsmc.2009.05.001

extracellular compartments. The neuron is also the only cell capable of rapidly conducting information from one part of the body to another. The neuron consists of structures specifically designed to accept and transfer electrical messages. This section focuses on the nature of the electrical signals that neurons use for intercellular communication and the mechanisms used to record those signals.[1]

The size, shape, and other characteristics of neurons can vary widely depending on the specialized tasks that they are able to carry out. The structure of the neuron is comprised of three parts: (1) the cell body that contains the cell's nucleus, (2) a single axon that extends from the cell body to other cells, and (3) multiple dendrites that conduct signals from other cells to the cell body. The cell bodies of neurons vary from 4 to 5 μm, to 50 to 100 μm (0.001 mm).[2] Electrical signals from the neuron are generated at the axon hillock between the cell body and the axon itself and transmitted down the axon and passed to the dendrites of the next neuron. At normal body temperature, nerve impulses can travel at speeds of 2 to 100 m/s (up to 260 mph) and are generally referred to as "action potentials."[1]

Axons are tube-like structures arising from the cell body that are covered in a myelin sheath. The myelin sheath is unusually rich in lipid and is formed by specialized cells called "oligodendrocytes" in the central nervous system (CNS). In the peripheral nervous system, nerve axons are myelinated by Schwann cells. Both oligodenrocytes and Schwann cells are supporting, or glial cells that surround and support nerve cells (neurons).

Although a myelin sheath surrounds most axons in the vertebrate nervous system, it is not strictly a part of the neuron but is considered critical for proper axonal function. In this regard it acts as an insulator of the axonal cytoplasm from the intracellular and extracellular conducting solutions. Myelin produced by the supporting glial cells wrap around the axon in concentric circles during neuronal development. The insulated axon is the "output cable" for the nerve cell.

The action potential of a neuron is an all-or-nothing phenomenon. If an electrical stimulus is delivered at intensities below the threshold (subthreshold) required to trigger a nerve impulse, there is a brief nonconducted response around the area of the stimulus on the nerve cell body called the "local process." The size and duration of the local process is proportional to the subthreshold stimulus.[2] Once the intensity of the stimulus reaches the threshold potential, the nerve cell's electrical polarity reverses, and becomes more positive inside than outside. This generates a nerve impulse, referred to as a "spike," which is conducted along the axon. Increasing a stimulus beyond the threshold level does not alter the amplitude or duration of the resulting spike, unlike subthreshold stimuli, which provoke a greater and greater local response until the threshold is reached. The neuron responds to the maximum of its capacity or it does not respond at all. Morphologic features of neuronal spikes are static as well following the all-or-nothing law.

At rest, when no electrical impulses are being conducted, the resting potential of the neuron reflects the balance of positive and negative charge on the inside (intracellular) and outside (extracellular) of the cell membrane. At rest, the extracellular space is positive (50–80 mV) relative to the intracellular space ($-40 - -90$ mV).[1,2] By convention, a negative membrane potential indicates that the inside of the cell membrane is more negative than the outside. When the membrane potential is less negative than the resting potential of the neuron it is said to be depolarized and when the membrane potential is more negative the neuron is said to be hyperpolarized.

Voltage differences are regulated by the neuron's semipermeable membrane, which allows different positively and negatively charged ions to move into and outside the cell. Along the axon covered with myelin insulation, there are short interruptions in the myelin called "nodes of Ranvier." Sodium (Na+) channels are concentrated in the node of Ranvier, whereas potassium (K^+) ions and various negatively charged ions, including chloride (Cl^-), are present in high densities in the juxtaparanodal region. Calcium (Ca^{2+}) is another important intracellular and extracellular fluid component (1 & 2).

Voltage-dependent ion channels regulating the flow of Na^+ and K^+ modulate the excitability of the axonal membrane at the nodes of Ranvier. The distribution of conducting ionic channels concentrated at the nodes allows saltatory conduction, in which an action potential leaps from node to node using a minimal expenditure of energy. Further neuronal energy efficiency is achieved through the action of the sodium-potassium ATPase (or sodium pump). The sodium pump maintains the ion concentration gradient by pumping Na^+ out of the cell and K^+ into the cell. By pumping more Na^+ out than K^+ in, the outside of the cell becomes more positive and the inside relatively more negative. This effectively charges the membrane battery. The sodium pump prevents the equalization of the ionic concentration gradients across the cell membrane, which would lead to an unexcitable cell membrane in ionic and electrical equilibrium.

Changes in charge across the neural membrane may be excitatory or inhibitory, depending on what neurotransmitter is released by an impinging neuron to affect the target neuron. Excitatory neurotransmitters depolarize the membranes of the cells they affect. In general, the connection between two neurons is called a "synapse," and the neuron that releases a stimulus (neurotransmitter) is considered "presynaptic," whereas the target neuron, which responds to the stimulus, is "postsynaptic."

An excitatory stimulus causes a net influx of positive charge on the target neuron. This tends to depolarize (reverse the charge on) the target neuron's membrane. In this condition, the target neuron is more likely to generate an action potential. The changes in the target neuron's membrane associated with a depolarizing stimulus are called the "excitatory postsynaptic potential."

Considered next is the effect of an inhibitory neurotransmitter. Here, the neuron becomes hyperpolarized (even more negative inside) because of an efflux of positive ions across the neuronal membrane caused by the action of the inhibitory neurotransmitter. This inhibits the neuron from reaching threshold and makes action potentials less likely. The postsynaptic membrane changes associated with an inhibitory stimulus is called "inhibitory postsynaptic potential."

For excitatory stimuli, an action potential is generated once the electrical threshold is reached. The semipermeable membrane of the neuron becomes much less selective because of the triggering of a rapid rearrangement of the proteins forming ion channels in the cell membrane by the excitatory stimuli, particularly at interruptions in the myelin covering of the axon. Current begins to flow when the new protein conformation of the ion channel is achieved. After an influx of positively charged ions lasting 1 to 2 milliseconds the neuron is definitively depolarized at that place. Already the wave of electrical activity is passing to the membrane just ahead of it, where similar changes occur. As this happens, the previous site of ionic influx resets itself toward the rest-state by means of active ionic pumping and the closing of ion channels that had been open.

For a short time following an action potential spike, the neuron is in an absolute refractory period and is incapable of responding to any additional stimuli. The absolute refractory period is then followed by a relative refractory period where the stimulus required for a spike is above the resting potential threshold (suprathreshold). The entire process from the stimulus that reaches the threshold to elicit a spike to the period when the relative refractory period returns to the actual level of the neuron's threshold is referred to as the "excitability cycle" of the neuron. The excitability cycle varies in time depending on the size and function of the neuron and the presence or absence of myelin surrounding the axon. Depending on these and other metabolic factors the entire excitability cycle of the neuron typically lasts 1 to 2 milliseconds.

As the action potential reaches the end of the axon, neurotransmitters are released into the synaptic cleft between the axon terminal and, most commonly, the dendrites of the target neuron. In this regard, synaptic transmission is unidirectional proceeding from the terminal ending of the axon (presynaptic release of neurotransmitter, which may be excitatory or inhibitory) to the following (postsynaptic) nerve cell. The extracellular fluid of the target neuron is infused with neurotransmitter molecules that bind to receptor proteins of the target neuron, effecting changes in the postsynaptic membrane as discussed.

If a group of neurons within the CNS become excitatory at relatively the same time through the activation of excitatory synapses, an additive change in the voltage of the extracellular fluid develops and the neuronal activity in that area of the CNS becomes synchronized. Although there are many factors that can influence this process, synchronization of neurons must occur within a window lasting approximately 10 milliseconds. Neurons within the surrounding neuronal network reinforce the excitatory activity of other neurons. This synchronization can produce significant voltage changes within the network. The greater the synchronization that occurs in local neurons the greater the voltage changes within that region.

RECORDING BIOPOTENTIALS

The propagation of the action potential along and between neurons creates an electrical current that spreads into surrounding tissues and can be detected on the surface of the body. Recording EEG parameters is done by placing a minimum of two electrodes on the scalp and amplifying the brain electrical activity generated by neurons in the cortex. The displayed electrical activity reflects electrical potentials at the surface created when the potential of many neurons change synchronously (either at the same time or sequentially) creating predictable rhythms of various types. The electrical activity recorded by a scalp electrode represents the collective activity of large numbers of neurons rather than a specific measurement of only several cells and can be the result of local changes beneath the electrode or alterations in neuronal activity in other parts of the cortex. Ultimately, the display for interpretation is the neuronal potential differences between the two scalp electrodes selected.

Recorded brain waves vary both in frequency (cycles per second, measured in hertz), and amplitude (height, expressed in voltage). The faster the rhythm the more frequent are the changes in electrical activity within the cortex. The greater the amplitude of the waveform the greater the potential differences between the groups of neurons measured by two compared electrodes. The voltages recorded are quite small and are measured in millionths of a volt referred to as "microvolts," and subsequently must be amplified for visualization. When recording the EEG during polysomnography, the different frequencies and amplitudes recorded not only indicate the stage of sleep but also may provide correlates to pathology.

The size of an electrode is quite large as compared with the size of a neuron. Depending on the type of cell, the size of a neuron is approximately 0.01 to 0.05 mm.[1] This means that roughly 5000 neurons could fit inside the cup of a standard electrode. What is monitored, however, is the synchronized neuronal activity of the cortex under the electrode. In general terms, the electrical activity recorded from an electrode placed on the scalp monitors the summed electrical activity from layers I to III of the six laminar layers of the cerebral cortex, an area comprised mostly of pyramidal neurons numbering literally in the millions. Electrodes used for monitoring electrophysiologic activity during a PSG are metal disks with shallow cups connected to wire inputs of varying lengths. These electrodes are usually made of gold or silver because these metals have electrical potentials that are optimal for recording cortical electrical activity.

Gold electrodes are actually silver electrodes that have been gold-plated and silver electrodes are a combination of silver-silver chloride. The combination of these materials contributes to minimal signal drift (stable materials); a long time constant (does not overreact to changes, smoothes the output); and optimal electrode resistance.

The electrode cup is filled with an electrolyte paste that contains free chloride ions. The ions can move, allowing a voltage to develop on the metal of the electrode. The formation of a layer of electrical charges on the metal electrode and another layer of opposite charges in the electrolyte paste allows the electrode to act as a charged capacitor when placed against the scalp. In this regard the electrode potential is called a half-cell potential because the electrical potential that develops on a single electrode acts as half of a battery. When two electrodes are connected and compared, these electrodes form a source of direct current (DC) potential.

When recording electrophysiologic signals, the electrode is not the only source of resistance to current. Other sources of resistance include an internal resistance from the electrical activity of the cortex; the resistance of other tissue including the dura mater, cranium, and scalp; and resistance within the amplifiers used to amplify the relatively low-voltage brain activity being recorded. Ideally, the capacitance and resistance of circuits are equal and the DC voltage at the two electrode inputs is equal. Differences in capacitance and resistance are small if the impedance of electrical activity entering the amplification system is small. One of the main functions of the sleep technologist applying electrode leads to the patient is the reduction in impedance, measured in kilo ohms (kΩ), of electrical activity between skin and electrode. Reducing and minimizing impedances of electrical activity to acceptable levels of under 5 kΩ is accomplished by using proper application techniques. For a more thorough explanation of the proper placement and application of electrodes, the reader is referred to the chapter entitled Recording Sleep; Electrodes, 10/20 Recording system and Sleep System Specifications, elsewhere in this issue. The topic is addressed here as an explanation of the methods of recording biopotentials.

THE ELECTROENCEPHALOGRAPHY OF SLEEP

Different patterns of EEG activity are recorded during a sleep study. Within the CNS, there are prominent features indicating whether a person is awake and asleep and the state or stage of sleep. During wakefulness, rapid eye movement (REM) sleep, and the lighter phases of non-REM (NREM) sleep, there is low-voltage desynchronized CNS activity. Desynchronization of electrical activity occurs because of the release of neurotransmitters called "neuromodulators," such as acetylcholine, serotonin, and norepinephrine, which support the generation of action potentials and activated CNS states. When neurons are desynchronized, positive ions enter some neurons and leave others. Large electrical changes in extracellular fluid are minimized to allow for the integration of sensory stimuli necessary for information processing within the CNS.[3]

In wakefulness with eyes closed, a prominent alpha rhythm (8–13 cps) is usually present in adults and older children.[2] Alpha activity is prominent in the occipital regions of the CNS but can also be seen more generally and at variable levels in other regions of the CNS. With the eyes open during wakefulness, frequencies faster than 13 cps (beta) are commonly seen in the frontal and central regions. Descent into sleep is commonly characterized by a waning of alpha activity, slow rolling of the eyes, and the emergence of a slower rhythmic low-voltage EEG activity called "theta" (4–7 cps), although nonrhythmic theta can also be seen in an adult who is awake. As sleep deepens, stage 2 sleep is characterized by higher voltages in the theta range along with K-complexes and sleep spindles. A K-complex is a biphasic sharp, slow wave often associated with sleep spindle bursts occurring predominately in the central region bilaterally in adults. The K-complex lasts at least 0.5 seconds and is characterized by a sharp negative (by convention, upward) deflection followed by a slower high-voltage positive component. There is no typical amplitude criterion for the K-complex. Both phases of the K-complex reflect synchronous excitation within large neuronal populations.[4] In adults, sleep spindles are 11.5 to 15 cps bursts of sinusoidal waves typically lasting 0.5 to 1.5 seconds with an amplitude usually less than 50 μV. As sleep deepens further and neuronal synchronization is at its maximum, delta waves, the depth of which depends on age and other factors, emerge in the EEG. Delta waves are high-voltage slow EEG activity. To qualify as delta, the waveform must be of 0 to 4 cps in duration and reach voltages of at least 75 μV.[5] Children can generate delta waves of 300 μV or more during the deeper phases of NREM sleep and these voltages decrease during the aging process. Finally, in REM, EEG activity again becomes desynchronized and is characterized by low-voltage fast activity and slower waveforms in the theta range that may present in a sawtooth pattern referred to as "sawtooth" waves. Sleep-state progression reflects the varying levels of neuronal synchronicity seen across the night and is dependent on many factors including age, pathology, medication regimens, chronobiology, and homeostatic pressure.

In recently updated guidelines for the description of sleep stages,[6] wakefulness is now referred to as stage W, stage 1 sleep is stage N1, stage 2 sleep is stage N2, deep NREM sleep is stage N3, and REM sleep is termed stage R. It should be noted that the recent changes in nomenclature eliminated the previously held distinction between the deepening phases of NREM sleep as sleep progresses through increasing levels of neuronal synchronicity. Although these changes still reflect increasing neuronal synchronicity as compared with the lighter phases of NREM sleep, levels of increased synchronicity vary with age and the lack of a distinction between the deeper phases of NREM sleep may be inappropriate for describing the sleep of children versus adults.

THE ELECTROMYOGRAM, ELECTRO-OCULOGRAM, AND EKG OF SLEEP

Other electrical activity monitored during a sleep study includes the electrical activity of the chin, intercostal, and leg muscles with an electromyogram (EMG), the electrical activity of the eye with an electro-oculogram, and the heart with an EKG. An EMG is possible because motor neurons stimulate muscle cells through the release of acetylcholine, which binds to receptor cells in the muscle cell membrane, which in turn has an excitatory effect on the muscle causing it to contract. In this regard, acetylcholine acts not as a modulator but opens ion channels in the muscle cell membrane and produces the action potential necessary for muscular contraction. To determine the presence of limb movements, a topic covered elsewhere in this issue, the EMG of the anterior tibialis is monitored. Monitoring the mentalis and submentalis chin muscles is done to determine the onset and offset of REM sleep. During waking and in NREM, muscle activity is variable. In REM sleep, however, the skeletal muscles are actively inhibited and this atonia is particularly evident in the facial muscles listed previously because the tone in these muscles is more variable in NREM sleep than other skeletal musculature. In this regard, the atonia of the chin muscles in REM stands in contrast to the variable tonicity seen in NREM and wakefulness. Using an intercostal EMG during a sleep study aids in the determination of central versus obstructive apnea because intercostal muscles are inactive during central apnea and show a distinct crescendo pattern during an obstructive apnea.

In addition to the desynchronization of EEG activity and loss of muscle tone of the facial muscles used in the determination of REM sleep, REM sleep includes, by definition, the presence of rapid eye movements. Additionally, sleep onset is characterized by slow rolling movements of the eyes. The electrical activity of the eyes is monitored with electro-oculogram channels of the eyes bilaterally. Electrodes are placed no more than 2 cm from the sclera of the eye at the outer canthi. There is a positive electropotential at the cornea and a negative electropotential at the retina called the "corneoretinal potential." The electro-oculogram shows eye movements according to the relative electropotential of each electrode as determined by the orientation of the eyes. Electrodes used to monitor the eyes are also commonly offset slightly above and below the eye to monitor vertical and horizontal movements. The electrodes placed near the eyes are commonly referenced to the ipsilateral mastoid, which is a relatively electrically inactive site used to achieve a signal free from the electrical activity at alternate sites. This is referred to as a "monopolar" or "referential" derivation because there is a single electrode at an active site. A bipolar derivation is when two equally active but dissimilar signals are referenced together and compared. The use of the monopolar derivation for the electro-oculogram serves three purposes: (1) to avoid electrical contamination; (2) to prevent the cross-contamination seen when referencing the eye leads to opposite mastoids that may appear as out-of-phase (disconjugate) eye movements; and (3) to aid in the determination and rectification of artifact in the eye channels.

The electrical activity of the heart is monitored using a standard lead II torso placement. The EKG is used to determine the presence of arrhythmias, such as premature beats, sinus pauses, heart blocks, atrial fibrillation, and other rhythms that can be determined using a lead II placement.

Although there are other electrophysiologic signals monitored during a sleep study, the previously mentioned channels represent endogenous electrical activity that can be monitored directly. The reader is encouraged to examine the available literature to determine the proper methods of monitoring respirations and breathing sounds, oxyhemoglobin saturation, end-tidal CO_2 values, plethysmography, and pH data.

THE DIFFERENTIAL AMPLIFIER AND ASSOCIATED FILTERS

To visualize any electrophysiologic signal appropriately, including the EEG, it is not only necessary to amplify these signals but to filter them appropriately. A differential amplification system, which takes the difference between two inputs and amplifies the difference, is used to boost the small electrophysiologic signals. The output of a differential amplifier is proportional to the differences in voltages received from those inputs and the sensitivity setting chosen by the polysomnographer. Through a process called "common mode rejection," the amplifier eliminates any electrical activity that is identical to both inputs. In this manner, the differential amplifier allows the polysomnographer to enhance only that electrical activity between two inputs. To process these

signals further, however, the appropriate use of filters is also necessary to eliminate expected but unwanted local signals intruding into the parameter being recorded.

Electrically, filters isolate and remove specific frequency bandwidths that either boost or attenuate (reduce the size) the signal. The use of a low and high filter is necessary appropriately to display the bandwidth of interest for each parameter (**Figs. 1** and **2**). For example, the frequency of respirations is quite slow as compared with EEG activity. The polysomnographer needs to display the slow activity and eliminate faster activity that may obscure the respiratory parameter. In the case of EEG data, the polysomnographer needs to display faster rhythms and eliminate slow activity that may obscure EEG data without attenuating or eliminating the slower features of sleep, such as K-complexes and delta waves mentioned previously. Further, filters serve to eliminate the effects of DC potentials from the skin, muscle activity near the recording site, or unwanted electrical activity from other devices on the patient or in the surrounding environment.

Isolating slow activity is done by applying a low-frequency filter (LFF) also known as a "high-pass" filter. A high-pass filter allows easy passage of high-frequency signals but difficult passage to low-frequency signals. The range of LFF is generally 0.1 to 15 Hz and the setting establishes the low-frequency recording limits of the polygraph. Isolating faster rhythms is done by the use of a high-frequency filter (HFF), also known as a "low-pass" filter, which allows easy passage of low-frequency signals and blocks high-frequency signals. The HFF setting establishes the high-frequency recording limits of the polygraph. The range of HFF is generally 15 to 100 Hz. Frequencies below and above 0.1 Hz and 100 Hz are virtually impossible in humans under normal circumstances, except perhaps for some EMG data above 100 Hz considered irrelevant for a sleep study or excessive high-frequency interference above 100 Hz that can obscure normal physiologic data.

Filters allow the polysomnographer to attenuate and appropriately display the slope of the curve (known as the "frequency response curve") of the parameter being recorded on the polygraph. Adjusting the filters, particularly the LFF, either up or down serves to define the lowest frequency recorded without significant attenuation and subsequent distortion of the activity below that setting. A LFF setting allows signals at or above this frequency to be linearly displayed without significant attenuation. The higher the LFF setting, the greater is the attenuation of the signal.

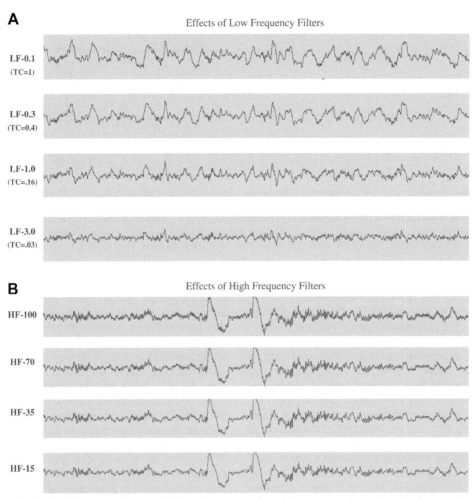

A Effects of Low Frequency Filters

LF-0.1
(TC=1)

LF-0.3
(TC=0.4)

LF-1.0
(TC=.16)

LF-3.0
(TC=.03)

B Effects of High Frequency Filters

HF-100

HF-70

HF-35

HF-15

Fig. 1. In this side-by side comparison of EEG data the practical usefulness of the filters is made clear. (*A*) Increasing the low-frequency filter shortens the time constant defined as the amount of time that it takes for the channel to return to 37% of the baseline of the channel and attenuates the slow activity of the EEG. The time constant is a function of the capacitance times the resistance. As the filter setting is increased, the time constant decreases, eliminating slower wave forms. This can be helpful with low-frequency artifact, such as respiratory motion arti- fact. Overuse of the filter may cause the true wave pattern to be misrepresented and interpreted as an incorrect sleep stage, as seen at the LF-3.0 setting. (*B*) In the second example, the high-frequency filter attenuates faster activity but has little appreciable effect on the amplitude of the waveform. The high-frequency filter can be help- ful in eliminating fast activity, such as high-frequency artifact, or fast physiologic activity, such as muscle tension, that may alter or obscure the intent of the channel. Overuse can lead to loss of appropriate fast wave forms, such as spindles. (*Adapted from* Amplifier Function and Calibration, Registry Review Course Lecture, Sleep Founda- tions, March, 2009.)

Although the filter attenuates all input frequencies to some degree, the attenuation of the frequency is 20% at the chosen setting. For example, a LFF of 0.3 Hz attenuates 0.3 Hz activity by 20%. The point on the frequency response curve at which output is reduced by 20% is known arbitrarily as the "cut-off frequency."[2]

Similar to the effect of the LFF on slow activity, there is an attenuation of output amplitude when a HFF is used. The higher the HFF, the less a signal with a known frequency input is attenuated. Again, the frequency at which the amplitude is attenuated by 20% by the HFF is the cut-off frequency. The HFF serves to isolate the higher frequency band- widths necessary to display the faster activities seen on a sleep study. For parameters with faster frequencies the HFF should be set at the upper limits. For channels where faster bandwidth activity is unwanted, a low setting for the HFF is desired. The polysomnographer must use caution not to attenuate inadvertently CNS discharges seen in epileptiform EEG activity indicating seizures or

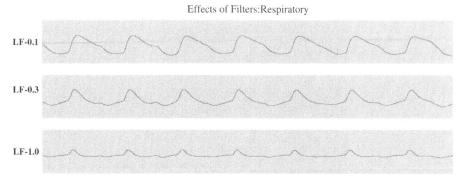

Fig. 2. Note the effects of the low-frequency filter on the waveforms of a respiratory channel. As the low-frequency filter is increased, the waveform is attenuated, there is a mild shift in the time axis, and there is also a loss of definition in the waveform. The figure shows that respiratory channels are best visualized using a low setting for the low-frequency filter and that using inappropriate filter settings may obscure useful data. (*Adapted from* Amplifier Function and Calibration, Registry Review Course Lecture, Sleep Foundations, March, 2009.)

other CNS pathology using inappropriate HFF filter settings that may blunt faster spike activity.

A thorough understanding of the effect of filters provides the polysomnographer with the theoretical underpinnings of the judicial use of these filters. Inappropriate excessive filtering of data to eliminate signal interference can change the appearance of the parameter being monitored to such a degree that the operator can no longer be certain that the parameter being recorded is physiologically accurate and the intent of the channel is lost. By convention, artifactual data should be eliminated by replacing the sensors rather than filtering the artifactual frequencies or turning down the sensitivity of the amplifier (**Table 1**).

Line frequency interference from the amplifier output can be eliminated with a special filter that is specifically designed to attenuate frequencies at or around 60 Hz. These notch filters, also referred to as 60-Hz filters, remove electrical noise at frequencies often found in electrically noisy recording sites, such as an ICU or in a sleep laboratory where ancillary equipment is often used. Although notch filters attenuate 60-Hz activity they also attenuate frequencies around this bandwidth to a lesser degree. Epileptiform activity may be attenuated because some of the components of discharge activity have frequency characteristics above the 30- to 40-Hz range.[2] The use of a notch filter is undesirable in most cases to avoid the attenuation of true physiologic data. High-quality amplification systems and appropriate electrode placement are usually sufficient to eliminate the need to use the notch filter. When optimal impedances are not possible because of existing skin conditions, the notch filter may be necessary to attenuate the resultant 60-Hz interference. For environments with stray frequencies in this bandwidth, the use of the notch filter on individual channels may be unavoidable until the source of the stray current is located. The notch filter should only be considered as a temporary solution, should be avoided particularly in EEG channels, and should not be used globally on all channels being recorded.

Table 1
Recommended filter settings for polysomnography

Routinely Recorded Filter Settings	Low-Frequency Filter (Hz)	High-Frequency Filter (Hz)
Electroencephalogram	0.3[a]	35[a]
Electro-oculogram	0.3	35
Electromyogram	10	100
Respiration	0.1	15
Snoring	10	100

[a] Note that the filter settings for the EEG may be increased to a low-frequency filter of 1 Hz and 70 Hz in children and other populations to attenuate more of the slow activity and allow the faster rhythms, such as EEG discharges, to be displayed more accurately.[6]

Data from Amplifier Function and Calibration, Registry Review Course Lecture, Sleep Foundations, March, 2009.

Previous discussions involved the use of parameters recorded as alternating current channels, although amplification systems manipulate voltages rather than current. An alternating current channel varies around a baseline of zero where signal excursions of the parameter recorded vary around a theoretical centerline. Previously, analog recorders required technologists to set both the mechanical and electrical baselines for all alternating current and DC channels. Digital acquisition systems no longer require manually setting and ensuring a baseline for alternating current channels. Conversely, digital systems still record some channels as DC channels where the output of a device does not vary around a centerline of zero but instead directly reflects output depending on the setting of a true zero and a maximum excursion set-point value. Devices that use DC channel inputs include external oximeters, continuous positive airway pressure machines, capnographs, some respiratory effort systems, and pH meters. Because a DC signal is a direct output from a device, filters, at least in the sense discussed previously, are not used in DC amplification systems. The DC channel is calibrated according to the specifications of the device being used. In simple terms, a constant zero is introduced into the DC amplifier from the device and the zero value is entered in the software of the recording instrument. A known maximum voltage is then sent into the recording instrument and this value corresponds to the maximum output of the device and is entered into the software of the recording instrument. In this manner, the recording instrument is calibrated according to a known set-point scale.

SUMMARY

Understanding the underlying science of the generation of electrophysiologic signals is necessary to monitor and interpret sleep studies accurately. There are many factors that can alter a signal observed on a PSG. These signals can be altered at the neuronal level because of the effects of medication or pathology. The proper use of the equipment used to monitor sleep can also have a significant impact on PSG interpretation and subsequent treatment decisions. Armed with the knowledge of how an electrophysiologic signal is generated and recorded, those who study sleep and its disorders are able to separate true from artifactual signals and know the difference between expected and unexpected alterations in these signals. At any step in the process the diagnostic accuracy of a PSG may be altered or unreliable, which if not detected and corrected, could adversely affect the care of the patient.

REFERENCES

1. Levitan I, Kaczmarek L. The neuron: cell and molecular biology. 3rd edition. New York: Oxford University; 2002.
2. Tyner F, Knott J, Mayer W. Fundamental of EEG technology: basic concepts and methods, vol. 1 & 2. New York: Raven Press; 1983.
3. Butlov N, Lee-Chiong T, editors. Fundamentals of sleep technology. Philadelphia: Lippincott Williams & Wilkins; 2007. Sections 6: 30 & 31.
4. Amzica F, Steriade M. The functional significance of K-complexes. Sleep Med Rev 2002;6(2):139–49.
5. Carney P, Berry R, Geyer D, editors. Clinical sleep disorders. Philadelphia: Lippincott Williams & Wilkins; 2005.
6. Iber C, Ancoli-Isreal S, Chesson A, et al. The AASM manual for the scoring of sleep and associated events: rules, terminology and technical specifications AASM. Westchester (IL): American Academy of Sleep; 2007.

Recording Sleep: The Electrodes, 10/20 Recording System, and Sleep System Specifications

Kelly A. Carden, MD, MBA

KEYWORDS

- Sleep • Electrodes • Recording • Monitoring
- Electroencephalography
- Electro-oculography • Electromyography • Airflow
- Respiratory effort • Electrocardiography

The core measurements of polysomnography have been stable for decades. In 1960, the inaugural meeting of the Association of the Psychophysiological Study of Sleep was convened for the purpose of adopting a standard scoring system for the stages of sleep. This meeting of experts then became an annual event. In 1967, because of concerns about the unreliability and variability of methodologies to record sleep, a special session on the scoring of sleep was held at the seventh annual meeting of the Association of the Psychophysiological Study of Sleep. Subsequently, an ad hoc committee of sleep experts was convened to develop terminology and procedures for recording and scoring sleep to be used universally by sleep researchers and clinicians. What came of those historic committee meetings was "A Manual of Standardized Terminology, Techniques, and Scoring System for Sleep Stages of Human Subjects."[1]

The editors of this landmark manual were Allan Rechtschaffen, PhD, and Anthony Kales, MD, which is why many sleep medicine practitioners refer to this manual as "the R and K manual." This manual served as the standard of practice from 1968 until 2007, at which time the American Academy of Sleep Medicine (AASM) published "The AASM Manual for the Scoring of Sleep and Associated Events: Rules, Terminology, and Technical Specifications" based on the body of evidence in the sleep medicine literature and the work of a steering committee and eight task forces appointed by the AASM.[2] This manual currently serves as the standard by which polysomnography is performed in the United States. The goal of this article is to review the current procedural standards for monitoring and evaluating sleep and wake in the clinical laboratory and research settings.

The standard parameters used to record sleep and wake are electroencephalography (EEG), electro-oculography (EOG), electromyography (EMG), airflow measurement, respiratory effort measurement, electrocardiography (ECG), oxygen saturation, snoring monitor, and sleep position evaluation. Each of these parameters is addressed in turn, including the application of the monitoring equipment, the derivations used, and the recommended specifications of the equipment.

ELECTROENCEPHALOGRAM AND THE 10-20 ELECTRODE SYSTEM

The signals derived from the EEG are fundamental to the evaluation of sleep and wake in human subjects. The EEG records local graded electric

Sleep Centers of Middle Tennessee, Sleep Center at StoneCrest, 300 Stonecrest Boulevard, Suite 370, Smyrna, TN 37167, USA
E-mail address: kcardenmd@gmail.com

Sleep Med Clin 4 (2009) 333–341
doi:10.1016/j.jsmc.2009.04.002

potentials generated by the cerebral cortex and other structures, including the thalamus. The EEG is thought to be the reflection of large apical dendrites of the pyramidal cell neurons and is not thought to reflect the action potentials of the neurons. The EEG signal is generated because of the relative difference in potential between the two electrodes used. A referential derivation includes an active signal and a passive one. A bipolar derivation includes two active signals. Most derivations used in routine polysomnography are referential in nature.

The quality and characteristics of the EEG tracing depend on the technique used to place the electrodes. Reliable EEG recording begins with accurate measurement of the human skull, as dictated by the International Federation 10–20 system of electrode placement (**Fig. 1**).[3] Each of the points on the 10–20 "map" indicates a possible electrode site. Each electrode site is designated with a letter or letters and a number. The letters FP, F, C, P, and O represent frontal pole, frontal, central, parietal, and occipital, respectively. M represents the mastoid process. Odd numbers are used to denote the left-sided electrode placements; even numbers are used to denote the right-sided electrode placements. "Z" denotes midline electrode placement sites.

The 10–20 map is derived by using four major landmarks: the nasion (the intersection of the frontal and two nasal bones, which is the depressed area between the eyes that is just superior to the bridge of the nose), the inion (the most prominent projection of the occipital bone in the lower rear part of the skull), and the left and right mastoid areas. The electrode locations are based on these landmarks. It should be noted that before

the publication of the 2007 AASM scoring manual, preauricular sites on the left and right sides of the head (A1 and A2 sites) were often used in the place of the M1 and M2 sites. The choice of the mastoid over the preauricular location was dictated by technical considerations because electrodes attached to the mastoid process are less likely to become detached during the recording.[4]

The "10" and "20" of the system's name indicate the distance between the adjacent electrodes as either 10% or 20% of the total front-to-back and mastoid-to-mastoid distance. To determine the potential electrode sites, the head circumference is measured with a tape measure. The normal adult circumference is 50 to 65 cm. This number is divided into the 10% and 20% measurements from the nasion to the inion on each side of the head. The nasion-to-mastoid distance is a total of 50% of the distance from the nasion to the inion (**Fig. 2**).

From the four major landmarks, the skull parameters are measured in the transverse and median planes. The CZ electrode location is determined by the intersection of the nasion to inion line with the left mastoid to right mastoid line. From there, the distance from the four major landmarks to the external ring of electrode sites is 10% of the total distance. For example, the distance between M1 and T3 is 10% of the distance between M1 and M2. The same is true of the right side such that the distance between M2 and T4 is

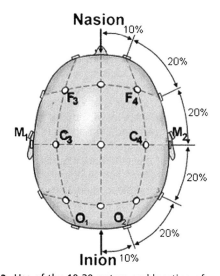

Fig. 2. Use of the 10-20 system and location of recommended electrode placement in polysomnography. (*From* Iber C, editor. The AASM manual for the scoring of sleep and associated events: rules, terminology, and technical specifications. Westchester, IL: American Academy of Sleep Medicine; 2007. p. 23; with permission).

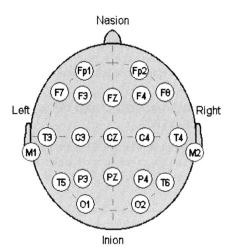

Fig. 1. Schematic representation of the 10-20 electrode placement system.

10% of the distance between M1 and M2. The 10% rule is used to help locate all of the electrode locations in the outer ring of electrodes, including the two FP sites, F7 and F8, T5 and T6, and O1 and O2. The distance between the midline structures and the outer ring of electrodes is 40% the distance from M1 to M2. By dividing that distance in half, the F3, F4, C3, C4, P3, and P4 placements are determined. This means that the distance between T3 and C3 is 20% of the distance between M1 and M2 as is the distance between C3 and CZ, and so on.

Prior to 2007, the standard electrode derivations for monitoring EEG activity during sleep and wake included C3/A2 or C4/A1 and O1/A2 or O2/A1.[1] A minimum of three EEG derivations is currently recommended to sample activity from the frontal, central, and occipital regions.[2] The current standard is to use F4-M1, C4-M1, and O2-M2 with back-up electrodes at F3, C3, O1, and M2 to allow the display of F3-M2, C2-M2, and O1-M2 if there is electrode malfunction with the primary electrodes during the study (see **Fig. 2**).[2] This recommendation is partly based on the fact that K complexes are maximally represented with frontal lobe electrodes, sleep spindles are maximally seen with central electrodes, and delta activity is maximally seen with frontal electrodes.[4] An occipital derivation is recommended because of predominant localization of alpha rhythm over the posterior head region. With an occipital derivation, sleep

onset determination might difficult. An accepted alternative is to use FZ-CZ, CZ-OZ, and C4-M1 with back-up electrodes at FPZ, C3, O1, and M2 for alternative electrode displays in case of primary electrode malfunction (**Fig. 3**).[2] If there is a concern about sleep-related epilepsy or other EEG abnormality, additional electrodes, including the full 10-20 electrode panel, may be used in an attempt to better capture the abnormality.

When measuring the human skull for electrode placement, a grease/wax pencil is used to mark the skull landmarks and electrode placement sites. Once the sites are determined, the hair is separated to expose the scalp. Initial scalp preparation and secure electrode application are important for optimal signal generation and reduction of the need for reapplication. Gentle abrading of the scalp with gauze or commercially available products before placement can improve adherence of the electrodes to the scalp; however, careful attention should be paid to avoid injury or infection. The scalp is cleaned and the electrodes are put into place. Gold cup electrodes are most commonly used. Several different media can be used to adhere the electrodes to the scalp. The use of collodion versus EEG paste is a cause of much debate among sleep technologists and clinicians. The collodion allows relatively stable adherence and fewer problems with impedance than other media; however, collodion is malodorous and is a toxic substance. Special care and attention must be used with application in light of this toxicity. A laboratory also must be able to appropriately handle and dispose of the toxic substance, maintain appropriate ventilation, and be mindful of the more time-consuming clean-up process.

ELECTRO-OCULOGRAPHY

The recording of eye movements, EOG, is a manifestation of the electrical potential that naturally exists across the eye. The cornea is positive relative to the retina. The EOG can reflect both horizontal and vertical eye movements. It should be noted that these are relative, not absolute movements. The R & K manual reports that at least two channels are necessary for recording eye movements accurately. The recommended location of the electrodes was 1 cm above and slightly lateral to the outer canthus of one eye, with a reference electrode on the ipsilateral earlobe or mastoid. The second eye movement channel was to be recorded from an electrode 1 cm below and slightly lateral to the outer canthus of the other eye, referred to as the contralateral ear or mastoid (both eyes referred to same reference electrode).[1] This arrangement produced the so-called "out of

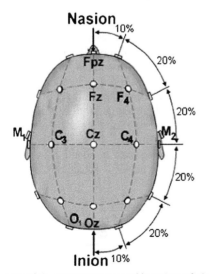

Fig. 3. Use of the 10-20 system and location of alternative electrode placement in polysomnography. (*From* Iber C, editor. The AASM manual for the scoring of sleep and associated events: rules, terminology, and technical specifications. Westchester, IL: American Academy of Sleep Medicine; 2007. p. 23; with permission).

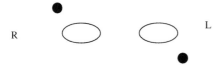

Fig. 4. Recommended EOG derivations. (*From* Iber C, editor. The AASM manual for the scoring of sleep and associated events: rules, terminology, and technical specifications. Westchester, IL: American Academy of Sleep Medicine; 2007. p. 24; with permission).

phase" deflections with most any conjugate eye movements, whereas EOG artifact produced in-phase or single-channel deflections.[1]

A modification of the R & K manual derivation is currently recommended because the term "slightly lateral" was removed to avoid variability in the placement of the electrodes. This derivation also produces out-of-phase deflections. The recommended EOG derivations are E1 (left eye)–M2 and E2 (right eye)–M2. E1 is placed 1 cm below the left outer canthus. E2 is placed 1 cm above the right outer canthus (**Fig. 4**). Using the recommended derivation, when a subject looks right-ward, a positive potential is generated as the cornea moves closer to the E2 electrode creating a downward deflection in E2-M2. At the same time, a negative potential is generated in the E1 electrode and the signal is upward in E1-M2. The same signal is generated when the subject looks upward. When the subject looks leftward or down-ward, the reverse occurs. Eye blinks result in a rapid upward rotation of the globe, which results in a positive deflection. It is especially prominent in the FP leads and visible in the EOG leads.

An alternative for the EOG derivations is provided in the 2007 AASM scoring manual. The left eye derivation is E1-FPZ, and the right eye derivation is E2-FPZ.[2] In this case, E1 is placed 1 cm below and 1 cm lateral to the outer canthus of the left eye, and E2 is placed 1 cm below and 1 cm lateral to the outer canthus of the right eye (**Fig. 5**). It is important to note that the alternative derivations record the direction of the eye movements. For example, vertical movements show

in-phase deflections and horizontal eye movements show out-of-phase deflections.

The EOG is important in the evaluation of sleep and sleep stages. Rapid eye movements (REMs) are one of the herald signs of REM sleep and are essential for the scoring of REM sleep. These movements are seen as sharp bursts of electrical activity. At the time of sleep onset, slow eye movement can be seen. By EOG, these movements are seen as undulating signals that are often described as "rolling" in nature. Of note, eye movements by EOG may be seen during the wake state as a subject watches television or reads before the start of the polysomnography. REMs, slow eye movements, and eye movements of wake are binocularly synchronous and register as out-of-phase deflections using the currently recommended derivation and register as in-phase deflections using the alternative EOG derivations described previously.

ELECTROMYOGRAM

The recording of muscle activity for the purposes of polysomnography is performed using surface electrodes instead of needle electrodes. The recording provides data about muscle areas or regions as opposed to specific muscles. The electrodes are usually held in place with short pieces of tape.

EMG recording from chin electrodes is used as one of the criteria for scoring REM sleep. Other skeletal muscles could be used for this purpose, but for convenience, the mentalis and submentalis muscle groups are used. It is recommended to use three electrodes to record the chin EMG. One electrode is placed in the midline 1 cm above the inferior edge of the mandible, another electrode is placed 2 cm below the inferior edge of the mandible and 2 cm to the right of the midline, and the last electrode is placed 2 cm below the inferior edge of the mandible and 2 cm to the left of the midline (**Fig. 6**).

EMG recording can be used to assess other areas of muscle activation during a

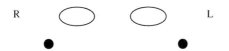

Fig. 5. Alternative EOG derivations. (*From* Iber C, editor. The AASM manual for the scoring of sleep and associated events: rules, terminology, and technical specifications. Westchester, IL: American Academy of Sleep Medicine; 2007. p. 24; with permission).

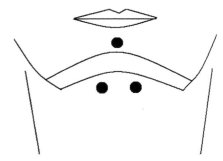

Fig. 6. Recommended chin EMG electrode placement.

polysomnogram. If there is a concern that the subject has significant bruxism, additional masseter electrodes may be placed in addition to the chin electrodes routinely used.[2] When determining the presence of periodic limb movements of sleep, surface electrodes are placed longitudinally and symmetrically around the middle of the anterior tibialis muscle such that the electrodes are 2 to 3 cm apart or one third the length of the muscle, whichever is shorter.[2] It is recommended that the legs be evaluated with separated channels. Monitoring of the upper extremities may be performed if clinically indicated. In the past, EMG has been used to monitor respiratory muscle activation and effort with the use of intercostal or diaphragmatic EMG electrode placement. This procedure is still considered an alternative for the detection of effort instead of esophageal manometry or inductance plethysmography.[2]

AIRFLOW MEASUREMENT

Body plethysmography and pneumotachography are considered the gold standard for the measurement of air flow; however, they are considered unsuitable for routine polysomnography.[5] Body plethysmography requires that the patient be enclosed in an airtight chamber, which is often referred to as a "body box." This technique is used most commonly during pulmonary function testing but is not feasible for polysomnography. Pneumotachometers require that a subject's nose and mouth be securely covered by a face mask, with the pneumotachometer attached to the mask. This is rather cumbersome for subjects and may not be tolerated well in the sleep laboratory. Pneumotachography also requires calibration at different air flows and frequent calibration to ensure linearity.[6] Pneumotachography continues to be commonly used in the research setting, and is described here briefly. The most commonly used pneumontachometer uses a differential pressure flow transducer that measures flow in terms of the proportional pressure drop across a resistance as measured by a manometer. A heated pneumotachometer is often used as the pressure-flow relationship is altered by the condensation that occurs on the resistance element.[7]

Airflow measurement in clinical polysomnography is determined by two different sensors. Thermal sensors, or thermistors, use the difference between the temperature of exhaled breath (heated by the human body) and the ambient air. These sensors are placed at the nose and mouth in the path of inspiratory and expiratory airflow. These sensors consist of temperature-sensitive resistors that are supplied with a constant current. Expiration heats the resistor, which increases resistance. Inspiration cools the resistor, which decreases resistance.[7] This alteration in resistance pattern is recorded and represents airflow. It is widely recognized that thermistry is a fairly reliable method to detect complete cessation of airflow, but it does not provide adequate quantitative measurement to accurately detect hypopneas.[7] Currently, use of an oronasal thermal sensor is recommended to detect the absence of airflow for the identification of an apnea but is to be used in conjunction with a nasal pressure transducer to allow the detection of hypopneas.[2]

Nasal pressure transducers monitor the pressure changes that occur with inspiration and expiration. Relative to the atmospheric pressure, the airway is negative with inspiration and positive with expiration. The signal obtained is used to estimate air flow and provides a breath-by-breath graphic representation of the size of each breath, i.e. flow amplitude. The ability of the nasal pressure transducer to adequately detect respiratory events is comparable to the "gold standard" approach of the pneumotachometer.[8,9] The signal obtained produces a nonlinear signal, thus a square root transformation of the signal is used as a means to convert the signal into a linear relationship between pressure change and air flow.[10,11] The nasal pressure signal has been used to detect airflow limitation even in the absence of hypopneas and apneas. The development of a plateau in the nasal pressure signal contour during inspiration parallels the changes seen in esophageal manometery.[12]

It is recommended that an oronasal thermal sensor be used to detect apnea events and a nasal air pressure transducer be used to detect hypopneas.[2] If degradation of one of the signals occurs, the alternative sensor may be used. For example, if the oronasal thermal sensor is unreliable, the nasal air transducer may be used to determine both types of events. If the nasal pressure transducer is unreliable, the scoring of hypopneas may be scored using inductance plethysmography or an oronasal thermal sensor.[2]

RESPIRATORY EFFORT MEASUREMENT

During human inspiration, there is contraction of the muscles of inspiration (including the intercostals muscles) and the diaphragm. In the resting position, the diaphragm is recoiled upward, which reduces the volume of the thoracic cavity. With active contraction, the diaphragm is displaced downward, which increases the thoracic volume. Contraction of the intercostal muscles lifts and expands the rib cage, which further increases the thoracic volume.

This is an active process that results in the generation of a negative pressure in the chest relative to the atmosphere. This change in pressure results in inspiration, and volume changes are seen in the lungs, rib cage, and abdomen. When the muscles of respiration relax there is also recoil of the fine structures of the lungs (alveoli) and as the chest volume diminishes, exhalation occurs.

Normally the expansion of the rib cage and enlargement of the abdomen occur at the same time or are "in phase." This is also true of the contraction of the rib cage and reduction in abdominal volume. "Out-of-phase" or so-called "paradoxic" motion of the thorax and abdomen can be seen with a loss of tone in the diaphragm or accessory muscles of respiration.[7] Of more clinical significance, paradoxic motion can be seen with partial and complete obstruction of the airway, more commonly with the latter. In the case of obstructive apnea events, the diaphragm contracts but no air movement occurs. As the diaphragm moves downward, the pressure generated in the abdomen expands the diameter of the abdomen. There is little chest expansion or even a slight contraction of the chest because of the high negative pressure generated by the contracting diaphragm. The volume changes occur in opposite directions, which is a classic finding in obstructive apnea events.

Various monitors have been used in the past to evaluate respiratory effort, most commonly determining both the chest and abdominal volume changes. Strain gauges are sealed tubes filled with an electrical conductor through which an electric current is passed.[7] When the length of the system is held constant, the resistance is stable. With stretching/lengthening of the system, the resistance increases because of a reduction in the cross-sectional area of the electrical conductor. Based on this property of strain gauges, they have been used in the past to monitor respiratory movements. Because of the qualitative rather than quantitative nature of these sensors, they are no longer recommended in the sleep laboratory setting.[5]

Piezoelectric transducers were used in the past to monitor chest and abdomen expansion and contraction. The use of these transducers is based on the ability of some materials (specifically some crystals) to generate an electric potential when mechanical stress is applied. Although sensitive to changes in length, these monitors are also qualitative in nature and are no longer recommended to be used to monitor respiratory effort during polysomnography.[7]

Impedance pneumography is an indirect method of monitoring ventilation based on the movement of the thorax. Impedance is the total opposition to an alternating current by an electrical conductor. In this case, the conductor is the thorax itself. Impedance is measured by applying a small current across the thorax using a pair of electrodes. Because of the properties of the system, inspiration increases impedance. Unfortunately, with apnea events, precise measurement of respiratory pattern and volume is unreliable;[7] therefore these monitoring devices are not used commonly in the laboratory setting.

It is currently recommended that either esophageal manometry or calibrated or uncalibrated inductance plethysmography be used to monitor and record respiratory effort, although an accepted alternative is diaphragmatic/intercostal EMG.[2] Esophageal manometry involves the passage of a thin flexible tube containing a pressure transducer through the nose or mouth, into the posterior pharynx, and into the esophagus. Diaphragmatic contraction during inspiration causes a drop in thoracic pressure that is transmitted to the esophagus and detected by the pressure transducer. The reverse occurs during expiration. Esophageal pressure measurements are a sensitive and qualitative index of inspiratory effort. Because esophageal manometry is not well accepted or tolerated by the average subject undergoing polysomnography, inductance plethysmography has become the method of choice in most sleep laboratories.

Respiratory inductance plethysmography measures respiratory effort from body surface movement. Inductance is the property of a circuit or circuit element that opposes a change in current flow. Bands that contain transducers (which consist of an insulated wire sewn onto an elasticized band in the shape of a horizontally oriented sinusoid) are placed around the rib cage and abdomen.[7] With inspiration and expiration, the changes in the cross-sectional area of the chest and abdomen cause a proportional change in the diameter of the transducer. This change in the diameter of the transducer alters the inductance. These monitors can be calibrated to a known volume, which provides both qualitative and quantitative analysis of breath volumes. Although likely less accurate, uncalibrated respiratory inductance plethysmography is more commonly used in the clinical setting.[5]

CARDIAC RHYTHM EVALUATION BY ELECTROCARDIOGRAPHY

During the recording of a routine ECG, a total of 12 leads is used, and lead II is determined by the use of electrodes on the extremities. Standard recording of the cardiac rhythm during polysomnography is by the use of a modified lead II electrograph. Leads are placed as shown in **Fig. 7**, with one lead just inferior to the right clavicle and the other on the left side at the level of the seventh rib. Modification of the electrode position and the use of additional leads to optimize signal and/or R-wave voltage are at the discretion of the practicing clinician.[13] Standard ECG electrode application minimizes artifact when compared with EEG gold cup electrodes.[2]

The prevalence of cardiac events seen in patients with obstructive sleep apnea is 18% to 48%.[14–16] In light of these data and the high proportion of patients who have sleep apnea studied by polysomnography, the current recommendations are that several cardiac parameters be reported in all sleep study interpretations. These include average heart rate during sleep, highest heart rate during sleep, highest heart rate during recording, bradycardia (and if observed, the lowest heart rate observed), asystole (and if observed, longest pause observed), sinus tachycardia during sleep (and if observed, the highest heart rate observed), narrow and/or wide complex tachycardia (and if observed, the highest heart rate observed), atrial fibrillation, and any other arrhythmia recorded.[2] The limitations of the use of a single lead should be noted. Because it is not possible for the practitioner to determine myocardial ischemia (ST segment changes) and

the origin of a wide complex QRS,[13] the current standards do not recommend report of these components.[2]

OXYGEN SATURATION

The use of invasive arterial monitoring of the oxygen of blood via indwelling arterial catheter is not recommended during routine polysomnography. Although considered the gold standard for accurately and directly determining the partial pressure of oxygen in the blood, the technique is limited by its invasive nature and its inability to provide continuous sampling. As in the hospital setting, the most commonly used noninvasive method for the continuous monitoring of blood oxygen is the use of pulse oximetry. In this method, the oxygen saturation of arterial blood (SaO_2) is determined by the passage of two wavelengths of light (650 nm and 805 nm) through a pulsating vascular bed from one sensor to another. The light is partially absorbed by the oxygen-carrying molecule, hemoglobin, depending on the percent of the hemoglobin saturated with oxygen. A processor calculates absorption at the two wavelengths and computes the proportion of hemoglobin that is oxygenated, giving it a numerical value.

Many pulse oximeters also provide a calculated heart rate. There are limitations to the use of pulse oximetry. A thin anatomic pulse site (such as the finger tip, ear lobe, nose, or toe) is required, as is proper alignment of the sensors. With movement in sleep, the device can become dislodged. Patient motion can cause significant artifact, although some oximeters have motion artifact detectors to compensate for this problem. The readings can also be affected by anemia, hemoglobinopathies, a high carboxyhemoglobin level, elevated methemoglobin level, anatomic abnormalities/previous injury to the site tested, sluggish arterial flow (due to hypovolemia or vasoconstriction), and the use of nail polish. Finally, the algorithm of the particular pulse oximeter device used can have profound effects on the signal produced. The most significant difference seen is in the averaging time of the signal. If the averaging time is too long or too short, the signal may not be accurate, thus proper selection of the device used is paramount.

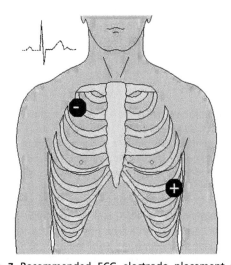

Fig. 7. Recommended ECG electrode placement for polysomnography. (*From* Iber C, editor. The AASM manual for the scoring of sleep and associated events: rules, terminology, and technical specifications. Westchester, IL: American Academy of Sleep Medicine; 2007. p. 39; with permission).

OTHER MONITORING DEVICES

In addition to the specified devices mentioned earlier, polysomnography also incorporates the use of a microphone, which is most commonly placed on the neck or upper chest, to record snoring sounds. The technologist may record his or her assessment of a subject's snoring by use of the video/sound monitoring system. Body position is also an important piece of information to monitor in the sleep laboratory. It is common to see a worsening of snoring and sleep apnea when a subject is in the supine position. If there is a positional difference, it may be important when determining treatment options. Body position is determined by a sensor, which is usually placed on the chest. The most common problem encountered with these monitors is a shift in position with subject movement such that the readings are erroneous. It is important for the technologist to monitor the subject's body position via camera/video monitoring to confirm accuracy of the body position monitor. If inaccuracy is encountered, the sensor can be repositioned or the technologist can separately log the body position digitally or in a written log.

SLEEP SYSTEM SPECIFICATIONS

The study of wake and sleep in humans began in 1924, when Hans Berger recorded the first human EEG. He was the first to describe the different waves and rhythms present in the normal brain, including alpha and beta rhythms. He published his work in 1929 as "Über das Elektrenkephalogramm des Menschen."[17] In the mid 1930s, Loomis, Harvey, and Hobart were the first to perform all-night polysomnography in humans using both EEG and EOG recording. A 44-inch drum rotated once per minute and recorded the data on huge paper sheets.[18,19] Although the technique for recording elements of human sleep improved, large polysomnography machines recorded the sleep study data with ink on paper for more than seven decades. For this reason, "paper speed" is often mentioned in the literature of sleep medicine. A paper speed of 10 mm/s resulted in one page consisting of 30 seconds of data. This 30-second measurement of data was classically designated as one epoch of recording and is still the period of time used in the scoring of sleep stages. In the current sleep medicine era, fully computerized polysomnography has replaced paper-based analog recording. Although it is still the standard to display 30 seconds of digital data on a computer screen, the digital equipment also allows compression of the time scale to allow viewing of 1 to 10 minutes of data at a time. This is particularly valuable when a bird's eye view is helpful in determining a subject's sleep-related breathing pattern.

As the digital era progressed, it became evident that standards were needed to ensure uniform data acquisition. These standards were born out of the AASM's Digital Task Force, and the data are summarized in its report.[20] The current recommendations by the AASM are outlined fully in the 2007 scoring manual.[2] These recommendations include the suggested sampling rates for each of the components of the polysomnogram, the maximum electrode impedances, the minimum digital resolution, and filter settings. Among other specifications, digital recording systems must also include separate filter controls for each channel, ability to select sampling rates for each channel, ability to display calibration signal, and a method to measure impedance of individual electrodes against a reference. It is recommended that the resolution of a digital screen and video card be at least 1600 × 1200, that a complete hypnogram be available on screen with time/cursor positioning, that the system have a variable time-scale viewing capability, and that there be video card synchrony with the raw polysomnography data. This article should be not considered the definitive source for the specifications for a digital system. It is suggested that the scoring manual be reviewed for details of the recommended and optional specifications of these systems.[2]

SUMMARY

It is an exciting time in the world of sleep medicine. The field has come a long way but has stayed true to its roots at the same time. As new technologies evolve, it is expected that the field will evolve as well. This article provides the basics of polysomnography set-up, but it is unclear what excitement the future holds for the field.

REFERENCES

1. Rechtschaffen A, Kales A, editors. A manual of standardized terminology, techniques, and scoring system for sleep stages of human subjects. Washington, DC: US Department of Health, Education, and Welfare Public Health Service - NIH/NIND; 1968.
2. Iber C, editor. The AASM manual for the scoring of sleep and associated events: rules, terminology, and technical specifications. Westchester (IL): American Academy of Sleep Medicine; 2007.
3. Jasper HH. (Committee Chairman) The ten twenty electrode system of the International Federation. Electroencephalogr Clin Neurophysiol 1958;10:371–5.
4. Silber MH, Ancoli-Israel A, Bonnet MH, et al. The visual scoring of sleep in adults. J Clin Sleep Med 2007;3(2):121–31.

5. Redline S, Budhiraja R, Kapur V, et al. The scoring of respiratory events in sleep: reliability and validity. J Clin Sleep Med 2007;3(2):169–200.

6. AARC clinical practice guideline. Respir Care 1995; 40(12):1336–43.

7. Kryger MH. Monitoring Respiratory and Cardiac Function. In: Kryger MH, Roth T, Dement WC, editors. Principles and practice of sleep medicine. 3rd edition. Philadelphia; 2004.

8. Heitman SJ, Atkar RS, Hajduk EA, et al. Validation of nasal pressure for the identification of apneas/hypopneas during sleep. Am J Respir Crit Care Med 2002;166:386–91.

9. Thurnherr R, Xie X, Bloch KE. Accuracy of nasal cannula pressure recordings for assessment of ventilation during sleep. Am J Respir Crit Care Med 2004;164:1914–6.

10. Farre R, Rigau J, Montserrat JM, et al. Relevance of linearizing nasal prongs for assessing hypopneas and flow limitation during sleep. Am J Respir Crit Care Med 2001;163:494–7.

11. Montserrat JM, Farre R, Ballester E, et al. Evaluation of nasal prongs for estimating air flow. Am J Respir Crit Care Med 1997;155:211–5.

12. Hosselet JJ, Norman RG, Ayappa I, et al. Detection of flow limitation with a nasal cannula/pressure transducer system. Am J Respir Crit Care Med 1998; 157(Pt 1):1461–7.

13. Caples SM, Rosen CL, Shen WK, et al. The scoring of cardiac events during sleep. J Clin Sleep Med 2007;3(2):147–54.

14. Guilleminault C, Connolly SJ, Winkle RA. Cardiac arrhythmia and conduction disturbances during sleep in 400 patients with sleep apnea syndrome. Am J Cardiol 1983;52:490–4.

15. Harbison J, O'Reilly P, McNicholas WT. Cardiac rhythm disturbances in the obstructive sleep apnea syndrome: effects of nasal continuous positive airway pressure therapy. Chest 2000;118: 591–5.

16. Mehra R, Benjamin EJ, Shahar E, et al. Association of nocturnal arrhythmias with sleep-disordered breathing: the Sleep Heart Health Study. Am J Respir Crit Care Med 2006;173(8):910–6.

17. Berger H. Über das elektrenkephalogramm des menschen. Archiv fur Psychiatrie und Nervenkrankheiten 1929;87:527–70.

18. Loomis AL, Harvey EN, Hobart GA. Potential rhythms of the cerebral cortex during sleep. Science 1935;81:597–8.

19. Loomis AL, Harvey EN, Hobart GA. Cerebral states during sleep, as studied by human brain potentials. J Exp Psychol 1937;21:127–44.

20. Penzel T, Hirshkowitz M, Harsh J, et al. Digital analysis and technical specifications. J Clin Sleep Med 2007;3(2):109–20.

Staging Sleep

Michael H. Silber, MBChB[a,b,*]

KEYWORDS
- Sleep scoring • Sleep staging • Polysomnography
- Non-REM sleep • REM sleep

Although a sleeper may perceive a night's sleep as a continuous uniform experience, it is clear that profound physiologic changes occur over the course of a night. Recognizing these alterations in state is essential for understanding the mechanisms of sleep, documenting the changes that occur with disease, and studying the consequences of experimental and clinical interventions. For more than 70 years it has been recognized that the changes in cortical electrical activity during sleep do not occur randomly but follow in a particular order in repeated cycles during the night. Transitions between recognizably different states of sleep are not usually abrupt, sometimes lasting even minutes. Quantitation of sleep stages requires clear, reliable definitions, however, even though these may be somewhat arbitrary, especially at the start and end of each stage.

This article reviews the historic development of human visual sleep staging and describes the current recommended American Academy of Sleep Medicine (AASM) classification of four sleep stages: N1, N2, N3, and R. The theoretical basis for the selection of specific staging criteria is discussed with particular emphasis on their biologic substrate and the evidence on which they are based. It should be clearly stated that the only authoritative sources for the actual rules of sleep staging are the official manuals published as free-standing monographs,[1,2] and physicians, scientists, and technologists learning sleep staging should consult these sources. A discussion of computerized analysis of sleep stages is beyond the scope of this article.

HISTORIC SURVEY

Barely 8 years after the discovery of the human scalp encephalogram (EEG),[3] Loomis and colleagues[4] published the first attempt to classify different brain rhythms during sleep. They described five stages (A–E), with stages A and B approximately corresponding to the current stage N1, stage C corresponding to stage N2, and stages D and E corresponding to stage N3. They recognized such phenomena as the fragmentation and fall-out of alpha rhythm, sleep spindles, and high-amplitude slow waves. Various modifications of this basic schema were suggested over the next 15 years,[5,6] and subsequently[7,8] with Gibbs and coworkers[6] describing a stage with an EEG pattern similar to wakefulness that they called "early morning sleep," probably an identification of the rapid eye movement (REM) state. It was the seminal discovery of periodic REM by Eugene Aserinsky, a graduate student working in the laboratory of Nathaniel Kleitman at the University of Chicago, however, that laid the groundwork for a more accurate classification of sleep stages.[9] In 1957, Dement and Kleitman[10] proposed the first classification based on an understanding that REM and non-REM (NREM) sleep alternate in successive cycles during the night. They suggested four stages (1–4), with stage 1 corresponding to stage N1 at the start of the night and stage R toward morning, stage 2 corresponding to stage N2, and stages 3 and 4 to stage N3. In the early 1960s, Williams and coworkers[11] developed a modified scoring system at the University of Florida based on 1-minute epochs and three EEG derivations.

In 1968, Rechtschaffen and Kales[12] led a team of sleep researchers in the production of the first sleep staging manual, based on expert consensus. The group made some fundamental prescient decisions that have deeply influenced the course of sleep research and sleep medicine. They recommended the recording of at least one

a Department of Neurology, Mayo Clinic, 200 1st Street SW, Rochester, MN 55905, USA
b Center for Sleep Medicine, Mayo Clinic, 200 1st Street SW, Rochester, MN 55905, USA
* Center for Sleep Medicine, Mayo Clinic, 200 1st Street SW, Rochester, MN 55905.
E-mail address: msilber@mayo.edu

Sleep Med Clin 4 (2009) 343–352
doi:10.1016/j.jsmc.2009.04.003

EEG derivation (C3 or C4 referenced to the opposite ear or mastoid), two electro-oculogram (EOG) derivations, and a channel recording submental electromyogram (EMG). They required that sleep be scored in arbitrary epochs of 20 to 30 seconds with a single stage being assigned to each epoch. They divided sleep into five stages: stages 1 through 4 of NREM sleep and stage REM sleep. Stage 1 consisted of relatively low-voltage mixed-frequency EEG activity with slow rolling eye movements. Stage 2 was defined by the appearance of K complexes, sleep spindles, or both. The presence of high-voltage (>75 μV) low-frequency (<2 Hz) EEG activity characterized stages 3 and 4 sleep: 20% to 50% of the epoch for stage 3 and greater than 50% of the epoch for stage 4. The EEG in stage REM showed low-voltage mixed-frequency activity in association with REM and low submental EMG activity.

Despite occasional suggestions for modifying the system,[13–18] the Rechtschaffen and Kales (R and K) manual remained the standard staging system for human sleep studies for almost 40 years. In 2004, the Board of Directors of the AASM commissioned the development of a new manual for the scoring of sleep, including not only sleep staging but also rules for the scoring of arousals, respiratory, cardiac, and movement events. This ambitious project was carried out through seven task forces overseen by a steering committee, led by Iber.[19] All proposals were peer reviewed and ultimately approved by the AASM Board of Directors. Published evidence was reviewed, followed by a rigorous consensus decision-making process. The Visual Task Force, consisting of 12 members, reviewed 128 relevant articles and voted on 71 questions before submitting its recommendations in late 2005. Input was also received from the Geriatric Task Force, and the Pediatric Task Force produced separate recommendations for modifying the proposed rules in children. The Visual Task Force followed certain general principles: rules should be compatible with published evidence; they should be based on biologic principles; they should be applicable to both normal and abnormal sleep; and they should be easily used by clinicians, technologists, and scientists.[20] The AASM *Manual for the Scoring of Sleep and Associated Events* and seven review papers, covering all aspects of sleep scoring, were published in 2007.[1] The AASM requires that the new scoring rules be followed in AASM-accredited sleep centers and laboratories. The manual steering committee continues to meet and publish answers to frequently asked questions and requests for clarification on the public portion of the AASM Web site (http://aasmnet.org/Resources/PDF/FAQsScoringManual.pdf).

DERIVATIONS AND MONTAGES

Based on the routine use of eight-channel electroencephalographs in the 1960s and the common practice of studying two subjects simultaneously with a single machine, the R and K manual recommended a single EEG derivation (C4-A1 or C3-A2).[12] With the availability of machines capable of recording 16 or more derivations, these limitations no longer apply. Studies have shown that K complexes and delta frequency slow waves are maximally represented frontally, with some K complexes not being evident with using central electrodes alone.[21,22] Sleep spindles occur maximally centrally,[22,23] whereas alpha rhythm of wakefulness arises from the occipital regions. Accordingly, three EEG derivations are currently required, sampling the frontal, central, and occipital regions (**Box 1**). One of two sets of derivations are selected at the discretion of the laboratory: the recommended montage with active electrodes referenced to the opposite mastoid process (M1 or M2); or the alternative montage with a combination of two bipolar derivations and a single referential derivation.[1]

Box 1
Polysomnogram montages

EEG

Recommended: F4-M1, C4-M1, O2-M1

Acceptable alternative: Fz-Cz, Cz-Oz, C4-M1

(Electrodes placed according to the International 10-20 system; M1 is left mastoid)

EOG

Recommended: E1-M2, E2-M2

(E1 1 cm below left outer canthus, E2 1 cm below right outer canthus; M2 is right mastoid)

Acceptable alternative: E1-Fpz, E2-Fpz

(E1 1 cm below and 1 cm lateral to left outer canthus, E2 1 cm below and 1 cm lateral to right outer canthus)

Chin EMG

Midline 1 cm above inferior edge of mandible; 2 cm below inferior edge of mandible, either 2 cm to right or 2 cm to left of midline

Data from Iber C, Ancoli-Israel S, Chessonn A, et al, for the American Academy of Sleep Medicine. The AASM Manual for the Scoring of Sleep and Associated Events: rules, terminology and technical specifications. Westchester (IL): American Academy of Sleep Medicine; 2007.

Two EOG derivations are required (see **Box 1**).[1] As with the EEG montages, laboratories may select from two different sets of EOG derivations. The recommended montage, referring the active electrodes to M2, records all eye movements as phase reversing deflections, making differentiation from volume conducted EEG potentials or electrode artifacts relatively simple. In contrast, the alternative montage (referring the active electrodes to a central forehead electrode [Fpz]) allows detection of eye movement direction by noting whether the deflections are in-phase or out-of-phase, and is especially useful when such distinction is deemed important. A single EMG derivation (see **Box 1**) with electrodes applied above and below the chin records EMG activity from the submental muscles.

STAGE TERMINOLOGY AND SCORING PRINCIPLES

The AASM manual classifies wake and sleep into the following stages: stage W (wakefulness); stage N1 (NREM stage 1 sleep); stage N2 (NREM stage 2 sleep); stage N3 (NREM stage 3 sleep); and stage R (REM sleep).[1] The change in abbreviations was instituted to differentiate the scoring rules from those of the R and K manual and allow other investigators and clinicians to determine easily which staging system was used. Older classifications, including that of R and K, arbitrarily divided the deeper portion of NREM sleep into two stages, depending on the amount of recorded slow wave activity.[12] This distinction has been eliminated in the AASM classification, because there is no biologic basis for such a demarcation.

The basic principle of sleep staging is that the night is divided into 30-second sequential periods known as "epochs." Each epoch is assigned a stage. If two or more stages can be identified during a single epoch, the stage comprising the greatest portion of the epoch is assigned. Although an assessment of the overall flow of sleep might be better obtained by relying on identifying the start and end of each stage irrespective of epochs, such a scoring method is intensely cumbersome in the presence of highly fragmented sleep such as may be seen in patients with obstructive sleep apnea.

WAKEFULNESS
Criteria for Stage W

The state of wakefulness is defined by the presence of alpha rhythm on the EEG (**Fig. 1**).[1] Alpha

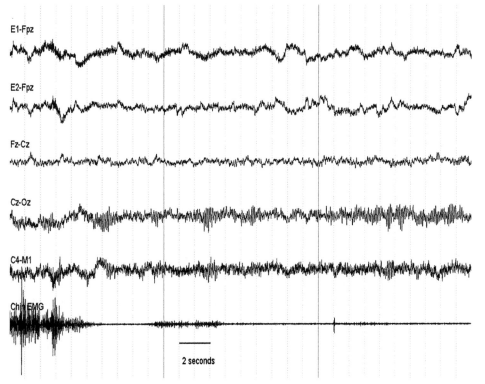

Fig. 1. Stage W. The Cz-Oz channel shows alpha rhythm, which defined the epoch as stage W, even though the EOG shows slow eye movements of drowsiness. See **Box 1** for electrode placements.

rhythm is defined as sinusoidal 8- to 13-Hz activity over the occipital head region with eye closure, attenuating with eye opening. Little or no alpha rhythm is generated by 10% to 20% of normal subjects.[24] When alpha rhythm is not clearly discernable by visual inspection of the EEG, wakefulness can still be scored if the EOG demonstrates any one of three markers of alertness. First, eye blinks with the eyes open or closed indicate the wake state. Blinking results in conjugate vertical eye movements at a frequency of 0.5 to 2 Hz (Bell's phenomenon), which are visible on the EOG, especially if the Fpz reference is used. Second, the presence of reading eye movements clearly indicates that the subject is awake. These conjugate movements, easily identifiable with experience, consist of a slow phase followed by a rapid movement in the opposite direction. Third, the presence of irregular conjugate eye movements with normal or high chin muscle tone suggests that the subject is awake and looking at the environment.

The Problem of Sleep Onset

When does sleep commence? Two valid alternative constructs can be used in considering the problem of defining sleep onset. First, there is electrophysiologic and psychophysiologic evidence that the change from wakefulness to sleep is a slow continuum best described by a period of drowsiness interspersed between full wakefulness and unequivocal sleep. The earliest electrophysiologic sign of drowsiness is reduction in the blink rate with the eyes closed.[24] This is followed by the development of slow eye movements, defined as conjugate, reasonably regular, sinusoidal eye movements with initial deflection usually lasting more than 500 milliseconds.[1] These EOG changes usually precede loss of alpha rhythm. EEG changes also precede fallout of alpha: alpha amplitude either decreases or increases, frontocentral spread of alpha occurs, and theta or delta transients become interspersed within alpha activity.[24] The stage of wakefulness or sleep in which subjects fail to respond to auditory stimuli varies between individual subjects. Some stop responding in R and K stage wake, most during R and K stage 1, and a few only during R and K stage 2.[25]

In contrast, there is also a body of evidence suggesting that it is valid to define a single point on this continuum as the moment of sleep onset. In some psychophysiologic experiments there is a 70% drop in responses to auditory stimuli at the transition between R and K stage wake and stage 1 NREM sleep.[25] Many physiologic processes undergo changes, some relatively abrupt, at the time alpha rhythm changes to slower theta frequencies. Minute ventilation,[26] phasic EMG activity in respiratory muscles,[27,28] and heart rate[29] fall, whereas upper airway resistance increases.[30] Cerebral blood flow falls in the frontal lobes and increases in the occipital lobes.[31,32]

Although the AASM manual recognizes that many signs of drowsiness are discernable before alpha rhythm is lost, it does specify a single time of sleep onset. This is defined as the start of the first epoch scored as any stage other than stage W, recognizing that in most subjects this is stage N1 (see later).[1]

NON–RAPID EYE MOVEMENT SLEEP
Stage N1 Sleep

Stage N1 sleep is defined by the presence of low amplitude, mixed frequency (predominantly 4–7 Hz) activity (**Fig. 2**).[1] The EOG generally shows slow eye movements and the chin EMG is often lower in amplitude than in stage W. The EEG may show vertex sharp waves, which are sharply contoured waves maximal over the central region, distinguishable from the background EEG and lasting less than 0.5 seconds. None of these additional features are required for scoring stage N1, although their presence may be helpful in equivocal situations. In subjects who do not generate alpha rhythm and show low-amplitude mixed-frequency activity with the eyes closed even in wakefulness, discerning sleep onset can be problematic. In these circumstances, stage N1 sleep should be scored when the first of the following phenomena is observed: slowing of background EEG frequencies by greater than or equal to 1 Hz, vertex sharp wave, or slow eye movements. The onset of slow eye movements antecedes the other changes in most subjects and is the criterion most likely to be applied. Because slow eye movements are usually seen while alpha rhythm is still present, the sleep latency is likely to be slightly shorter in subjects who do not generate alpha rhythm.

Stage N2 Sleep

Stage N2 sleep is defined by the presence of one or more K complexes without associated arousals or one or more trains of sleep spindles in the first half of the epoch or in the second half of the prior epoch (**Fig. 3**).[1] A K complex is a well-defined biphasic wave easily discernable from the background EEG with total duration greater than or equal to 0.5 seconds, usually maximal frontally. A sleep spindle is a train of waves with frequency 11 to 16 Hz, but usually 12 to 14 Hz, with duration greater than or equal to 0.5 seconds, usually

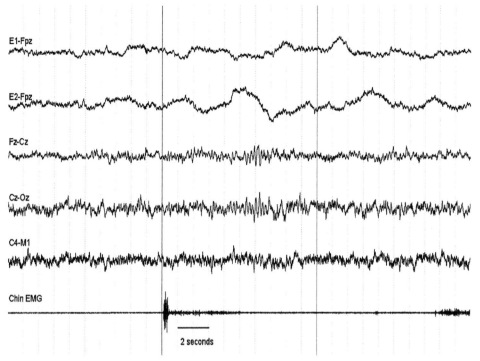

Fig. 2. Stage N1. The EEG shows low-amplitude mixed frequency (predominantly 4–7 Hz) activity. Slow eye movements persist. See **Box 1** for electrode placements.

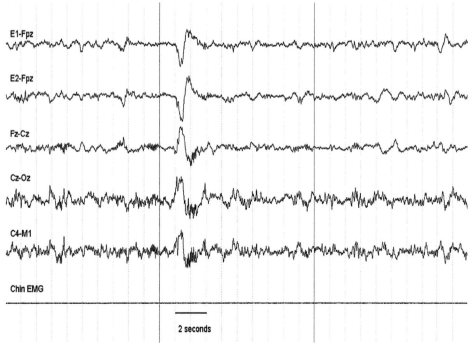

Fig. 3. Stage N2. The EEG shows sleep spindles and K complexes. Eye movements have ceased. See **Box 1** for electrode placements.

maximal centrally. There are no defined amplitude criteria for a K complex or a sleep spindle. K complexes can be associated with arousals induced by environmental stimuli or by phenomena, such as obstructive apneas. In some patients with obstructive sleep apnea sleep can be highly fragmented by repeated apnea-induced arousals with frequent K complexes. K complexes with associated arousals do not represent a deeper level of sleep and so cannot be used to designate stage N2 sleep, unless a spontaneous K complex or sleep spindle is also present in the same epoch. Because K complexes and sleep spindles are intermittent phenomena, they may not always be present in successive epochs. Their absence does not indicate that the sleep stage has reverted to stage N1 unless an arousal occurs or a major body movement (see later) followed by slow eye movements is present. Stage N2 sleep also terminates when there is a transition to stages W, N3, or R.

Stage N3 Sleep

Several lines of evidence indicate that slow wave sleep is sufficiently distinct from lighter stages of NREM sleep to warrant being defined as a separate stage. The neurophysiologic genesis of slow waves differs from that of K complexes.[33] Growth hormone is maximally released during slow wave sleep rather than stage N2.[34,35] Evening exercise

and passive body heating increase slow wave sleep but not N2 sleep.[36,37] During the first recovery night after total sleep deprivation, there is rebound of slow wave, but not N2 sleep.[38]

Stage N3 sleep is scored when greater than or equal to 20% of an epoch consists of slow wave activity, defined as waves of frequency 0.5 to 2 Hz with peak-to-peak amplitude greater than 75 μV recorded over the frontal regions (**Fig. 4**).[1] The frequency band is a subset of the classically defined delta frequency range (<4 Hz) and the term "delta sleep" should not be used. Sleep spindles may persist in stage N3 sleep, but are not required for scoring. The amplitude of slow waves falls with age but similar age-related drops in amplitude also occur in other sleep-related waves and frequency bands.[39] Although the choice of greater than 75 μV as the amplitude criterion for all ages of subjects is arbitrary, many experiments have demonstrated that changes in slow wave percentage can be measured in subjects of any age in response to a wide range of interventions, including sleep deprivation,[40–42] sleep fragmentation,[42,43] and forced desynchronization.[44]

RAPID EYE MOVEMENT SLEEP

REM sleep is scored if an epoch includes low-amplitude, mixed-frequency EEG; REMs; and low chin EMG tone (**Fig. 5**).[1] The EEG resembles that of stage N1, but some subjects have more

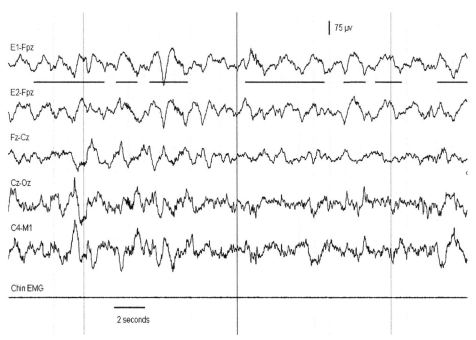

Fig. 4. Stage N3. The EEG shows slow waves with frequency <2 Hz and amplitude, measured frontally, >75 μV (*underlined*) for more than 20% of the epoch. See **Box 1** for electrode placements.

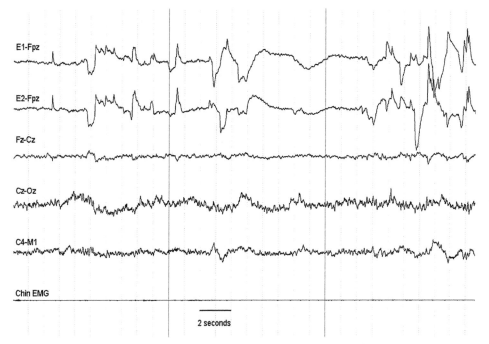

E1-Fpz

E2-Fpz

Fz-Cz

Cz-Oz

C4-M1

Chin EMG

2 seconds

Fig. 5. Stage R. The EEG shows low-amplitude, mixed frequency activity. The EOG shows conjugate, irregular rapid eye movements. Chin EMG shows low tone. See **Box 1** for electrode placements.

prominent alpha frequencies, often at a frequency somewhat slower than that of their alpha rhythm while awake. REMs are defined as conjugate, irregular, sharply peaked eye movements with the duration of the initial deflection usually less than 500 milliseconds. Low chin EMG tone implies that the chin EMG amplitude is no higher than in any other stage and is usually at the lowest level of the entire polysomnogram. Certain other phenomena, if present, may support scoring stage R but are not required. These include sawtooth waves (2–6 Hz sharply contoured or triangular, often serrated waves maximal over the central head regions and frequently preceding bursts of REM) and transient muscle activity, previously known as "phasic muscle twitches" (burst of EMG activity lasting <0.25 seconds superimposed on low tone, which may be present in the chin, anterior tibial, or EEG-EOG derivations).

Detailed rules have been established defining when a period of stage R sleep ends.[1] In broad outline, once stage R has been scored, subsequent epochs should continue to be scored as stage R until there has been a definite change to another stage, an arousal or major body movement is followed by slow eye movements, or K complexes or sleep spindles occur in the absence of REMs, even if chin EMG tone remains low. If an epoch contains REMs and the chin EMG tone is low, stage R should be scored even if K complexes

or sleep spindles are present. This latter situation frequently occurs during the first REM period of the night when REM and NREM phenomena intermix. There are also rules concerning the scoring of transition epochs between epochs of definite stage N2 and definite REM sleep. In outline, stage R should be scored if chin EMG tone is low and K complexes and sleep spindles are absent, even if REM has not yet commenced. If K complexes or sleep spindles are present in the transition epochs without rapid eye movements, however, these should be scored as stage N2, even if chin muscle tone is low.

MAJOR BODY MOVEMENTS

The term "movement time" was used in the R and K manual to classify epochs when more than 50% of the EEG was obscured by body movements and muscle artifact.[12] The AASM manual eliminated this term, replacing it with the concept of major body movements. Epochs with major body movements are scored as stage W if any alpha rhythm, even comprising less than half the epoch, is present, or if the preceding or following epoch is scored as stage W. Otherwise, the epoch is given the same stage as the epoch that follows.[1] The logic behind this rule is that major body movements generally result in an arousal or at least a change to a lighter stage of sleep.

PEDIATRIC CONSIDERATIONS

Maturational changes in the EEG with age make staging more challenging in children, especially in the first year of life. The AASM manual provides modifications for the staging of sleep in children from 2 months postterm upward. For infants less than 2 months old, the 1971 Anders manual for the scoring of states of sleep and wakefulness in newborn infants is recommended.[2] Standard montages are used, but the distances between chin EMG electrodes and between EOG electrodes and the eyes may need to be reduced in infants and younger children.

Infant sleep should be scored using information derived from the EEG, eye movements, muscle tone, respiration, and behavior, including movements and vocalization. Three stages of sleep are recognized: (1) active sleep believed the precursor of REM sleep, (2) quiet sleep representing the precursor of NREM sleep, and (3) indeterminate sleep.[2] The EEG patterns of quiet sleep include high-voltage slow activity, trace alternant, and mixed rhythms. Trace alternant consists of bursts of moderate- to high-voltage delta frequency activity lasting 3 to 8 seconds, alternating with 4- to 8-second periods of lower-amplitude mixed-frequency rhythms.

After 2 months of age, staging largely follows adult terminology. An undifferentiated stage N (NREM sleep), however, is used for appropriate epochs in records in which no K complexes and sleep spindles or no slow waves are present.[1] Sleep spindles usually develop at 2 to 3 months postterm and K complexes at 4 to 6 months.[45] Occipital alpha rhythm develops slowly with time, preceded by slower rhythms that attenuate with eye opening. The term "alpha rhythm" is replaced by the concept of "dominant posterior rhythm," which increases in frequency with age and can be as slow as 3.5 Hz in 3-month postterm infants. The patterns of drowsiness are also more varied in children. Stage N1 sleep can be characterized by hypnagogic hypersynchrony (paroxysmal bursts of high-amplitude 3–4.5 Hz sinusoidal waves maximal frontocentrally most common before age 5 years) or rhythmic anterior theta activity (runs of 5–7 Hz activity frontally most common in adolescents).[1,45]

FUTURE TRENDS

Although great care was taken to ensure that the new AASM staging system is compatible with published data and based on biologic principles, it is essentially a set of rules developed by expert consensus. Studies determining the interrater and intrarater reliability of human scorers need to be performed, using records of normal and abnormal sleep at different ages. Previous studies of the R and K staging system revealed substantial reliability for complete studies, whereas the reliability of scoring stage 1 NREM sleep was lowest and REM sleep was highest.[20] Validity studies may not be possible because there is no accepted gold standard for human sleep staging. Studies comparing the AASM with the R and K scoring method, however, allow differences to be highlighted and better understood.

The AASM rules may need modification when dealing with certain pathologic conditions, such as REM sleep behavior disorder, in which the atonia of REM sleep is lost.[46] In patients with advancing dementia, sleep architecture may deteriorate, resulting in an intermixture of wake rhythms and different states of sleep.[47] The phenomenon of alpha intrusion into sleep[48] may also result in scoring difficulties, especially in the transition from wake to sleep. The rules do not address issues regarding the microstructure of sleep. Subpatterns of different stages, known as "cyclic alternating patterns," have been described and an atlas with scoring rules published.[49] Although these concepts have resulted in insights into the nature of sleep and its disturbance by various disorders, the clinical benefit of scoring cyclic alternating patterns is still uncertain.

The computerized scoring of sleep is beyond the scope of this article. Commercial systems based on digital algorithms largely using R and K rules are available and reliability data compared with human subjects have been published.[50,51] These algorithms need to be adapted to the AASM rules and their reliability tested. Further work is needed to determine if computerized scoring, with or without human revision, may one day reliably replace visual scoring in normal and abnormal sleep. At a research level, more sophisticated analyses, including quantitative EEG, spectral analysis, and period amplitude analysis, may provide novel insights into sleep and its disorders.[52] New hardware technology may also change the way physiologic signals are recorded, such as the use of direct current eye movement monitors, to record changes of drowsiness.[53]

REFERENCES

1. Iber C, Ancoli-Israel S, Chessonn A, et al, for the American Academy of Sleep Medicine. The AASM manual for the scoring of sleep and associated

events: rules, terminology and technical specifications. 1st edition. Westchester (IL): American Academy of Sleep Medicine; 2007.

2. Anders T, Emde R, Parmelee A. A manual of standardized terminology, techniques and criteria for scoring states of sleep and wakefulness in newborn infants. Los Angeles (CA): UCLA Brain Information Service, NINDS Neurological Information Network; 1971.

3. Berger H. Uber das elektroenkephalogramm des mensen. Arch Psychiatr Nervenkr 1929;87:527–70 [in German].

4. Loomis AL, Harvey EN, Hobart GA. Cerebral states during sleep, as studied by human brain potentials. J Exp Psychol 1937;1:24–38.

5. Blake H, Gerard R, Kleitman N. Factors including brain potentials during sleep. J Neurophysiol 1939;2:48–60.

6. Gibbs E, Lorimer F, Gibbs F, editors. Atlas of Encephalography, Volume 1, Methodology and Controls. 2nd edition. Reading, MA: Addison-Wesley Publishing Company; 1950.

7. Roth B. The clinical and theoretical importance of EEG rhythms corresponding to states of lowered vigilance. Electroencephalogr Clin Neurophysiol 1961;13:395–9.

8. Simon EW, Emmons WH. EEG, consciousness, and sleep. Science 1956;124:1066–9.

9. Aserinsky E, Kleitman N. Regularly occurring periods of eye motility and concomitant phenomena during sleep. Sleep 1953;118:273–4.

10. Dement W, Kleitman N. Cyclic variations in EEG during sleep and their relation to eye movements, body motility, and dreaming. Electroencephalogr Clin Neurophysiol 1957;9:673–90.

11. Williams RL, Karacan I, Hursch CJ. Electroencephalography (EEG) of human sleep: clinical applications. New York: John Wiley & Sons; 1974.

12. Rechtschaffen A, Kales A. A manual of standardized terminology, techniques, and scoring system for sleep stages of human subjects. Bethesda (MD): National Institute of Neurological Disease and Blindness; 1968.

13. Himanen S-L, Hasan J. Limitations of Rechtschaffen and Kales. Sleep Med Rev 2000;4:149–67.

14. Hirshkowitz M. Standing on the shoulders of giants: the Standardized Sleep Manual after 30 years. Sleep Med Rev 2000;4:169–79.

15. McGregor P, Thorpy MJ, Schmidt-Nowara WW, et al. T-sleep: an improved method for scoring breathing-disordered sleep. Sleep 1992;15:359–63.

16. Shepard JW. Atlas of sleep medicine. Armonk (NY): Futura Publishing Company; 1991.

17. Van Sweden B, Kemp B, Kamphuisen HAC, et al. Alternative electrode placement in (automatic) sleep scoring (Fpz-Cz/Pz-Oz versus C4-A1). Sleep 1990; 13:279–83.

18. Hori T, Sugita Y, Koga E, et al. Proposed supplements and amendments to "A manual of standardized terminology, techniques and scoring system for sleep stages of human subjects", the Rechtschaffen and Kales (1968) standard. Psychiatry Clin Neurosci 2001;55:305–10.

19. Iber C, Ancoli-Israel S, Chambers M, et al. The new sleep scoring manual: the evidence behind the rules. J Clin Sleep Med 2007;3:107.

20. Silber MH, Ancoli-Israel S, Bonnet MH. The visual scoring of sleep in adults. J Clin Sleep Med 2007; 3:121–31.

21. Happe S, Anderer P, Gruber G, et al. Scalp topography of the spontaneous K-complex an dof delta-waves in human sleep. Brain Topogr 2002;15: 43–9.

22. McCormick L, Nielsen T, Nicolas A, et al. Topographical distribution of spindles and K-complexes in normal subjects. Sleep 1997;20:939–41.

23. De Gennaro L, Ferrara M, Bertini M. Topographical distribution of spindles: variations between and within NREM sleep cycles. Sleep Res Online 2000; 3:155–60.

24. Santamaria R, Chiappa KH. The EEG of drowsiness in normal adults. J Clin Neurophysiol 1987;4:327–82.

25. Ogilvie RD, Wilkinson RT. Behavioral versus EEG-based monitoring of all night sleep/wake patterns. Sleep 1988;11:139–55.

26. Trinder J, Whitworth F, Kay A, et al. Respiratory instability during sleep onset. J Appl Phys 1992;73: 2462–9.

27. Mezzanotte WS, Tangel DJ, White DP. Influence of sleep onset on upper-airway muscle activity in apnea patients versus normal controls. Am J Respir Crit Care Med 1996;153:1880–7.

28. Worsnop C, Kay A, Pierce R, et al. Activity of respiratory pump and upper airway muscles during sleep onset. J Appl Phys 1998;85:908–20.

29. Burgess HJ, Kleiman J, Trinder J. Cardiac activity during sleep onset. Psychophysiology 1999;36: 298–306.

30. Fogel RB, White DP, Pierce RJ, et al. Control of upper airway muscle activity in younger versus older men during sleep onset. J Physiol 2003; 553:533–44.

31. Kjaer TW, Law I, Wiltschiotz G, et al. Regional cerebral blood flow during light sleep: a H15 O-PET study. J Sleep Res 2002;11:201–7.

32. Spielman AJ, Zhang G, Yang C, et al. Intracerebral hemodynamics probed by near infrared spectroscopy in the transition between wakefulness and sleep. Brain Res 2000;866:313–25.

33. Steriade M, Amzica F. Slow sleep oscillations, rhythmic K-complexes, and their paroxysmal developments. J Sleep Res 1998;7(Suppl 1):30–5.

34. Holl RW, Hartmann ML, Veldhuis JD, et al. Thirty-second sampling of plasma growth hormone in man: correlation with sleep stages. J Clin Endocrinol Metab 1991;72:854–61.

35. Van Cautier E, Plat L, Copinschi G. Interrelations between sleep and the somatotrophic axis. Sleep 1998;21:553–66.

36. Bunnell DE, Agnew JA, Horvath SM, et al. Passive body heating and sleep: influence of proximity to sleep. Sleep 1988;11:210–9.

37. Horne JA, Staff LH. Exercise and sleep: body-heating effects. Sleep 1983;6:36–46.

38. Aeschbach D, Cajochen C, Landolt H, et al. Homeostatic sleep regulation in habitual short sleepers and long sleepers. Am J Phys 1996;270:R41–53.

39. Tan X, Campbell IG, Feinberg I. Inter-night reliability and benchmark values for computer analyses of non-rapid eye movement (NREM) and REM EGG in normal young adult and elderly subjects. Clin Neurophysiol 2001;112:1540–52.

40. Brendel DH, Reynolds CF, Jennings JR. Sleep stage physiology, mood, and vigilance responses to total sleep deprivation in healthy 80-year-olds and 20-year-olds. Psychophysiology 1990;27:667–85.

41. Carskadon MA, Dement WC. Sleep loss in elderly volunteers. Sleep 1985;8:207–21.

42. Reynolds CF, Kupfer DJ, Hoch CC, et al. Sleep deprivation in healthy elderly men and women: effects on mood and on sleep during recovery. Sleep 1986;9:492–501.

43. Reynolds CF, Kupfer DJ, Hoch CC, et al. Sleep deprivation as a probe in the elderly. Arch Gen Psychiatry 1987;44:982–90.

44. Dijk DJ, Duffy JF, Riel E, et al. Ageing and the circadian and homeostatic regulation of human sleep during forced desynchrony of rest, melatonin and temperature rhythms. J Physiol 1999;516:611–27.

45. Grigg-Damberger M, Gozal D, Marcus CL, et al. The visual scoring of sleep and arousal in infants and children. J Clin Sleep Med 2007;3:201–40.

46. Olson EJ, Boeve BF, Silber MH. Rapid eye movement sleep behavior disorder: demographic, clinical and laboratory findings in 93 cases. Brain 2000;123:331–9.

47. Mahowald MW, Schenck CH. Status dissociates: a perspective on states of being. Sleep 1991;14:69–79.

48. Hauri P, Hawkins DR. Alpha-delta sleep. Encephalogr Clin Neurophysiol 1973;34:233–7.

49. Terzano MG, Parrino L, Sherieri A, et al. Atlas, rules and recording techniques for the scoring of cyclic alternating pattern (CAP) in human sleep. Sleep Med 2001;2:537–53.

50. Anderer P, Gruber G, Parapatics S, et al. An E-health solution for automatic sleep classification according to Rechtschaffen and Kales: validation study of the Somnolyzer 24 × 7 utilizing the Siesta database. Neuropsychobiology 2005;51:115–33.

51. Prinz PN, Larsen LH, Moe KE, et al. C STAGE, automated sleep scoring: development and comparison with human sleep scoring for healthy older men and women. Sleep 1994;17:711–7.

52. Penzel T, Hirshkowitz M, Harsh J, et al. Digital analysis and technical specifications. J Clin Sleep Med 2007;3:109–20.

53. Atienza M, Cantero JL, Stickgold R, et al. Eyelid movements measured by Nightcap predict slow eye movements during quiet wakefulness in humans. J Sleep Res 2004;13:25–9.

Respiratory Monitoring Equipment and Detection of Respiratory Events

Jahan Naghshin, MD[a], Patrick J. Strollo, Jr., MD, FCCP, FAASM[b,c,d],*

KEYWORDS

- Respiratory monitoring • Nasal pressure
- Inductance plethysmography • Pneumotachograph
- Esophageal pressure • Oximetry • Gas exchange

This article examines the current sleep laboratory tools available for diagnosing sleep-disordered breathing (SDB). The authors discuss the advantages and disadvantages of each modality. It is important to consider that in identifying an SDB event, the use of more than one device may be required (ie, to measure airflow, effort, or gas exchange). This consideration frequently is critical when trying to discriminate obstructive from central events or to assess hypoventilation. The authors focus on the current state of monitoring in adults. The precision of classifying a given event is dependent on the accuracy of the data generated by a given monitor and how those data are integrated by the scoring algorithm that is employed. The authors also provide a brief discussion of advanced signal processing in existing and emerging technology. In 2007, the American Academy of Sleep Medicine published a new manual that included new definitions and scoring criteria for respiratory events.[1]

MEASUREMENT OF AIRFLOW
Thermal Technology

Thermocouples and thermistors are small sensors used for semiquantitative measurement of airflow. The electrical characteristics of these sensors (ie, voltage and resistance) depend on temperature. They detect changes in the temperature as a surrogate for measuring airflow. The sensor is a temperature-sensitive resistor and is generally composed of semiconductor materials.

To detect airflow, the sensor should be placed at the airway openings close to both nostrils and the mouth. A change in the airflow causes a change in the sensor's electrical properties. Depending on the exact position of the sensor, the amount of airflow, and the temperature, a semiquantitative signal is collected to represent the airflow. Currently, many sleep centers use this thermal technology as an adjunctive method to detect the airflow or mouth breathing.

> Advantages: These devices are small in size, comfortable to the patient, relatively inexpensive, and reusable. Thermocouples and thermistors are good for detecting apnea.
>
> Disadvantages: These thermal devices have poor dynamic response, relatively slow response times, and a curvilinear response

Work supported in part by HL076379-01, HL077785, HL076852-1, HL082610-01A1, 1UL1RR024153-01.

[a] University of Pittsburgh, PA, USA
[b] Department of Medicine, University of Pittsburgh, PA, USA
[c] Clinical and Translational Science, University of Pittsburgh, PA, USA
[d] UPMC Sleep Medicine Center, University of Pittsburgh, UPMC Montefiore, Suite S639.11, 3459 Fifth Avenue, Pittsburgh, PA 15213-2582, USA
* Corresponding author. UPMC Sleep Medicine Center, University of Pittsburgh, UPMC Montefiore, Suite S639.11, 3459 Fifth Avenue, Pittsburgh, PA 15213-2582.
E-mail address: strollopj@upmc.edu (P.J. Strollo).

to temperature change that flattens as airflow increases. Moreover, the thermal sensor's signal has a poor correlation with actual airflow or minute ventilation. This thermal technology is unable to accurately measure airflow and is not accurate for detecting hypopneas.[2,3]

Polyvinylidene fluoride film airflow sensors

These thermal sensors are an alternative to thermistors and thermocouples. The polyvinylidene fluoride film signal is proportional to the temperature difference detected on the two sides of the film.

> Advantages: A single device can detect nasal and oral airflow. Preliminary data suggest that these sensors have faster response times than thermistors and thermocouples and have a more linear response when compared with that of a pneumotachograph.[4]
> Disadvantage: Currently, these sensors are more expensive than other thermal sensors.

Pneumotachograph

This device accurately measures airflow during breathing. The device is organized to cause airflow to become laminar, allowing the recording of pressure differences across a straight tube of fixed-flow resistance that has known pressure-flow characteristics. A pneumotachograph has been considered the gold standard for measuring airflow.[4]

> Advantages: The airflow and volume of individual breaths can be precisely calculated.
> Disadvantages: It is a cumbersome piece of equipment that requires an oronasal seal. Except in the setting of research studies, quantitative measures of airflow are not routinely used.

Nasal Pressure Cannula

This monitoring device consists of a standard nasal cannula that is connected to a simple pressure transducer. The sensitivity of this device is close to that of the thermal sensors used for detecting apnea, but it is more accurate for detecting hypopneas and flow-limited events.[5]

> Advantages: These devices are simple, inexpensive, and convenient for the patient to wear. The response time of the signal is sufficient to allow for accurate assessment of hypopneas and airflow limitation by examining the shape of the breath.
> Disadvantages: The relationship between nasal pressure and airflow is not linear.[6]

However, this signal can be made linear through mathematical conversion.[3,7] A linear pressure signal from nasal prongs has been shown to closely correlate with a flow signal from a pneumotachograph.[3,7] The signal amplitude depends on the location of the sensor and the pattern of breathing. Because these two parameters change constantly throughout the night, the airflow signal during a respiratory event can be compared only with the signal during the normal cycle just before the event. These devices cannot measure the airflow during mouth breathing.

As a technical note, nasal pressure measurement can be performed using either AC or DC electrical input.

> DC input: The best way to measure nasal pressure is to use a DC amplifier or input. Using this type of input signal avoids any concern about the setting of low-frequency filters.
> AC input: When using an AC amplifier and input, the configuration of the nasal pressure tracing depends on the low-frequency filter setting. The optimal setting uses a cutoff filter of 0.01 Hz (time constant of approximately 5 seconds) or at least the capability of establishing a low-frequency cutoff-filter setting of 0.05 Hz or less (or a time constant of approximately 3 seconds). If the cutoff is set at higher frequencies, the flow signal could be significantly underestimated during the airflow limitation. Some older sleep systems do not have sufficient DC channels to add the additional nasal pressure signal. However, by using AC channels at the correct setting, nasal pressure waveforms can be recorded that are essentially identical to those from a DC signal.[8]

MEASUREMENT OF EFFORT

This section summarizes different techniques used to measure the respiratory effort during the use of polysomnographic equipment.

Respiratory Inductance Plethysmography

When using respiratory inductance plethysmography (RIP) technology, bands with inductive coils are placed on the chest and abdomen (ie, the two compartments of respiration). Changes in the electromagnetic properties of these coils during breathing are recorded as an electric signal. The sum of the two signals, when calibrated, correlates with the tidal volume of the breath.[9,10] RIP technology is widely used at sleep centers across the world.

> Advantages: Using calibration bags (such as a Spiro bag), this signal can be calibrated to measure the tidal volume. This technique can easily detect abnormal patterns of breathing such as paradoxical respiration. The thoracic and abdominal channels can be combined into an additional "sum" channel. RIP is noninvasive and convenient for the patient.
>
> Disadvantages: RIP can only semiquantitatively measure the tidal volume during sleep. The relationship between the tidal volume and RIP changes with changing body positions during the sleep period.[11] The RIP sensors can slip and change position during the sleep period, which can cause inaccuracy in the measurement of respiratory efforts. The sensors are more expensive than piezoelectric belts.

Piezoelectric Sensors

In a technique similar to that of the RIP method, piezoelectric sensors or belts are placed around the thoracic and abdominal compartments to measure the tension and change in each belt as a surrogate for measuring respiratory effort. Unlike inductance plethysmography sensors, the piezo-based effort sensors measure the tension only in a single location—where a sensor crystal is pulled by the band during chest or abdominal movement. Patient movement and loss of tension, such as when a patient turns on his side, can affect the accuracy of the results. Piezo belts also can produce false results indicative of paradoxical respiratory effort.

> Advantages: The technology is inexpensive and convenient for the patient.
>
> Disadvantages: The signal cannot be calibrated. Unlike the RIP sensors, the signals from the thoracic and abdominal belts cannot be combined into an additional sum channel. If the piezoelectric belt is stretched beyond its limit, it can switch polarity, which could mistakenly be interpreted as indicative of paradoxical breathing. Similar to RIP sensors, these belts can also move during sleep, which can cause inaccuracy in their measurements. Moreover, the loss of tension on the belt can cause signal deterioration or loss.

Esophageal Pressure Measurement

Esophageal pressure (P_{es}) is measured using different methods and reflects pleural pressure variations. Regardless of the method used, P_{es} has been considered the gold standard for measurement of respiratory effort. Studies have demonstrated that the effects of monitoring P_{es} on sleep architecture are minimal.[12,13]

Esophageal balloons

High-compliance esophageal balloons have been used widely in sleep research and to some degree in the clinical setting to record P_{es} as a measure of respiratory effort. The correlation between the measurement of respiratory effort and esophageal pressure would depend on factors such as the location of the catheter and the lung and chest wall mechanics.

Millar catheters

Millar catheters are also used for P_{es} measurement. They have been used mainly to measure the supraglottic pressure in research settings. Transpulmonary pressure can be calculated by subtracting the P_{es} from the supraglottic pressure. These devices are accurate but expensive.

Fluid-filled catheters

In measuring P_{es} using fluid-filled catheters, a small-bore tube (frequently a pediatric feeding tube) is used. Some patients find these catheters more comfortable than standard esophageal balloons. They have a lower tendency to fail because of the ability to maintain the signal using a constant flow of saline through the system and the opportunity to sample changes in pressure at more than one site.

> Advantage: P_{es} measurement determined by this method can provide an excellent estimate of respiratory effort.
>
> Disadvantages: This monitoring technique is relatively more invasive, inconvenient to the patient, and can be displaced during the study.

Diaphragmatic EMG

If the EMG leads are placed properly, this technique can identify diaphragmatic activation as a surrogate for measuring respiratory effort.

> Advantages: It is noninvasive and relatively inexpensive
>
> Disadvantages: The signal cannot be calibrated and mainly reflects the activation of intercostal muscles rather than the diaphragm. It is less accurate in obese individuals.

MEASUREMENT OF GAS EXCHANGE
Oxygen

The measurement of oxygen saturation is an important part of respiratory monitoring during the use of polysomnography. A decrease in hemoglobin oxygen saturation by 4% or more is one of the current criteria for defining hypopnea. Moreover, nocturnal oxygen desaturation without airflow limitation is an important finding in subjects who have sleep hypoventilation disorders or structural lung diseases such as chronic obstructive pulmonary disease with or without sleep apnea. The presence of oxygen saturation can be assessed using two techniques: pulse oximetry and transcutaneous oximetry.

Pulse oximetry

Pulse oximetry is based on the principle that oxygenated and deoxygenated blood absorbs light differently when light is shined through the blood. Two different wavelengths of light, red and infrared light, are shined by an emitter through a translucent part of the skin, usually the fingertip, and a photodetector on the opposite side determines the amount of passed light. The red-to-infrared ratio, determined using a calibration table, is used to estimate the oxygenation of the blood that the light beam has passed through. This technique, although less accurate than directly measuring the arterial partial pressure of oxygen in an arterial blood gas, is more practical, noninvasive, and the most commonly used method for measuring hemoglobin oxygenation in clinical practice, including during polysomnography. It is important to pay attention to the averaging time of the oximeter. Most current oximeters have an averaging time of 3 seconds. An averaging time greater than three seconds can result in underestimation of the number of respiratory events, including hypopnea and oxygen desaturation.[14] Furthermore, the choice of the oximeter may potentially affect the results using the apnea-hypopnea index (AHI), even when the averaging time is the same, because of the variability of oximeters' measurement of saturation.[15]

Transcutaneous oximetry

Transcutanous oximetry is similar to the transcutaneous carbon dioxide (CO_2) measurement that is described below. Similar to pulse oximetry, transcutaneous oximetry is also noninvasive and easy to use. However, problems with calibration and adjustment for increased skin temperature have limited the use of this method.

Arterial blood gas

Determining the levels of arterial blood gas is the most accurate way of measuring blood oxygenation. However, because of the more invasive nature of the test, it has not been widely used in the sleep laboratory setting.

Carbon Dioxide

The arterial partial pressure of carbon dioxide ($PaCO_2$) can be affected by many factors, such as alveolar ventilation, alveolar-capillary diffusion capacity for CO_2, cardiac output, tissue perfusion, and metabolism. Under steady-state conditions, the $PaCO_2$ is mainly a reflection of alveolar ventilation.

End tidal carbon dioxide

The measurement of end tidal carbon dioxide (CO_2), measured either mainstream or sidestream at the steady state and in hemodynamically stable individuals, closely reflects the measurement of $PaCO_2$.

Transcutaneous carbon dioxide

For the measurement of transcutaneous CO_2, a noninvasive method for continuous or spot monitoring of $PaCO_2$ is used. The transcutaneous electrode used for the assessment of CO_2 consists of a glass electrochemical sensor that has been modified for transcutaneous use by incorporating a thermostatically controlled heater unit. Transcutaneous measurements of CO_2 are based on the principle that a heating element in the electrode raises the skin temperature. This increases the capillary blood flow and the partial pressure of carbon dioxide, and thus makes the skin permeable to gas diffusion. This technique may result in overestimation of the partial pressure of CO_2 because of the increase in CO_2 production at a higher tissue temperature. The measured value then should be normalized for the temperature. Depending on the technology that had been used, studies suggest that the measurement of transcutaneous CO_2 has a better correlation with the measurement of $PaCO_2$ than with the measurement of end tidal CO_2 during wakefulness.[16,17] This technique, however, has not been widely used in polysomnography.

Arterial blood gas

Determining the levels of arterial blood gas is the most accurate and most invasive way of measuring the $PaCO_2$. This method is infrequently used in clinical polysomnography.

NEW APPLICATIONS OF OLD TECHNOLOGY
Advanced Signal Processing of Pulse Oximetry

In addition to its use in polysomnography, pulse oximetry has been used to independently diagnose obstructive sleep apnea (OSA). Magalang and colleagues[18] showed that the Delta index (ie, the average of the absolute differences in oxygen saturation between successive 12-s intervals) produced accurate results that are comparable with those produced using the oxygen desaturation index for predicting OSA. Their data suggested that using a combination of these two indices may increase the precision of predicting the AHI results. Advances in computer-assisted analysis of the pulse oximetry signal in conjunction with newer technology such as multiwavelength pulse oximetry[19] may allow oximetry to have a more promising role in the future.

Advanced Signal Processing of ECG

ECG recording using Holter monitoring has been studied as a diagnostic or screening tool for OSA. Roche and colleagues[20] used heart-rate variability, the power spectral density of the interbeat interval increment of very-low frequencies, and its percentage over the total power spectral density as diagnostic tools in patients who were suspected clinically of having OSA. They reported a diagnostic sensitivity of 87% for the total power spectral density and a strong association with disease status for both percentage over the total power spectral density and power spectral density of the interbeat interval increment of very-low frequencies. de Chazal and colleagues[21] introduced an algorithm for using a single-channel ECG to calculate an ECG-derived respiratory signal. They created a 74-member vector of features for each 1-minute epoch. Recently, the same group used the same algorithm to study the value of the ECG signal as a screening tool for SDB.[22] They showed a strong correlation between the ECG-derived signal and AHI scores, as measured using polysomnography (r = 0.88 and P<.001). However, they admitted that the Holter monitoring signal underestimated the true AHI scores for high AHI values and overestimated the true AHI scores at lower AHI values.

Advantages: The test is inexpensive and noninvasive.

Disadvantages: The results are influenced by factors such as thoracic impedance, skin humidity, temperature, and other artifacts that may affect ECG recordings. More important, these algorithms[22] have not been studied in women and individuals who take beta-blockers or have cardiovascular diseases. The correlation between the ECG-derived signals and

polysomnography data cannot be generalized to the other patient populations.

In summary, this technology could potentially be promising but requires further research.

NEW TECHNOLOGY
Pulse Transit Time

The measurement of pulse transit time (PTT) is an innovative method that can be used to assess SDB. The measurement of PTT can be used to detect the changes in respiratory effort in a noninvasive way and only requires the use of a conventional pulse oximeter, EKG leads, and a computational system. By definition, PTT is the time that it takes for the pulse wave to travel from the aortic valve, as detected from the R wave on the EKG, to the peripheral arteries, where it is detected by the pulse oximeter sensor. When a person is breathing regularly, this transit time is within a relatively narrow range, as indicated by the arrows in **Fig. 1**. However, during episodes of obstructive apnea or hypopnea, increased blood pressure from either an increase in sympathetic nerve activity or changes in the intrathoracic pressure can change the arterial wall stiffness and, therefore, increase the PTT, as represented by the higher amplitude in the PTT signal.[23] PTT may be used to detect micro-arousals.[23] It can also be useful in differentiating obstructive from central SDB events.

Advantages: PTT technology is noninvasive and relatively inexpensive.

Disadvantages: It has limited use in patients who have cardiac arrhythmias or advanced peripheral vascular disease. To date, this technique has not been widely used in clinical practice.

Peripheral Arterial Tonometry

Autonomic nervous system hyperactivity plays an important role in the pathophysiology of the cardiovascular consequences of SDB. Peripheral arterial tonometry (PAT), which was first introduced in 1999 by Lavie and colleagues,[24] is a noninvasive method of assessment of vasoconstriction in the finger as a marker of sympathetic nerve activity at the level of the peripheral vasculature.[24–26] Increased sympathetic nerve activity during obstructive episodes is believed to be related to hypoxia,[27,28] hypercapnia,[27,29] or arousals.[30,31] PAT technology has been incorporated into an ambulatory device that uses a specially designed finger pneumo-optic plethysmograph. The pulse waveform of the PAT signal

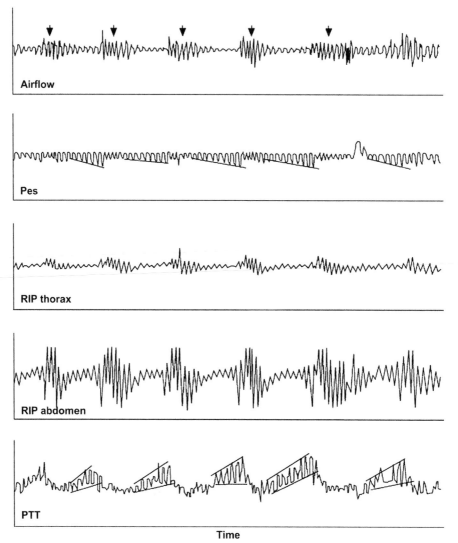

Fig. 1. EKG pulse transit time. (*Modified from* Farré R, Montserrat JM, and Navajas D. Noninvasive monitoring of respiratory mechanics during sleep. Eur Respir J 2004;24:1052–60; with permission.)

decreases transiently following an episode of obstructive apnea or hypopnea in patients who have OSA. By detecting these physiologic changes during sleep-related apnea and hypopnea, PAT can be used as a tool to examine respiratory events during the sleep.

>   Advantages: PAT-based technology is noninvasive.
>   Disadvantages: PAT has limited use in patients who have cardiac arrhythmias such as atrial fibrillation or in patients who are on peripheral alpha-blocking agents. There have been a limited number of outcome studies comparing the PAT

devices with conventional, laboratory-based polysomnography.

DEFINITIONS

The reason for measuring airflow, effort, and gas exchange is to identify the physiologic events that cause the symptoms and consequences of SDB and to determine the severity of the disorder. As the study of sleep progressed, it was necessary to standardize the terminology and definitions of the different events that were being recorded. The American Academy of Sleep Medicine recommendations related to scoring respiratory events have recently been published.

REFERENCES

1. Iber C, Ancoli-Israel S Jr, Chesson A, et al. The AASM manual for the scoring of sleep and associated events: rules, terminology and technical specification. American Academy of Sleep Medicine; 2007.

2. Berg S, Haight JS, Yap V, et al. Comparison of direct and indirect measurements of respiratory airflow: implications for hypopneas. Sleep 1997;20(1):60–4.

3. Farre R, Montserrat JM, Rotger M, et al. Accuracy of thermistors and thermocouples as flow-measuring devices for detecting hypopnoeas. Eur Respir J 1998;11(1):179–82.

4. Berry RB, Koch GL, Trautz S, et al. Comparison of respiratory event detection by a polyvinylidene fluoride film airflow sensor and a pneumotachograph in sleep apnea patients. Chest 2005; 128(3):1331–8.

5. Norman RG, Ahmed MM, Walsleben JA, et al. Detection of respiratory events during NPSG: nasal cannula/pressure sensor versus thermistor. Sleep 1997;20(12):1175–84.

6. Montserrat JM, Farre R, Ballester E, et al. Evaluation of nasal prongs for estimating nasal flow. Am J Respir Crit Care Med 1997;155(1):211–5.

7. Thurnheer R, Xie X, Bloch KE. Accuracy of nasal cannula pressure recordings for assessment of ventilation during sleep. Am J Respir Crit Care Med 2001;164(10 Pt 1):1914–9.

8. Rapoport D, Norman R, Nielson M. Nasal pressure airflow measurement: an introduction. Mukilteo (WA): Protech Primer; 2001.

9. Zimmerman PV, Connellan SJ, Middleton HC, et al. Postural changes in rib cage and abdominal volume-motion coefficients and their effect on the calibration of a respiratory inductance plethysmograph. Am Rev Respir Dis 1983;127(2):209–14.

10. Sackner MA, Watson H, Belsito AS, et al. Calibration of respiratory inductive plethysmograph during natural breathing. J Appl Physiol 1989;66(1): 410–20.

11. Whyte KF, Gugger M, Gould GA, et al. Accuracy of respiratory inductive plethysmograph in measuring tidal volume during sleep. J Appl Physiol 1991; 71(5):1866–71.

12. Skatvedt O, Akre H, Godtlibsen OB. Nocturnal polysomnography with and without continuous pharyngeal and esophageal pressure measurements. Sleep 1996;19(6):485–90.

13. Chervin RD, Aldrich MS. Effects of esophageal pressure monitoring on sleep architecture. Am J Respir Crit Care Med 1997;156(3 Pt 1):881–5.

14. Farré R, Montserrat JM, Ballester E, et al. Importance of the pulse oximeter averaging time when measuring oxygen desaturation in sleep apnea. Sleep 1998;21(4):386–90.

15. Zafar S, Ayappa I, Norman RG, et al. Choice of oximeter affects apnea-hypopnea index. Chest 2005; 127(1):80–8.

16. Casati A, Squicciarini G, Malagutti G, et al. Transcutaneous monitoring of partial pressure of carbon dioxide in the elderly patient: a prospective, clinical comparison with end-tidal monitoring. J Clin Anesth 2006;18(6):436–40.

17. Reid CW, Martineau RJ, Miller DR, et al. A comparison of transcutaneous end-tidal and arterial measurements of carbon dioxide during general anaesthesia. Can J Anaesth 1992;39(1):31–6.

18. Magalang UJ, Dmochowski J, Veeramachaneni S, et al. Prediction of the apnea-hypopnea index from overnight pulse oximetry. Chest 2003;124(5): 1694–701.

19. Aoyagi T, Fuse M, Kobayashi N, et al. Multiwavelength pulse oximetry: theory for the future. Anesth Analg 2007;105(6 Suppl):S53–8 [tables of contents].

20. Roche F, Duverney D, Court-Fortune I, et al. Cardiac interbeat interval increment for the identification of obstructive sleep apnea. Pacing Clin Electrophysiol 2002;25(8):1192–9.

21. de Chazal P, Heneghan C, Sheridan E, et al. Automated processing of the single-lead electrocardiogram for the detection of obstructive sleep apnoea. IEEE Trans Biomed Eng 2003;50(6): 686–96.

22. Heneghan C, de Chazal P, Ryan S, et al. Electrocardiogram recording as a screening tool for sleep disordered breathing. J Clin Sleep Med 2008;4(3): 223–8.

23. Pitson DJ, Sandell A, van den Hout R, et al. Use of pulse transit time as a measure of inspiratory effort in patients with obstructive sleep apnoea. Eur Respir J 1995;8(10):1669–74.

24. Schnall RP, Shlitner A, Sheffy J, et al. Periodic, profound peripheral vasoconstriction—a new marker of obstructive sleep apnea. Sleep 1999; 22(7):939–46.

25. Lavie P, Shlitner A, Sheffy J, et al. Peripheral arterial tonometry: a novel and sensitive non-invasive monitor of brief arousals during sleep. Isr Med Assoc J 2000;2(3):246–7.

26. Lavie P, Schnall RP, Sheffy J, et al. Peripheral vasoconstriction during REM sleep detected by a new plethysmographic method. Nat Med 2000; 6(6):606.

27. O'Donnell CP, Schwartz AR, Smith PL, et al. Reflex stimulation of renal sympathetic nerve activity and blood pressure in response to apnea. Am J Respir Crit Care Med 1996;154(6 Pt 1):1763–70.

28. Schneider H, Schaub CD, Chen CA, et al. Neural and local effects of hypoxia on cardiovascular responses to obstructive apnea. J Appl Physiol 2000;88(3):1093–102.

29. Somers VK, Mark AL, Zavala DC, et al. Contrasting effects of hypoxia and hypercapnia on ventilation and sympathetic activity in humans. J Appl Physiol 1989;67(5):2101–6.

30. O'Donnell CP, Ayuse T, King ED, et al. Airway obstruction during sleep increases blood pressure without arousal. J Appl Physiol 1996; 80(3):773–81.

31. Schneider H, Schaub CD, Chen CA, et al. Effects of arousal and sleep state on systemic and pulmonary hemodynamics in obstructive apnea. J Appl Physiol 2000;88(3):1084–92.

Differentiating Nocturnal Movements: Leg Movements, Parasomnias, and Seizures

Anil Natesan Rama, MD, MPH[a],*, Rajive Zachariah, BA[b],
Clete A. Kushida, MD, PhD[c,d,e]

KEYWORDS
- Differentiating • Nocturnal • Movements
- Parasomnias • Seizures

The need to evaluate nocturnal movements is a common clinical problem in the practice of sleep medicine. Because reports of the movements occurring during sleep typically cannot be relayed by the patients themselves, the event descriptions often become secondhand during the evaluation by a sleep medicine clinician. Use of polysomnography, at times with use of specialized techniques, becomes an integral part of the diagnosis of these movements. This article describes the clinical steps involved in the diagnostic plan and reviews the most common sleep-related movements and their polysomnographic findings.

APPROACHING THE DIAGNOSIS OF NOCTURNAL MOVEMENTS
First Step: Clinical History

Obtaining a complete clinical history from the patient, bed partner, parent, or caregiver is the first and most important step in the diagnosis of nocturnal movements. The onset, duration, frequency, pattern, and description of nocturnal movements should be elicited. Reviewing the patient's past medical, family, and social history along with current medications and allergies may also unmask an underlying cause of the nocturnal movements for which a specific therapy can be implemented. For instance, if the patient has been told that he or she has staring spells or the patient reports episodes of loss of consciousness, then a seizure disorder is suspected.

Second Step: Physical Examination

A general physical examination is necessary but often overlooked by many physicians treating nocturnal movements. The examination should include an evaluation of the mental status. For instance, is the patient alert, demented, depressed, or anxious? The upper airway should be carefully assessed for evidence of sleep-related breathing disorders. Specifically, is the nasal septum deviated, are the nasal turbinates enlarged, are the nasal valves collapsing, is the hard palate high and arched, is the soft palate low, is the tongue large, or is the mandible recessed? A cardiovascular and pulmonary examination should be conducted. For example, is there evidence of congestive heart failure, pulmonary hypertension, or restrictive or obstructive lung disease? A neurologic examination should also

a Division of Sleep Medicine, The Permanente Medical Group, 275 Hospital Parkway, Suite 425, San Jose, CA 95119, USA
b 7777 Bates Road, Tracy, CA 95304, USA
c Stanford University Medical Center, Stanford Sleep Medicine Center, Stanford, CA, USA
d Stanford Center for Human Sleep Research, Palo Alto, CA, USA
e Stanford Sleep Disorders Clinic, 401 Quarry Road, Suite 3301, Stanford, CA 94305–5730, USA
* Corresponding author.
E-mail address: anil.rama@kp.org (A.N. Rama).

Sleep Med Clin 4 (2009) 361–372
doi:10.1016/j.jsmc.2009.04.004

be performed. In particular, is there evidence of spinal disease or a neurodegenerative disorder, such as Parkinson's disease? A comprehensive physical examination can often elicit clues to the underlying etiology of the patient's nocturnal movements.

Third Step: Actigraphy and Polysomnogram

Sleep testing for nocturnal movements should be considered but ordered only after obtaining a comprehensive clinical history and performing a meticulous physical examination. Actigraphy involves wearing a motion-sensing device on the wrist or ankles that may help define circadian rhythm disorders and periodic limb movements of sleep. Polysomnography involves the use of video and a variety of sensors that record variables including muscle tone, electroencephalogram (EEG) potentials, EKG potentials, electromyogram (EMG) potentials, electro-oculographic potentials, esophageal pressure, acid or nonacid gastro-esophageal reflux, nasal-oral airflow, and thoracic-abdominal excursions. Polysomnography may be used to help differentiate various nocturnal movements, such as limb movements associated with obstructive apneas, periodic limb movements of sleep, epilepsy, sleep starts, and rhythmic movement disorder.

CONSTRUCTING A DIFFERENTIAL DIAGNOSIS OF NOCTURNAL MOVEMENTS

A physician's approach to nocturnal movements should be similar to how he or she approaches any symptom: a differential diagnosis should be constructed and various disease states need to be ruled in or out. One of the goals of this article is to present a straightforward differential diagnosis for the patient complaining of nocturnal movements. By methodically evaluating each potential etiology in the context of the patient's medical history and physical examination, a cause for most cases of nocturnal movements can be determined. Once a diagnosis is established, disease-specific treatments can then be used.

When evaluating a patient with nocturnal movements, various categories of disease states should be considered. **Box 1** contains a general list of

categories used to classify nocturnal movements derived from the *International Classification of Sleep Disorders, 2nd Edition*.[1] These include sleep-related movement disorders, parasomnias, sleep-related epilepsies, and miscellaneous medical conditions. By formulating a differential diagnosis in the context of the patient's medical history and physical examination, one or more etiologies for the patient's nocturnal movements can be determined. The remainder of the article reviews in detail the sleep-related movement disorders, parasomnias, sleep-related epilepsies, and miscellaneous conditions comprising the differential diagnosis of nocturnal movements.

IMPORTANT DIAGNOSTIC FEATURES AND CRITERIA TO DISTINGUISH NOCTURNAL MOVEMENTS
Sleep-Related Movement Disorders

Sleep-related movement disorders involve either simple movements, such as periodic limb movements of sleep, or complex movements, such as body rocking, that occur on entry into sleep or during sleep. The movements are involuntary and usually stereotyped. The stereotyped nature of these movements allows them to be differentiated from parasomnias, which can involve more complex and seemingly goal-oriented movements. A diagnosis of a sleep-related movement disorder additionally requires that the movements impair sleep or daytime function and that they cannot be explained by any underlying condition. **Box 2** outlines the various sleep-related movement disorders, which are described in more detail next.

Periodic limb movement disorder

Clinical information Periodic limb movement disorder is characterized by limb movements occurring during sleep that may result in a complaint of insomnia and excessive daytime sleepiness. Periodic limb movements affecting the lower extremities can be described as intermittent extensions of the big toe and dorsiflexion of the ankle with occasional flexion of the knee and hip.[2] The movements are

---

Box 1
Nocturnal movements: differential diagnosis

- Sleep-related movement disorders
- Parasomnias
- Sleep-related epilepsies
- Miscellaneous

Box 2
Sleep-related movement disorders

- Periodic limb movement disorder
- Leg cramps
- Bruxism
- Rhythmic movement disorder
- Sleep-related movement disorder caused by drugs
- Sleep-related movement disorder caused by medical condition

often bilateral but may predominate in one leg or alternate between legs.[3] Periodic limb movements may affect the upper extremity and manifest as intermittent flexion at the elbow. Periodic limb movements of sleep are predominant in the first half of the night and show a typical pattern of progressive decline through the course of the night.[4]

When symptoms of insomnia and excessive daytime sleepiness exist, the diagnosis of idiopathic periodic limb movement disorder can be made if no other medical, psychiatric, or sleep disorders can be found to account for these symptoms. Periodic limb movement disorder may also occur in association with certain medications or with a variety of other conditions, such as narcolepsy and obstructive sleep apnea (OSA).[5,6] These limb movements can be differentiated from hypnic jerks, normal phasic rapid eye movement (REM) activity, and fragmentary myoclonus, all of which occur with less regular periodicity. Periodic limb movements of sleep must be clearly distinguished from upper airway resistance syndrome.[7,8] With technologic advancements in polysomnographic and respiratory monitoring, it is now recognized that some periodic limb movements of sleep may be triggered by subclinical hypopneas or respiratory effort–related arousals and these movements generally improve after nasal continuous positive airway pressure is administered.

Polysomnographic findings The diagnosis of periodic limb movement disorder is made by polysomnography using EMG recordings from the tibialis anterior muscles, as demonstrated in **Fig. 1**. Movements are counted if they last 0.5 to 10 seconds and occur in a series of four or more at intervals of 5 to 90 seconds. The minimum EMG amplitude of the nocturnal limb movements must be an 8-μV increase in EMG voltage above resting EMG.[9] Alternatively, the diagnosis can be made using automated limb actigraphic recordings, although discrepancies are observed in patients with sleep-related breathing disorders or insomnia and in children.[10,11]

Sleep-related leg cramps

Clinical information Sleep-related leg cramps are characterized by nonperiodic, painful, and involuntary contractions that typically occur in the calf or foot muscles during sleep or wakefulness. Predisposing factors include metabolic disorders, neuromuscular disorders, peripheral vascular disease, vigorous exercise, certain medications, and pregnancy. Restless leg syndrome can also be associated with painful sensations, but can be differentiated from leg cramps. Leg cramps involve actual muscle spasms, are typically restricted to certain muscle groups, and are only alleviated by stretching and not by simple movement.[12]

Polysomnographic findings Polysomnography demonstrates nonperiodic bursts of gastrocnemius EMG activity.

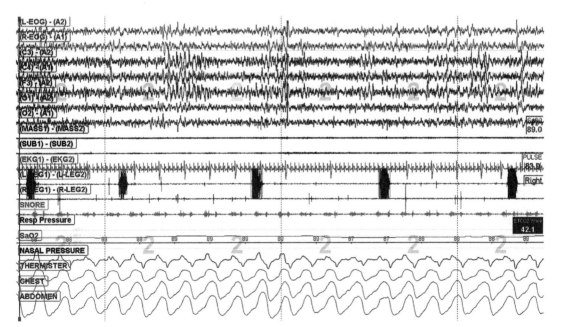

Fig. 1. This 90-second polysomnography epoch demonstrates repetitive limb movements seen in the left leg EMG lead (L-LEG1-L-LEG2). At least four repetitive leg movements are required to score a series of periodic limb movements.

Sleep-related bruxism

Clinical information Sleep-related bruxism is characterized by grinding of the teeth and is associated with brief arousals from sleep. The disorder can be idiopathic or secondary to sleep-disordered breathing or mental retardation.[13] The jaw contractions are most frequent in sleep stages N1 and N2 and may be either sustained (tonic contractions) or repetitive (phasic contractions). Temporomandibular joint pain, tooth wear, and disturbing sounds are typical symptoms of bruxism.

Polysomnographic findings Polysomnography demonstrates phasic or tonic elevation of activity in the masseter EMG (**Fig. 2**), and is often confirmed by audio and video. Phasic contractions occur at a frequency of 1 Hz for 0.25 to 2 seconds, and sustained contractions can last longer or follow a mixed pattern.

Sleep-related rhythmic movement disorder

Clinical information Rhythmic movement disorder is a nocturnal disorder involving stereotyped and repetitive movements within large muscle groups. These movements occur most often at sleep onset and may persist into light sleep. The disorder is typically classified into three subtypes: (1) head rolling, (2) head banging, and (3) body rocking. The disorder is common in infants, occasionally persisting into childhood, and rarely persisting into adulthood. The diagnosis should only be made if the movements are predominantly nocturnal and impair normal sleep or daytime function.[14]

Polysomnographic findings Polysomnography demonstrates that rhythmic movements occur most frequently during drowsiness and stage 2 sleep with normal EEG activity between episodes.

Drugs and Substances

Sleep-related movement disorders may be precipitated by a drug or substance. For example, akathisia is an inner sense of restlessness accompanied by a desire to move usually found associated with neuroleptic medications. In addition, many antidepressants (with the exception of bupropion) and dopamine receptor antagonists can precipitate periodic limb movements. Furthermore stimulants, such as cigarettes and caffeine, can be associated with sleep-related bruxism.

Medical Conditions

Nocturnal movement disorders may be precipitated by medical, neurologic, or psychiatric conditions. For example, Parkinson's disease is associated with REM sleep behavior disorder. Neurologic disorders, such as narcolepsy, can be associated with periodic limb movements during sleep. Sleep-related rhythmic movement disorder can be associated with underlying developmental diseases in children, such as autism and mental retardation.

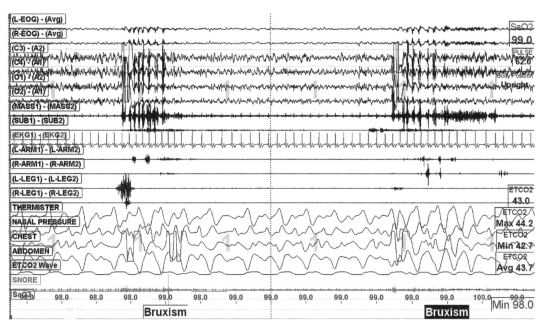

Fig. 2. This 60-second polysomnographic epoch demonstrates repetitive masseter chin EMG lead (MASS1-MASS2) bursts with synchronous muscle artifact in the EEG leads above. This is a typical image of bruxism.

SLEEP DISORDERS
Parasomnias

Parasomnias comprise a variety of complex behaviors and undesirable events that occur during entry into sleep, within sleep, or during arousals from sleep (**Box 3**). Parasomnias involve abnormal sleep-related movements, behaviors, emotions, perceptions, dreaming, and autonomic nervous system functioning. The resulting injury, sleep disruption, adverse health effects, and negative psychosocial effects may cause individuals to seek medical attention. Individuals may suffer from multiple, overlapping parasomnias (eg, sleepwalking, confusional arousals, and sleep terrors). Parasomnias can also be exacerbated by other sleep disorders, most notably OSA.[15] They can be differentiated from simple sleep-related movement disorders, which are not typically associated with goal-directed behaviors or dream mentation. Polysomnography demonstrates that episodes of sleepwalking, confusional arousals, and night terrors arise from slow wave sleep; whereas nightmares and REM sleep behavior disorder arise from REM sleep.

Sleepwalking

Clinical information Sleepwalking is characterized by arousal from non-REM (NREM) sleep and walking out of bed in an altered state of consciousness. Like confusional arousals and sleep terrors, episodes of sleepwalking typically occur in the first third of sleep (when NREM sleep predominates). Episodes are common in children, with the disorder usually disappearing spontaneously around adolescence when slow wave sleep diminishes.[16] The behavior of the sleeper in these episodes can be confused, inappropriate, and belligerent, with the patient engaged in complicated tasks, such as walking, running, driving, leaping out windows, blow-drying hair, and so forth. These actions are in contrast to REM sleep behavior disorder in which the patient is enacting a dream and is typically unable to navigate far from the bed because of bumping into obstacles in the room.

Box 3
Parasomnias

- Sleepwalking
- Confusional arousal
- Sleep terrors
- REM sleep behavior disorder
- Nightmare disorder
- Sleep-related eating disorder

Polysomnographic findings Polysomnography demonstrates spontaneous or pathologic (eg, apneas, periodic limb movements, gastroesophageal reflux, seizures) arousals from slow wave sleep in association with tachycardia and tachypnea.[17] **Fig. 3** demonstrates an example of a respiratory effort–related arousal from slow wave sleep. EEG readings include diffuse, rhythmic delta activity; diffuse delta and theta activity; mixed delta, theta, alpha, and beta activity; or alpha and beta activity. Time-synchronized video monitoring is essential to the diagnosis.

Confusional arousals

Clinical information Confusional arousals involve confused behavior and disorientation following arousals from NREM sleep. The benign forms of the disorder are common in children and episodes can be precipitated by forced awakenings. The sleeper does not leave the bed during confusional arousals, but can exhibit varying levels of behavioral complexity and aggression.

Polysomnographic findings Polysomnography demonstrates arousals from slow wave sleep. EEG findings of brief episodes of delta activity, stage 1 theta patterns, repeated microsleeps, or a diffuse alpha rhythm may also be observed. As with sleep walking, video recording of the behavior can support the diagnosis.

Sleep terrors

Clinical information Sleep terrors are characterized by arousals from slow wave sleep accompanied by autonomic discharge and behavioral manifestations of fear. Like sleepwalking and confusional arousals, the episodes are associated with amnesia and typically disappear spontaneously during adolescence. Sleep terrors can be differentiated from nightmare disorder, in which the patient rapidly becomes alert, usually arouses from REM sleep, and can recount his or her dreams and nightmares.

Polysomnographic findings Polysomnography findings of sleepwalking are similar to that of sleep terrors.

Rapid eye movement sleep behavior disorder

Clinical information REM sleep behavior disorder (RBD) is characterized by abnormal behavior and dream enactment that occurs during REM sleep. This parasomnia is more prominent in the latter half of the night, when REM sleep becomes more frequent. Episodes are marked by unpleasant dreams and sometimes violent behavior, which can result in injury to the patient or their bed partner. RBD is related to various underlying conditions,

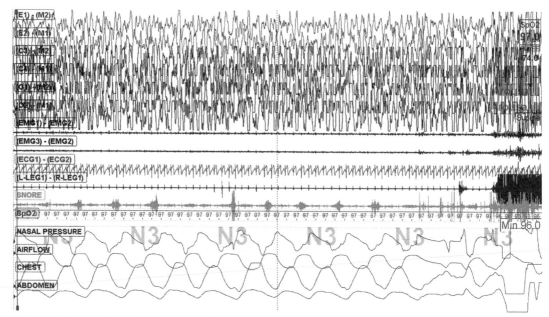

Fig. 3. This 60-second epoch demonstrates frequent slow wave activity in the EEG leads (C3-M2, C4-M1, O1-M2, O2-M1), with an arousal at the end of the epoch (noted by the increased EMG and EEG activity). The arousal is respiratory-related as signified by the flattening of the airflow (nasal pressure and nasal-oral thermistor) signal before the arousal.

particularly synucleinopathies, such as Parkinson's disease and Lewy body dementia.[18] RBD can also be exacerbated by most antidepressant medications. RBD should be differentiated from disorders of arousal, such as sleepwalking and sleep terrors, which occur during NREM sleep earlier in the night. Unlike sleepwalking, the patient's eyes usually remain closed during the RBD episode, and the patients typically become fully alert rapidly following the end of the episode. Patients with RBD typically are engaged in dream-like behavior and they do not navigate far from the bed because they are typically stumbling into furniture. This behavior is in contrast to sleepwalkers, who can stray quite far from the bed and usually engage in more complex activities.

Polysomnographic findings Diagnosis can be made by polysomnographic findings of excessive sustained EMG activity or intermittent loss of REM atonia, or excessive phasic muscle twitch activity of the submental or limb EMG during REM sleep (**Fig. 4**). As in the case of disorders of arousal, video monitoring of abnormal behavior is essential.

Nightmare disorder

Clinical information Nightmare disorder is characterized by recurrent nightmares that occur during REM sleep. The disorder is associated with acute stress disorder; posttraumatic stress disorder; and the use of drugs affecting

neurotransmitters norepinephrine, serotonin, and dopamine. Unlike sleep terrors, which occur in stage N3 sleep and are associated with amnesia, patients with nightmare disorder rapidly become alert and have full recall. Nightmare disorder is not associated with violent movements or injury as are characteristic of RBD.

Sleep-related eating disorder

Clinical information Sleep-related eating disorder is characterized by chronic, recurrent episodes of involuntary eating and drinking during NREM sleep. Sleep fragmentation, injury, and ingestion of inedible substances can be associated with the disorder and episodes are often accompanied with partial to complete amnesia.[19] Sleep-related eating disorder can be idiopathic, but is often associated with sleepwalking. Sleep-related eating disorder should be distinguished from nocturnal eating syndrome, in which the individual is fully alert while eating.

Polysomnographic findings Polysomnography demonstrates fragmentation of all NREM sleep stages, but most typically stage N3 sleep, and only rare arousals from REM sleep.

Neurologic Disorders

Sleep-related epilepsies

Seizures can manifest extensively during sleep in patients with certain epileptic syndromes. Seizures are caused by excessive discharge of

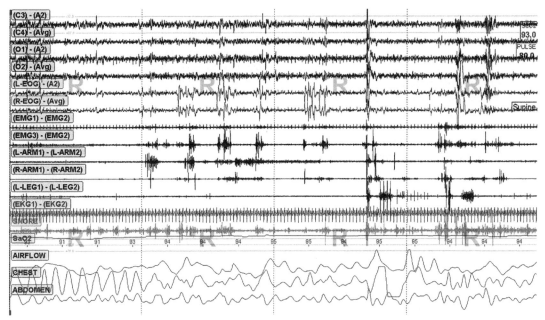

Fig. 4. This 120-second polysomnographic epoch demonstrates increased phasic activity during REM sleep. The behavior is observed in the leg (L-LEG1-L-LEG2), arm (L-ARM1-L-ARM2, R-ARM1-R-ARM2), and chin (EMG1-EMG-2, EMG3-EMG-2). This epoch of increased EMG tone is consistent with, but not necessarily diagnostic of, REM sleep behavior disorder.

neurons of the cerebral cortex resulting in either complex or simple movements. Seizures occurring predominantly during sleep can mimic parasomnias or simple sleep-related movements (**Box 4**). Sleep-related epilepsy can be differentiated from these disorders by the presence of interictal epileptiform activity. Polysomnography using a complete seizure montage and video recording can help categorize a questionable nocturnal movement as epileptic or nonepileptic.

Nocturnal frontal lobe epilepsy
Clinical information Nocturnal frontal lobe epilepsy is a paroxysmal sleep-related disturbance associated with seizures of variable intensity and duration, manifesting as four different subtypes: (1) a complex behavioral disorder mimicking disorders of arousal, (2) repetitive stereotyped behavior, (3) nocturnal paroxysmal dystonia, or (4) nocturnal paroxysmal arousals.[20] Unlike disorders of arousal, episodes of nocturnal frontal lobe epilepsy are typically of shorter duration, cluster, have associated stereotyped motor activity, and are not always associated with amnesia.[21]

Polysomnographic findings The characteristic ictal and interictal epileptiform EEG pattern further differentiates nocturnal frontal lobe epilepsy from simple sleep-related movement disorders. Autonomic activation (tachycardia and modified breathing patterns) is a common feature during seizures. Nocturnal frontal lobe epilepsy episodes occur most frequently during NREM sleep and should be differentiated from disorders of arousal using video monitoring.[22] Episodes of nocturnal frontal lobe epilepsy also occur more frequently than those characteristic of disorders of arousal.

Box 4
Sleep-related epilepsies

- Nocturnal frontal lobe epilepsy
- Benign epilepsy of childhood with centro-temporal spikes
- Juvenile myoclonic epilepsy
- Early or late onset occipital epilepsy
- Landau-Kleffner syndrome
- Continuous spike waves during REM sleep

Benign epilepsy of childhood with centrotemporal spikes
Clinical information Benign epilepsy of childhood with centrotemporal spikes is characterized by predominantly nocturnal partial seizures consisting of unilateral convulsions of the facial, pharyngeal, and laryngeal muscles. Generalized seizures are observed at a lower frequency and children may also show cognitive impairment during the active phase of the disease.[23]

Polysomnographic findings Seizures are more common during sleep and drowsiness than waking. The EEG demonstrates centrotemporal spikes.

Juvenile myoclonic epilepsy

Clinical information Juvenile myoclonic epilepsy is characterized by bilateral synchronous myoclonic jerks, most frequently occurring on awakening. Myoclonic seizures involving the arms are common in juvenile myoclonic epilepsy and tonic-clonic seizures and absence seizures may also occur.

Polysomnographic findings EEG demonstrates a generalized polyspike-and-wave pattern.[24]

Early or late onset occipital epilepsy

Clinical information Childhood epilepsy with occipital paroxysms is characterized by occipital epileptic discharges during sleep on an EEG and is classified according to early (Panayiotopoulos) or late (Gastaut) onset syndrome subtypes.[25] Panayiotopoulos syndrome presents with infrequent and prolonged seizures with ictal vomiting, whereas Gastaut syndrome presents with frequent seizures and visual ictal manifestations and migraine headaches. The rigidity of this classification is debated and various mixed clinical phenomena have been observed.[26]

Polysomnographic findings EEG demonstrates occipital epileptic discharges.

Landau-Kleffner syndrome

Clinical information Landau-Kleffner syndrome is an epileptic aphasia disorder characterized by severe and regressive impairment in verbal skills and comprehension with abnormal epileptiform activity. Kleffner-Kleffner syndrome can be associated with behavioral disorders and is frequently accompanied by nocturnal seizures.[27]

Polysomnographic findings EEG demonstrates variable epileptiform abnormalities with predominant bilateral spike-and-wave patterns in NREM sleep.[28] Specific EEG readings include bilateral independent temporal or temporoparietal spikes, bilateral 1- to 3-Hz slow wave maximally temporal activity, generalized sharp or slow wave discharges, and multifocal or unilateral spikes.[29]

Continuous spike waves during non–rapid eye movement sleep

Clinical information Continuous spike waves during NREM sleep is an epilepsy associated with cognitive and motor impairment, but clinical seizures are not necessarily present during sleep. Continuous spike waves during NREM sleep

typically disappear before adulthood, but may persist into adolescence.

Polysomnographic findings EEG demonstrates nearly continuous spike-wave discharges in slow wave sleep, usually with a frequency of 1.5 to 3 Hz on an EEG.[30]

MISCELLANEOUS SYMPTOMS AND CONDITIONS

Miscellaneous sleep-related symptoms and conditions that cannot be classified into definite pathologies or that could be considered benign are outlined in **Box 5**.

Sleep Starts

Clinical information

Sleep starts (hypnic jerks) are characterized by a brief, single contraction of the body or one or more body segments that occur typically at sleep onset.[31] The jerks must be associated with a subjective feeling of falling, a sensory flash, or a hypnagogic dream. The course is typically benign but sleep deprivation and related injury can occasionally occur. Sleep starts can be differentiated from physiologic partial hypnic myoclonus, which consists of small contractions of distal muscles resembling fasciculations particularly during stage N1 and REM sleep. Hypnic jerks can also be separated from excessive fragmentary myoclonus, which involves small, asynchronous, and bilateral distal muscle twitches, and which is seen at sleep onset and in all sleep stages. Another disorder in the differential diagnosis of sleep starts is propriospinal myoclonus, which is characterized by jerks slowly propagated from spinally innervated axial muscles of the trunk, neck, or abdomen to rostral and caudal muscles. Sleep starts can be further differentiated from periodic limb movements, which are characterized by muscle contractions that are much longer in duration, demonstrate periodicity, occur primarily during NREM sleep, and usually involve the lower extremities.

Box 5
Miscellaneous symptoms and conditions associated with nocturnal movements

- Sleep starts
- Benign sleep myoclonus of infancy
- Hypnagogic foot tremor and alternating leg muscle activation
- Propriospinal myoclonus at sleep onset
- Excessive fragmentary myoclonus
- Sleep-disordered breathing
- Sleep-related abnormal swallowing, choking, and laryngospasm

Polysomnographic findings

Polysomnography demonstrates EMG recordings of short 75- to 250-millisecond, high-amplitude potentials. EEG demonstrates drowsiness or stage 1 sleep patterns. Autonomic discharge, such as tachycardia and irregular breathing, may follow intense jerks.

Benign Sleep Myoclonus of Infancy

Clinical information

Benign sleep myoclonus of infancy is characterized by repetitive, bilateral, large myoclonic jerks of the face, trunk, or limbs during sleep and is limited to the neonatal period.[32] This disorder is different from infantile spasms, which are associated with a hypsarrhythmic EEG pattern and are characterized by sudden head and lower-extremity flexion and arm extension.

Polysomnographic findings

EMG demonstrates paroxysmal muscle activity, without ictal or interictal EEG abnormalities. Muscle jerks are typically 40 to 300 milliseconds in duration and occur in clusters of four or five jerks per second. Gentle rocking of the infant stimulates the myoclonus as demonstrated by EEG.

Hypnagogic Foot Tremor and Alternating Leg Muscle Activation During Sleep

Clinical information

Hypnagogic foot tremor is characterized by rhythmic movement of the feet that occurs at the transition from wake to sleep or during stage N1 and N2 NREM sleep. Alternating leg movement activation is characterized by anterior tibialis contractions alternating between the legs and occurs during NREM sleep and frequently during arousals from sleep.[33]

Polysomnographic findings

Hypnagogic foot tremor polysomnography (**Fig. 5**) demonstrates EMG bursts occurring at a frequency of 0.3 to 4 Hz with a minimum four burst train.[34] Alternating leg movement activation may represent the same disorder as hypnagogic foot tremor and produces EMG potentials similar to hypnagogic foot tremor with a frequency ranging from 0.5 to 3 Hz and also requires a four burst train for the diagnosis. Both disorders are considered benign and should be differentiated from periodic leg movements in sleep, which occur at longer intervals (from 5–90 seconds).

Propriospinal Myoclonus at Sleep Onset

Clinical information

Propriospinal myoclonus at sleep onset is a chronic condition characterized by spontaneous or evoked sudden muscular jerks of spinally innervated muscles of the neck, chest, or abdomen that slowly propagate to rostral and caudal muscles.[35] The muscle jerks may vary in intensity, frequency, and duration, and usually involve flexion, although extension is possible. Propriospinal myoclonus is

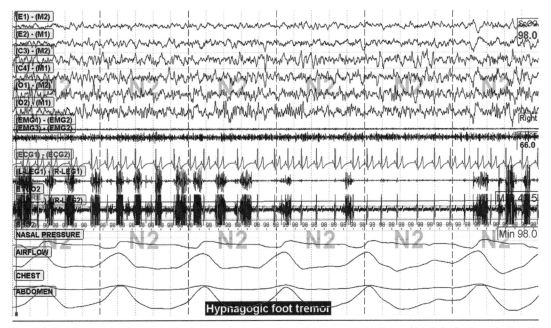

Fig. 5. This 180-second polysomnography epoch demonstrates frequent activation of both limbs (seen below the EKG lead), particularly notable in the first half of the epoch. These EMG bursts are indicative of hypnagogic foot tremor.

present during relaxed wakefulness and disappears with sleep onset. Propriospinal myoclonus can be differentiated from sleep starts, periodic limb movements, and fragmentary myoclonus by the variable and slow propagation of movements and the disappearance of the events by mental activation.

Polysomnographic findings

Polysomnography demonstrates nonperiodic and brief myoclonic EMG bursts with an alpha pattern on the EEG. EMG activity originates in muscles innervated by thoracic or cervical spinal segments, propagating to rostrally and caudally innervated muscles in 2 to 16 milliseconds.

Excessive Fragmentary Myoclonus

Clinical information

Excessive fragmentary myoclonus is characterized by involuntary small muscle twitches in the fingers, toes, or corners of the mouth that can occur in wakefulness and sleep.[36] The condition and course are considered benign and often no visible movement is observed. Unlike other sleep-related movement disorders, excessive fragmentary myoclonus occurs during all stages of sleep and does not occur synchronously or in clusters, as in hypnagogic foot tremor or alternating leg movement activation, or specifically during transitions between sleep stages as in sleep starts. Excessive fragmentary myoclonus can be further differentiated from sleep starts, which are characterized by large jerks.

Polysomnographic findings

Polysomnography demonstrates brief (<150 milliseconds), asynchronous, and asymmetrical EMG bursts present for 20 minutes, with at least five bursts per minute. Episodes may begin at sleep onset and continue through NREM and REM sleep.

Sleep-Related Breathing Disorders

Clinical information

Sleep-disordered breathing caused by OSA, central sleep apnea (CSA), sleep-related hypoventilation-hypoxemia, and chronic lung diseases may manifest as restless sleep or body movements associated with respiratory-related arousals.

OSA is characterized by repetitive partial (ie, hypopneas) or complete (ie, apneas) obstruction of the upper airway with subsequent increased ventilatory effort (eg, snoring, gasping, choking) resulting in cortical arousals or oxygen desaturations. OSA is associated with excessive daytime sleepiness, hypertension, stroke, and cardiovascular morbidity.[37–39] OSA should be considered in those with excess body weight but also in thin individuals or children with abnormal anatomic features.[40,41]

CSA is characterized by cessation of respiration caused by repetitive lapses in ventilatory effort resulting in sleep fragmentation and restless sleep.[42] Unlike OSA, an increased ventilatory response to carbon dioxide is a predisposing factor to the development of CSA. Patients with CSA sometimes have a lower than normal carbon dioxide level (ie, hypocapnia) caused by hyperventilation, and a small increase in carbon dioxide levels may result in cessation of ventilation. CSA is often idiopathic (ie, primary CSA), but can be triggered by drug use (ie, opioids); high altitude (ie, high-altitude periodic breathing); congestive heart failure (Cheyne-Stokes breathing pattern); or dysfunctions in the renal or central nervous systems.[43]

Hypoventilation syndromes are characterized by an elevation of the arterial carbon dioxide tension to above 45 mm Hg caused by an imbalance between the metabolic production, circulation, and elimination of carbon dioxide through exhaled gas.[44] Sleep-related hypoventilation syndromes most commonly stem from pulmonary parenchymal or vascular pathologies, lower airway obstructions, or neuromuscular and chest wall disorders.[45] Hypoventilation disorders are generally distinguishable from OSA and CSA because the oxygen desaturation level is consistent and sustained throughout the nocturnal period, whereas in CSA and OSA, the oxygen desaturation level may fluctuate in accordance with altered airflow during the apneic episodes.

Chronic lung diseases, such as chronic obstructive pulmonary disease, cystic fibrosis, and asthma, can disrupt sleep.[46,47] For example, patients with chronic obstructive pulmonary disease may have disrupted sleep because of cough, excess mucous production, arousals from sleep caused by hypercapnia, and secondary to medications used to manage the lung disease.[48,49]

Polysomnographic findings

Polysomnography in OSA demonstrates recurrent episodes (more than five per hour) of breathing cessation followed by oxygen desaturation and arousal during sleep. CSA is associated with more than five events per hour of respiratory events with absent airflow in the setting of no respiratory effort. Patients with hypoventilation demonstrate low baseline oxygen saturations and elevated carbon dioxide levels in the absence of OSA or CSA.

Sleep-Related Abnormal Swallowing, Choking, and Laryngospasm

Clinical information

Sleep-related abnormal swallowing, choking, and laryngospasm can result in abrupt awakenings from sleep. Sleep-related abnormal swallowing is characterized by pooling of the saliva in the upper airway, resulting in choking. Sleep-related laryngospasm is characterized by tracheal muscle dysfunction or paratracheal soft tissue swelling that interrupts breathing. The blockage is often followed by a period of stridor. Sleep-related choking is associated with awakenings without stridor. These disorders should be differentiated from OSA by polysomnographic findings.

Polysomnographic findings

Polysomnography may demonstrate frequent awakenings, tachypnea, and abnormal swallowing on a cricothyroid muscle EMG.

SUMMARY

A multitude of sleep-related movement disorders, parasomnias, epilepsies, and miscellaneous conditions may cause nocturnal movements. A physician should approach nocturnal movements by formulating a differential diagnosis and systematically evaluating it in the context of the patient's medical history and physical examination. The etiology of the patient's nocturnal movements can then be elucidated, often by the use of polysomnography with or without a full seizure montage. At that time, appropriate treatment can be instituted.

REFERENCES

1. American Academy of Sleep Medicine. International classification of sleep disorders 2005; Westchester (IL): American Academy of Sleep Medicine.
2. Smith RC. Relationship of periodic limb movements in sleep (nocturnal myoclonus) and the Babinski sign. Sleep 1985;8(3):239–43.
3. Stiasny K, Oertel WH, Trenkwalder C. Clinical symptomatology and treatment of restless legs syndrome and periodic limb movement disorder. Sleep Med Rev 2002;6(4):253–65.
4. Sforza E, Jouny C, Ibanez V. Time course of arousal response during periodic leg movements in patients with periodic leg movements and restless legs syndrome. Clin Neurophysiol 2003;114(6):1116–24.
5. Montplaisir J, Godbout R. Nocturnal sleep of narcoleptic patients: revisited. Sleep 1986;9(1 Pt 2):159–61.
6. Fry JM, DiPhillipo MA, Pressman MR. Periodic leg movements in sleep following treatment of obstructive sleep apnea with nasal continuous positive airway pressure. Chest 1989;96:89–91.
7. Baran AS, Richert AC, Douglas AB, et al. Change in periodic limb movement index during treatment of obstructive sleep apnea with continuous positive airway pressure. Sleep 2003;26(6):717–20.
8. Exar EN, Collop NA. The association of upper airway resistance with periodic limb movements. Sleep 2001;24(2):188–92.
9. Iber C, Ancoli-Israel S, Chesson A, et al, for the American Academy of Sleep Medicine. The AASM Manual for the Scoring of Sleep and Associated Events: rules, terminology and technical specifications. Westchester (IL): American Academy of Sleep Medicine; 2007.
10. Montgomery-Downs HE, Crabtree VM, Gozal D. Actigraphic recordings in quantification of periodic leg movements during sleep in children. Sleep Med 2005;6(4):325–32 [Epub 2005 April 1].
11. Sforza E, Johannes M, Claudio B. The PAM-RL ambulatory device for detection of periodic leg movements: a validation study. Sleep Med 2005; 6(5):407–13 [Epub 2005 April 1].
12. Walters AS. Clinical identification of the simple sleep-related movement disorders. Chest 2007; 131:1260–6.
13. DiFrancesco RC, Junqueira PA, Trezza PM, et al. Improvement of bruxism after T & A surgery. Int J Pediatr Otorhinolaryngol 2004;68(4):441–5.
14. Hoban TF. Rhythmic movement disorder in children. CNS Spectr 2003;8(2):135–8.
15. Walters AS, Lavigne G, Hening W, et al. The scoring of movements in sleep. J Clin Sleep Med 2007;3(2): 155–67.
16. Szelenberger W, Niemcewicz S, Dabrowska AJ. Sleepwalking and night terrors: psychopathological and psychophysiological correlates. Int Rev Psychiatry 2005;17(4):263–70.
17. Poyares D, Almeida CM, Silva RS, et al. [Violent behavior during sleep]. Rev Bras Psiquiatr 2005; 27(Suppl 1):22–6 [Epub 2005 July 28], [in Portuguese].
18. Hickey MG, Demaerschalk BM, Caselli RJ, et al. Idiopathic rapid-eye-movement (REM) sleep behavior disorder is associated with future development of neurodegenerative diseases. Neurologist 2007;13(2):98–101.
19. Najjar M. Zolpidem and amnestic sleep related eating disorder. J Clin Sleep Med 2007;3(6):637–8.
20. Provini F, Plazzi G, Tinuper P, et al. Nocturnal frontal lobe epilepsy: a clinical and polygraphic overview of 100 consecutive cases. Brain 1999;122(Pt 6): 1017–31.
21. Eisenman NL, Attarian HP. Sleep epilepsy. Neurologist 2003;9(4):200–6.
22. Zucconi M, Ferini-Strambi L. NREM parasomnias: arousal disorders and differentiation from nocturnal

frontal lobe epilepsy. Clin Neurophysiol 2000; 111(Suppl 2):S129–35.

23. Wolff M, Weiskopf N, Serra E, et al. Benign partial epilepsy in childhood: selective cognitive deficits are related to the location of focal spikes determined by combined EEG/MEG. Epilepsia 2005;46(10): 1661–7.

24. Alfradique I, Vasconcelos MM. Juvenile myoclonic epilepsy. Arq Neuropsiquiatr 2007;65(4B):1266–71.

25. Shahar E, Genizi J. Childhood epilepsy with occipital paroxysms: variations on the theme. Clin Pediatr (Phila) 2008;47(3):224–7 [Epub 2007 December 5].

26. Genizi J, Zelnik N, Ravid S, et al. Childhood epilepsy with occipital paroxysms: difficulties in distinct segregation into either the early-onset or late-onset epilepsy subtypes. J Child Neurol 2007;22(5): 588–92.

27. Mikati MA, Shamseddine AN. Management of Landau-Kleffner syndrome. Paediatr Drugs 2005; 7(6):377–89.

28. Pearl PL, Carrazana EJ, Holmes GL. The Landau-Kleffner syndrome. Epilepsy Curr 2001;1(2):39–45.

29. Gomez MR, Klass DW. Epilepsies in childhood: the Landau-Kleffner syndrome. Dev Med Child Neurol 1990;32:270–4.

30. Van Hirtum-Das M, Licht EA, Koh S, et al. Children with ESES: variability in the syndrome. Epilepsy Res 2006; 70(Suppl 1):S248–58 [Epub 2006 June 23].

31. Fusco L, Pachatz C, Cusmai R, et al. Repetitive sleep starts in neurologically impaired children: an unusual non-epileptic manifestation in otherwise epileptic subjects. Epileptic Disord 1999;1(1):63–7.

32. Paro-Panjan D, Neubauer D. Benign neonatal sleep myoclonus: experience from 38 infants. Eur J Paediatr Neurol 2008;12(1):14–8 [Epub 2007 June 18].

33. Chervin RD, Consens FB, Kutluay E. Alternating leg muscle activation during sleep and arousals: a new sleep-related motor phenomenon? Mov Disord 2003;18(5):551–9.

34. Berry RB. A woman with rhythmic foot movements. J Clin Sleep Med 2007;3(7):749–51.

35. Montagna P, Provini F, Vetrugno R. Propriospinal myoclonus at sleep onset. Neurophysiol Clin 2006; 36(5–6):351–5 [Epub 2007 January 26].

36. Vetrugno R, Plazzi G, Provini F, et al. Excessive fragmentary hypnic myoclonus: clinical and neurophysiological findings. Sleep Med 2002;3(1):73–6.

37. Caples SM, Kara T, Somers VK. Cardiopulmonary consequences of obstructive sleep apnea. Semin Respir Crit Care Med 2005;26(1):25–32.

38. Baguet JP, Narkiewicz K, Mallion JM. Update on hypertension management: obstructive sleep apnea and hypertension. J Hypertens 2006;24(1): 205–8.

39. Collop NA. Obstructive sleep apnea: what does the cardiovascular physician need to know? Am J Cardiovasc Drugs 2005;5(2):71–81.

40. Ryan CM, Bradley TD. Pathogenesis of obstructive sleep apnea. J Appl Physiol 2005;99(6):2440–50.

41. Deane S, Thomson A. Obesity and the pulmonologist. Arch Dis Child 2006;91(2):188–91.

42. White DP. Pathogenesis of obstructive and central sleep apnea. Am J Respir Crit Care Med 2005; 172(11):1363–70.

43. Caples SM, Wolk R, Somers VK. Influence of cardiac function and failure on sleep-disordered breathing: evidence for a causative role. J Appl Physiol 2005; 99(6):2433–9.

44. Krachman S, Criner GJ. Hypoventilation syndromes. Clin Chest Med 1998;19(1):139–55.

45. Annane D, Chevrolet JC, Chevret S, et al. Nocturnal mechanical ventilation for chronic hypoventilation in patients with neuromuscular and chest wall disorders. Cochrane Database Syst Rev 2000;(2): CD001941.

46. Kutty K. Sleep and chronic obstructive pulmonary disease. Curr Opin Pulm Med 2004;10(2):104–12.

47. Henry Benitez M, Morera Fumero AL, Gonzalez Martin IJ, et al. [Insomnia in asthmatic patients]. Actas Luso Esp Neurol Psiquiatr Cienc Afines 1994; 22(4):164–70 [in Spanish].

48. George CF. Perspectives on the management of insomnia in patients with chronic respiratory disorders. Sleep 2000;23(Suppl 1):S31–5 [discussion: S36–8].

49. Weitzenblum E, Chaouat A. Sleep and chronic obstructive pulmonary disease. Sleep Med Rev 2004;8(4):281–94.

Cardiac Monitoring During Sleep

Conrad Iber, MD[a,b],*, Kyuhyun Wang, MD[c]

KEYWORDS

- Cardiac • Rhythm • Sleep • Tachycardia
- Bradycardia • Asystole • Monitoring

Sleep alters cardiac rate and rhythms. The increased parasympathetic activity accompanying non rapid eye movement (NREM) sleep[1] is associated with heart rate slowing and changes in heart rate variability. Sleep permits the increased expression of second-degree atrioventricular block and brief cardiac asystole in some individuals, even in the absence of heart disease.[2] During polysomnographic monitoring, cardiac rhythm disturbances may reflect underlying comorbid cardiovascular disease or may be an expression of sleep disorders. Obstructive sleep apnea (OSA) produces cyclical cardiac slowing and acceleration and an increased occurrence of asystoles, tachydysrhythmias, and ectopic atrial and ventricular activity.[3,4] Other sleep disorders producing arousal also may be associated with an increased prevalence of cardiac rhythm disturbances. Despite the rather common occurrence of cardiac rhythm changes during polysomnography, serious consequences of these changes are rare. In one multicenter survey of 16,084 polysomnographies, adverse events occurred in 0.35% of studies, and mortality occurring within 2 weeks of an adverse event was noted in only 0.006% of studies.[5]

In ambulatory settings, standardization of 24-hour and longer electrocardiographic recording has been devised by the American Heart Association (AHA) and American College of Cardiology (ACC).[6–8] Despite the importance of recognizing cardiac dysrhythmias during sleep, standardization of methods for monitoring cardiac rhythm during polysomnography lagged behind polysomnographic methods for staging sleep and identifying respiratory events. Before 2007, standards for polysomnography had not included standardized methods for the monitoring and scoring of cardiac rhythms.[9–12] More recently, the American Academy of Sleep Medicine (AASM) has recommended methods for ECG acquisition and for the scoring and reporting of cardiac rhythms during polysomnography.[13,14]

As compared with multiple-lead monitoring of cardiac rhythm over prolonged periods employed as part of patient care strategies in patients with suspected heart disease,[6,15] the single bipolar lead 2 that is recommended for the monitoring of cardiac rhythm during polysomnography is understandably insufficient for qualitative measures such as ischemia and hypertrophy,[14] or for identifying originating focus for some dysrhythmias. Despite these limitations, many dysrhythmias common to sleep disorders and comorbid conditions should be identifiable employing lead 2 during standard polysomnographic recordings. Specifically, sinus bradycardia, sinus tachycardia, narrow and wide complex tachycardias, atrial fibrillation, and cardiac asystole should be scored routinely when present during polysomnography.[14] Other cardiac rhythms that are recognizable within the context of the sleep study should be reported. Sleep medicine practitioners should be familiar with routine methods, limitations, and scoring of cardiac events during polysomnography. Interventions for identified cardiac rhythms should be conditioned by the nature of the dysrhythmia, risks identified by patient characteristics and comorbidities, and prevailing patient care strategies in managing heart disease.

---

[a] Department of Medicine, Hennepin County Medical Center, 701 Park Avenue South, Minneapolis, MN 55415, USA
[b] University of Minnesota, Minneapolis, MN, USA
[c] Division of Cardiology, Department of Medicine, University of Minnesota, Mayo Mail Code 508, 420 Delaware Street Southeast, Minneapolis, MN 55455, USA
* Corresponding author. Department of Medicine, Hennepin County Medical Center, 701 Park Avenue South, Minneapolis, MN 55415.
E-mail address: iberx001@umn.edu (C. Iber).

Sleep Med Clin 4 (2009) 373–384
doi:10.1016/j.jsmc.2009.04.005
1556-407X/09/$ – see front matter © 2009 Published by Elsevier Inc.

NORMAL CARDIAC RHYTHM CHANGES DURING SLEEP

NREM sleep alters balance of the autonomic nervous system, resulting in consistent slowing of cardiac rate. Additional circadian influences may govern reductions in heart rate and blood pressure at night.[16] Although there are modest gender differences in heart rate during sleep, limited data from cross-sectional studies suggest that the appropriate lower confidence interval for normal heart rate during sleep is approximately 40 beats/min, and the upper limit for the

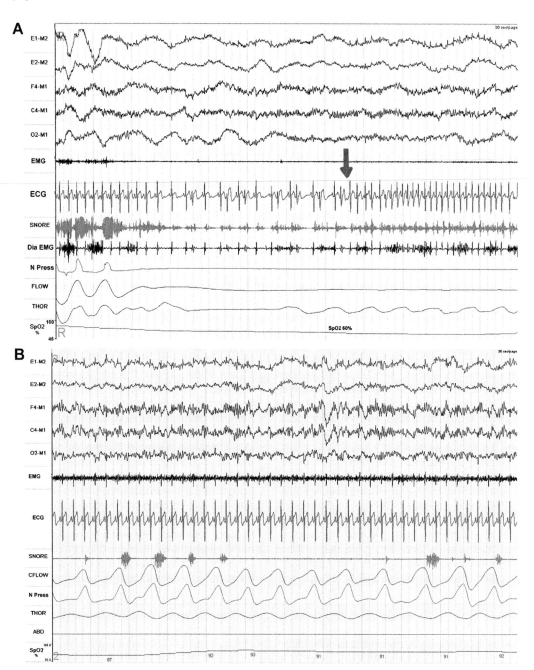

Fig. 1. Thirty-second epochs of polysomnography in an obstructive sleep apnea patient with previously unrecognized sleep-associated dysrhythmias. Before treatment (*A*), ECG demonstrates cyclical acceleration and slowing of heart rate, ventricular premature beats, and abrupt onset of narrow complex tachycardia (*arrow*). Following continuous positive airway pressure (*B*), cyclical changes in rate, ventricular premature beats, and narrow complex tachycardia have resolved.

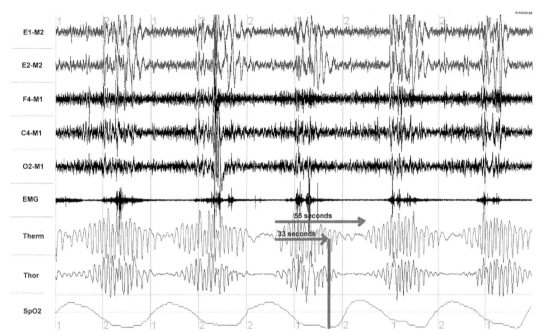

Fig. 2. Cheyne-Stokes crescendo–decrescendo breathing with prolonged hyperpnea, prolonged cycle length (55 seconds), and prolonged lung-to-ear circulation time (33 seconds). This patient had unrecognized right heart failure and tricuspid insufficiency following heart transplant and was referred initially for suspected sleep apnea. Subsequent to sleep studies, a cardiac catheterization led to tricuspid valvular repair. Iber published detailed information concerning standardized scoring of Cheyne-Stokes breathing.[14]

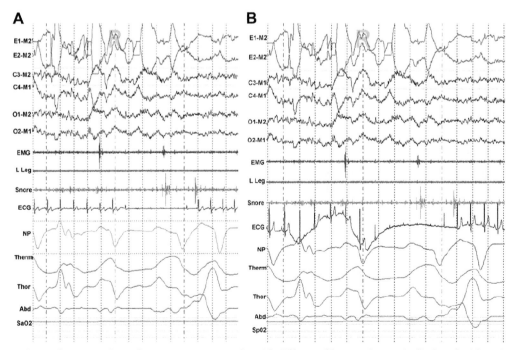

Fig. 3. Identical 15-second rapid eye movement epochs with different filter settings. *A* is displayed with an incorrect low-frequency filter setting of 3 Hz, and *B* is shown with a correct low-frequency setting of 0.3 Hz. ECG event from *A* was identified incorrectly as an asystole until filter setting error was corrected, revealing large artifact from electrode movement causing dampening of r wave.

confidence interval is approximately 90 beats/min for heart rate in adults.[13]

Activity of the autonomic nervous system is altered by sleep state and stage whether measured by heart rate variability[17–21] or muscle sympathetic nerve activity.[22] Compared with wakefulness, NREM sleep increases parasympathetic activity, whereas sympathetic activity is variably restored during rapid eye movement (REM) sleep.[1] Gender differences in autonomic balance are more prominent during REM.[23] Because of the effects of cardiovascular fitness and parasympathetic tone during sleep, substantial bradycardia and even atrioventricular

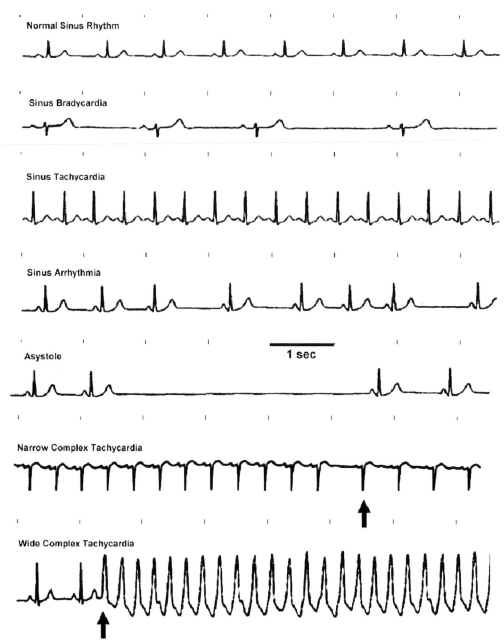

Fig. 4. Representative tracings of normal sinus rhythm, sinus tachycardia, sinus bradycardia, asystole, narrow complex tachycardia, and wide complex tachycardia. Note that unlike sustained sinus mechanisms, both narrow and wide complex tachycardias are characterized by abrupt onset and offsets (*arrows*). Short vertical lines are 1-second intervals.

block may be noted in young or even older endurance athletes.[2,24] The presence of frequent type 2 atrioventricular block during REM also may reflect a failure to increase sympathetic activity during REM.[18,25] Time of night additionally may affect likelihood of changes in cardiac rhythm. In otherwise healthy individuals, the occurrence of sleep-associated paroxysmal supraventricular tachycardias peaks between 4 a.m. and 6 a.m.[26]

Rapid changes in heart rate also may promote dysrhythmias. In normal individuals, over 80% of the instances of atrioventricular block, sinus pauses, and ventricular ectopy accompany rapid changes in heart rate.[27] Heart rate changes linked to sympathetic activity may precede arousal from sleep.[20] Heart rate increases also may occur following environmental stimuli whether or not arousal occurs.[28]

CLINICAL SCENARIOS
Risk of Sudden Cardiac Death

At-risk populations for sudden cardiac death usually are defined by common clinical comorbidities such as coronary artery disease, cardiomyopathy, and heart failure or more rare familial risks, including[29]:

Wolf Parkinson White syndrome
Long QT syndrome
Polymorphic ventricular tachycardia with normal QT[30]
Brugada syndrome
Congenital short QT syndrome

Controversy exists over the utility of identifying the complexity and frequency of ventricular premature beats in otherwise normal individuals, with the balance of evidence favoring increased risk of sudden cardiac death primarily in individuals who have known heart disease. In one large and often-cited study, the presence of ventricular premature beats (at least two beats over 2 minutes) in otherwise healthy individuals conferred a fourfold increased risk of sudden cardiac death.[31]

Although patients at risk for sudden death may express wide complex tachycardia, atrial fibrillation, and abnormal QT interval, evaluation usually requires detailed electrocardiographic or electrophysiologic analysis[32] that is beyond the scope of lead 2 employed in the setting of polysomnography. Even resting 12-lead electrocardiogram is far superior to lead 2 alone in detecting repolarization variant[33] and Brugada syndrome.[34] Certainly Brugada syndrome has been recognized to present with clinical symptoms at night[35] in individuals from Southeast Asia, although prevalence of this syndrome is sufficiently rare that occurrence of symptoms during polysomnography is unlikely.[5]

Obstructive Sleep Apnea

OSA is associated with cyclic slowing and acceleration of heart rate that mirrors the timing of respiratory events.[36–38] Heart rate slowing during OSA is more prominent than in central sleep apnea.[39] Modest cyclical changes in heart rate also have been noted with periodic leg movements.[40,41] In sleep apnea, cyclical ECG changes have been used to identify respiratory events, and spectral analysis of ECG has been used to segregate different respiratory events in preliminary studies.[42] Derived signals incorporating pulse and oxygen saturation have been used to identify

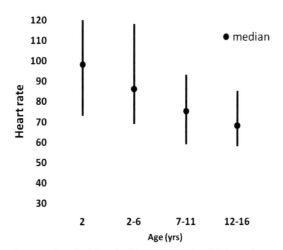

Fig. 5. The median (*circle*) and range (*vertical lines*) of heart rates in children decrease with age.[13,61–63]

respiratory events, arousals, and changes in sleep stage.[43–48]

OSA is the most common cause for abnormal cardiac rhythms in patients undergoing polysomnography. In addition to cyclical changes in ECG, the occurrence of asystole, tachyarrhythmias, and recurrent atrial fibrillation/flutter is more common in patients who have OSA.[3,4,26,49–53] Up to 48% of patients with OSA have been observed to have cardiac rhythm abnormalities including asystoles of 2.5 to 13 seconds in 11% and ventricular tachycardia in 2% of 400 patients in an early case series.[3] The severity of measures of sleep apnea have not correlated consistently with the occurrence of cardiac events,[3] although the severity and frequency of oxygen desaturation have been implicated in the incidence of atrial fibrillation.[50] The direct role of respiratory events in the genesis of cardiac rhythm changes has been inferred from the response of these dysrhythmias to continuous positive airway pressure **(Fig. 1)**.[51]

Cheyne-Stokes Breathing

Cheyne-Stokes breathing (CSB) is a respiratory pattern that is relatively unique to heart disease, and its presence may useful in identifying patients who have unrecognized heart failure. Heart failure frequently is associated with this characteristic crescendo/decrescendo breathing pattern **(Fig. 2)**, which can be distinguished from the breathing pattern seen in OSA patients without

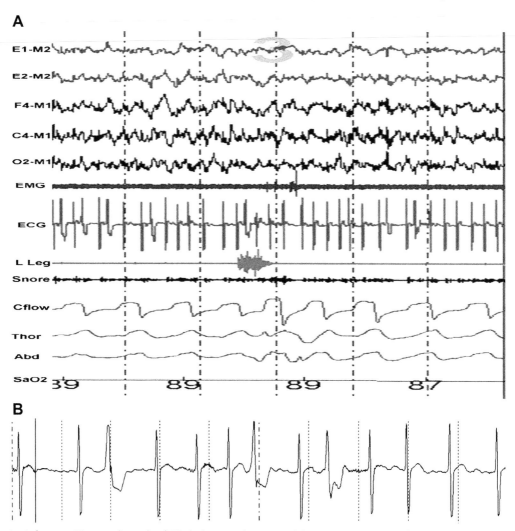

Fig. 6. *A* shows a 30-second epoch of N3 during continuous positive airway pressure administration in a patient with an irregularly irregular ventricular rhythm. Displaying a magnified version of a portion of the epoch in *B* reveals an irregularly irregular ventricular rhythm. There is replacement of p waves with activity of variable timing and morphology compatible with atrial fibrillation. Single wide complex beats are compatible with ventricular ectopic beats or conduction delay.

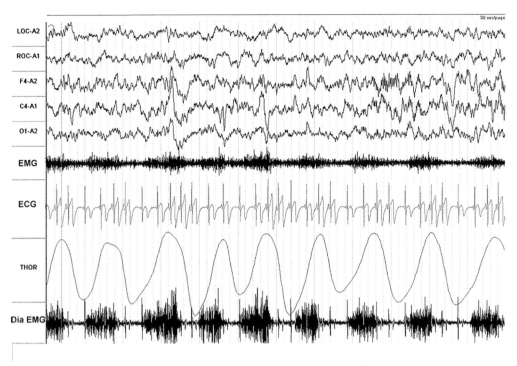

Fig. 7. A 30-second epoch of N2 with a regularly irregular rhythm in a 14 year-old boy. Sinus arrhythmia is evident with heart rate acceleration during inspiration. The inspiratory phase can be identified by phasic diaphragm contraction (Dia electromyogram) and prominent phasic chin electromyogram.

heart failure.[14] Although CSB has been associated most consistently with decreased left ventricular ejection fraction, heart failure is not always captured by measurement of ejection fraction. Thus, CSB may occur in isolated right ventricular disease[54] or valvular disease.

Heart failure patients may have components of both OSA and CSB. Two retrospective studies have identified a prevalence of either predominantly CSB or OSA (based on an AHI of greater than or equal to 15) of 51% to 61%[55,56] of individuals who have heart failure. A recent prospective study found that 53% of stable heart failure patients with ejection fractions of 22% plus or minus 8% had obstructive sleep apnea as defined as greater than10 events per hour.[57] The presence of sleep apnea in this study was associated with higher rates of atrial fibrillation, sleep disruption, and higher sympathetic activation. Obstructive events outnumbered central events 3:1.

Does CSB on polysomnography predict heart failure? The inference from the relatively unique and frequent association of CSB with heart failure is that the incidental finding of CSB during polysomnography might be used to illuminate an unsuspected diagnosis of heart failure in a patient referred for evaluating a breathing disorder during sleep (as in **Fig. 2**). Both the shape of the sinusoidal breathing pattern and the timing of respiratory parameters are somewhat specific to heart failure and likely are dictated by the presence of pulmonary congestion or a delay in systemic circulation time. The coexistence of OSA and CSB may occur in the same patient with variability in distribution of each component over time.[58] When OSA occurs in the setting of heart failure, the respiratory pattern and estimates of circulation time may be altered substantially by the heart failure. As compared with uncomplicated OSA patients, during obstructive events, heart failure patients with OSA have:

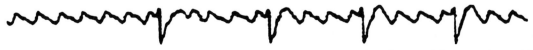

Fig. 8. Irregularly irregular ventricular rhythm with regular atrial activity identifies atrial flutter with variable atrioventricular block.

Box 1
Activities requiring reporting

Average heart rate during sleep

Highest heart rate during sleepHighest heart rate during recording

Occurrence of the following arrhythmias (yes/no). If present, list arrhythmia and heart rate or duration of pause:

Bradycardia—report lowest heart rate observed

Asystole—report longest pause observed

Sinus tachycardia during sleep—report highest heart rate observed

Narrow complex tachycardia—report highest heart rate observed

Wide complex tachycardia—report highest heart rate observed.

Atrial fibrillation

Occurrence of the other arrhythmias (yes/no). If present, list arrhythmia.

Longer hyperpnea (26 plus or minus 8 seconds versus 18 plus or minus 6 seconds)

Delayed lung-to-ear circulation (15 plus or minus 3 seconds versus 9 plus or minus 2 seconds)

Longer cycle duration (49 plus 11 seconds versus 39 plus 10 seconds)[59]

In patients who have CSB or those who have OSA with features suggestive of heart failure (such as delayed circulation, long cycle duration, and long hyperpnea), confirmatory tests for heart failure should be considered. Prospective studies are needed to determine if CSB found incidentally on polysomnography is a clinically useful predictor of heart disease.

STANDARDIZED METHODS
Data Acquisition and Display

The standard practice of polysomnography recording has employed a single bipolar ECG derivation that is insufficient for analysis of myocardial

Box 2
Example of portion of polysomnographic report incorporating cardiac event summary

Study no. 07-0000		No. of previous studies: 0	
DOB: 5/7/1980		Age: 27 y	
Height: 5'6"		Weight: 124 lb	
BMI: 20			
Medications: none			
Sleep parameters			
Lights out time	20:51:36	Wake after sleep onset	95.0
Lights on time	06:48:07	Total sleep time (min)	501.5
Total recording time (min)	596.5	Sleep efficiency	84.1%
Latency to sleep (min)	0.0	Latency to R (min)	255.0
N1 (min)	22	% N1	4.4
N2 (min)	250	% N2	49.9
N3 (min)	165	% N3	32.9
R (min)	66	% R	12.9
Arousal events			
Arousals	19	Arousals/hr	2.3
Cardiac			
Average rate/min during sleep	52	Highest rate/min recorded	80
Highest rate/min during sleep	60		

Cardiac events		Rate	*Cardiac events*		Rate
Bradycardia	Y	38	Narrow complex tachycardia	N	
Asystole	N		Wide complex tachycardia	N	
Sinus tachycardia	N		Atrial fibrillation	N	
Other arrhythmia	N	List			

ischemia and does not sample all topographic areas of the myocardium. Given the constraints of this practice standard, lead 2 provides sufficient information to identify atrial and ventricular activity for simple rhythm analysis.[13] Most computer analysis software now contains options for caliper measurement of time intervals and capability for display enlargement to assist in more careful visual inspection of cardiac rhythm and intervals.

The AHA previously recommended a sampling frequency of 500 Hz[60] to capture detailed electrocardiographic analysis. Mirroring these recommendations, AASM specifications for data acquisition during polysomnography include a minimum sampling rate of 200 Hz and a desirable sampling rate of 500 Hz. Sampling rates of 500 Hz may demonstrate pacer spikes better. The low-frequency filter setting of 0.3 Hz recommended by AASM is felt to better detect respiratory, movement, and sweat artifact in the setting of polysomnography as opposed to standard multiple-lead ECG (**Fig. 3**). A wide bandwidth with a high-frequency filter setting of 70 Hz also is recommended.

Scoring of Cardiac Events

The AASM recently recommended scoring of cardiac events employing a single lead 2 derivation. Additional scoring of events that may be interpreted within the context of single or multiple lead is left to the discretion of the responsible physician, although routine scoring of events should include at least the following:

Sinus tachycardia during sleep: a sustained sinus heart rate of greater than 90 beats per minutes lasting more than 30 seconds in adults (**Fig. 4**). Sinus rates vary according to age in children, with faster rates in young children as compared with adults (**Fig. 5**).[13,61–63] Maturation effects on sleep sinus rates preclude a common threshold for sinus tachycardia in all children, and readers are referred to a recent review for typical sinus rates by age in children.[13]

Bradycardia during sleep: a sustained heart rate of less than 40 beats per minute lasting more than 30 seconds in age 6 through adult (see **Fig. 4**)

Asystole: a cardiac pause greater than 3 seconds for ages 6 through adult (see **Fig. 4**)

Wide complex tachycardia: a rhythm lasting a minimum of three consecutive beats at a rate greater than 100 beats per minute with QRS duration of greater than or equal to 120 milliseconds (see **Fig. 4**). An abrupt

onset and offset characterize wide and narrow complex tachycardias.

Narrow complex tachycardia: a rhythm lasting a minimum of three consecutive beats at a rate of greater than 100 per minute with QRS duration of less than 120 milliseconds (see **Fig. 4**)

Atrial fibrillation: an irregularly irregular ventricular rhythm associated with replacement of consistent p waves by rapid oscillations that vary in size, shape, and timing (**Fig. 6**)

The specification of 30seconds for sustained sinus rhythm abnormalities was developed by the AASM Cardiac Task Force[13] and published in Scoring Manual FAQs.[64]

The irregular rhythm of atrial fibrillation can be distinguished easily from other irregular narrow complex rhythms by careful attention to p wave morphology and pattern. In sinus arrhythmia, the presence of p waves and the characteristic cyclical inspiratory acceleration are diagnostic (**Fig. 7**). In atrial flutter with variable block, the presence of regular atrial (f wave) activity at a rate of approximately 300 beats per minute is diagnostic (**Fig. 8**).

Reporting Cardiac Activity

AASM recommendations specify the routine reporting of certain cardiac activities and events during polysomnographic documents provided in the medical record (**Box 1**).

These events may be included in tabular format in the context of the polysomnographic report with additional comments in summary statements (**Box 2**).

REFERENCES

1. Trinder J, Kleiman J, Carrington M, et al. Autonomic activity during human sleep as a function of time and sleep stage. J Sleep Res 2001;10(4):253–64.

2. Viitasalo MT, Kala R, Eisalo A. Ambulatory electrocardiographic recording in endurance athletes. Br Heart J 1982;47(3):213–20.

3. Guilleminault C, Connolly SJ, Winkle RA. Cardiac arrhythmia and conduction disturbances during sleep in 400 patients with sleep apnea syndrome. Am J Cardiol 1983;52(5):490–4.

4. Roche F, Xuong AN, Court-Fortune I, et al. Relationship among the severity of sleep apnea syndrome, cardiac arrhythmias, and autonomic imbalance. Pacing Clin Electrophysiol 2003;26(3):669–77.

5. Mehra R, Strohl KP. Incidence of serious adverse events during nocturnal polysomnography. Sleep 2004;27(7):1379–83.

6. Kadish AH, Buxton AE, Kennedy HL, et al. ACC/AHA clinical competence statement on electrocardiography and ambulatory electrocardiography. A report of the ACC/AHA/ACP-ASIM Task Force on Clinical Competence (ACC/AHA Committee to Develop a Clinical Competence Statement on Electrocardiography and Ambulatory Electrocardiography). J Am Coll Cardiol 2001;38(7):2091–100.

7. Kadish AH, Buxton AE, Kennedy HL, et al. ACC/AHA clinical competence statement on electrocardiography and ambulatory electrocardiography: A report of the ACC/AHA/ACP-ASIM task force on clinical competence (ACC/AHA Committee to develop a clinical competence statement on electrocardiography and ambulatory electrocardiography) endorsed by the International Society for Holter and Noninvasive Electrocardiology. Circulation 2001;104(25):3169–78.

8. Crawford MH, Bernstein SJ, Deedwania PC, et al. ACC/AHA guidelines for ambulatory electrocardiography: executive summary and recommendations. A report of the American College of Cardiology/American Heart Association Task Force on Practice Guidelines (Committee to Revise the Guidelines for Ambulatory Electrocardiography) developed in collaboration with the North American Society for Pacing and Electrophysiology. Circulation 1999; 100(8):886–93.

9. Anonymous. Indications and standards for cardiopulmonary sleep studies. American Thoracic Society. Medical Section of the American Lung Association. Am Rev Respir Dis 1989;139(2):559–68.

10. Anonymous. Standards and indications for cardiopulmonary sleep studies in children. American Thoracic Society. Am J Respir Crit Care Med 1996; 153(2):866–78.

11. Block AJ, Cohn MA, Conway WA, et al. Indications and standards for cardiopulmonary sleep studies. Sleep 1985;8(4):371–9.

12. George CF. Standards for polysomnography in Canada. The Standards Committees of the Canadian Sleep Society and the Canadian Thoracic Society. CMAJ 1996;155(12):1673–8.

13. Caples SM, Rosen CL, Shen WK, et al. The scoring of cardiac events during sleep. J Clin Sleep Med 2007;3(2):147–54.

14. Iber C, Chesson A, Ancoli-Israel S, et al. The scoring of sleep and associated events: rules, terminology, and technical specifications. 1st edition. Westchester (IL): American Academy of Sleep Medicine; 2007.

15. Crawford C. Sleep recording in the home with automatic analysis of results. Eur Neurol 1986;25(Suppl 2): 30–5.

16. Carrington M, Walsh M, Stambas T, et al. The influence of sleep onset on the diurnal variation in cardiac activity and cardiac control. J Sleep Res 2003;12(3):213–21.

17. Cajochen C, Pischke J, Aeschbach D, et al. Heart rate dynamics during human sleep. Physiol Behav 1994;55(4):769–74.

18. Janssens W, Willems R, Pevernagie D, et al. REM sleep-related brady–arrhythmia syndrome. Sleep Breath 2007;11(3):195–9.

19. Elsenbruch S, Harnish MJ, Orr WC. Heart rate variability during waking and sleep in healthy males and females. Sleep 1999;22(8):1067–71.

20. Bonnet MH, Arand DL. Heart rate variability: sleep stage, time of night, and arousal influences. Electroencephalogr Clin Neurophysiol 1997;102(5):390–6.

21. Vanoli E, Adamson PB, Ba L, et al. Heart rate variability during specific sleep stages. A comparison of healthy subjects with patients after myocardial infarction. Circulation 1995;91(7):1918–22.

22. Okada H, Iwase S, Mano T, et al. Changes in muscle sympathetic nerve activity during sleep in humans. Neurology 1991;41(12):1961–6.

23. Valladares EM, Eljammal SM, Motivala S, et al. Sex differences in cardiac sympathovagal balance and vagal tone during nocturnal sleep. Sleep Med 2008;9(3):310–6.

24. Northcote R, Canning G, Ballantyne D. Electrocardiographic findings in male veteran endurance athletes. Br Heart J 1989;61(2):155–60.

25. Viola AU, Simon C, Doutreleau S, et al. Abnormal heart rate variability in a subject with second-degree atrioventricular blocks during sleep. Clin Neurophysiol 2004;115(4):946–50.

26. Coccagna G. Cardiac arrhythmias during sleep. Somnologie 2000;4(3):103–10.

27. Viitasalo M, Halonen L, Partinen M, et al. Sleep and cardiac rhythm in healthy men. Ann Med 1991;23(2): 135–9.

28. Griefahn B, Brode P, Marks A, et al. Autonomic arousals related to traffic noise during sleep. Sleep 2008;31(4):569–77.

29. Behr E, Wood DA, Wright M, et al. Cardiological assessment of first-degree relatives in sudden arrhythmic death syndrome. Lancet 2003; 362(9394):1457–9.

30. Wever EF, Robles de Medina EO. Sudden death in patients without structural heart disease. J Am Coll Cardiol 2004;43(7):1137–44.

31. Abdalla IS, Prineas RJ, Neaton JD, et al. Relation between ventricular premature complexes and sudden cardiac death in apparently healthy men. Am J Cardiol 1987;60(13):1036–42.

32. Zipes DP, Camm AJ, Borggrefe M, et al. ACC/AHA/ESC 2006 guidelines for management of patients with ventricular arrhythmias and the prevention of sudden cardiac death—executive summary: a report of the American College of Cardiology/American Heart Association Task Force and the European Society of Cardiology Committee for Practice Guidelines (Writing

Committee to Develop Guidelines for Management of Patients with Ventricular Arrhythmias and the Prevention of Sudden Cardiac Death) developed in collaboration with the European Heart Rhythm Association and the Heart Rhythm Society. Eur Heart J 2006;27(17):2099–140.

33. Haissaguerre M, Derval N, Sacher F, et al. Sudden cardiac arrest associated with early repolarization. N Engl J Med 2008;358(19):2016–23.

34. Marill KA, Ellinor PT, Marill KA, et al. Case records of the Massachusetts General Hospital. Case 372005. A 35-year-old man with cardiac arrest while sleeping. N Engl J Med 2005;353(23):2492–501.

35. Parrish RG, Tucker M, Ing R, et al. Sudden unexplained death syndrome in Southeast Asian refugees: a review of CDC surveillance. MMWR CDC Surveill Summ 1987;36(SS-1):43SS–53SS.

36. Guilleminault C, Connolly S, Winkle R, et al. Cyclical variation of the heart rate in sleep apnoea syndrome. Mechanisms, and usefulness of 24 h electrocardiography as a screening technique. Lancet 1984; 1(8369):126–31.

37. Gula LJ, Krahn AD, Skanes A, et al. Heart rate variability in obstructive sleep apnea: a prospective study and frequency domain analysis. Ann Noninvasive Electrocardiol 2003;8(2):144–9.

38. Stein PK, Duntley SP, Domitrovich PP, et al. A simple method to identify sleep apnea using Holter recordings. J Cardiovasc Electrophysiol 2003;14(5):467–73.

39. Spicuzza L, Bernardi L, Calciati A, et al. Autonomic modulation of heart rate during obstructive versus central apneas in patients with sleep-disordered breathing. Am J Respir Crit Care Med 2003;167(6): 902–10.

40. Gosselin N, Lanfranchi P, Michaud M, et al. Age and gender effects on heart rate activation associated with periodic leg movements in patients with restless legs syndrome. Clin Neurophysiol 2003;114(11): 2188–95.

41. Sforza E, Juony C, Ibanez V. Time-dependent variation in cerebral and autonomic activity during periodic leg movements in sleep: implications for arousal mechanisms. Clin Neurophysiol 2002; 113(6):883–91.

42. Thomas RJ, Mietus JE, Peng CK, et al. Differentiating obstructive from central and complex sleep apnea using an automated electrocardiogram-based method. Sleep 2007;30(12):1756–69.

43. Pittman SD, Pillar G, Berry RB, et al. Follow-up assessment of CPAP efficacy in patients with obstructive sleep apnea using an ambulatory device based on peripheral arterial tonometry. Sleep Breath 2006;10(3):123–31.

44. Pepin JL, Delavie N, Pin I, et al. Pulse transit time improves detection of sleep respiratory events and microarousals in children. Chest 2005;127(3): 722–30.

45. Bar A, Pillar G, Dvir I, et al. Evaluation of a portable device based on peripheral arterial tone for unattended home sleep studies. Chest 2003;123(3): 695–703.

46. Freimark D, Adler Y, Sheffy J, et al. Oscillations in peripheral arterial tone in congestive heart failure patients: a new marker for Cheyne-Stokes breathing. Cardiology 2002;98:21–4.

47. Smith RP, Argod J, Pepin JL, et al. Pulse transit time: an appraisal of potential clinical applications. Thorax 1999;54(5):452–7.

48. Bresler M, Sheffy K, Pillar G, et al. Differentiating between light and deep sleep stages using an ambulatory device based on peripheral arterial tonometry. Physiol Meas 2008;29(5):571–84.

49. Chen LY, Shen WK. Epidemiology of atrial fibrillation: a current perspective. Heart Rhythm 2007;4(Suppl 3):S1–6.

50. Gami AS, Hodge DO, Herges RM, et al. Obstructive sleep apnea, obesity, and the risk of incident atrial fibrillation. J Am Coll Cardiol 2007;49(5):565–71.

51. Harbison J, O'Reilly P, McNicholas WT. Cardiac rhythm disturbances in the obstructive sleep apnea syndrome: effects of nasal continuous positive airway pressure therapy. Chest 2000;118(3):591–5.

52. Kanagala R, Murali NS, Friedman PA, et al. Obstructive sleep apnea and the recurrence of atrial fibrillation. Circulation 2003;107(20):2589–94.

53. Mooe T, Gullsby S, Rabben T, et al. Sleep-disordered breathing: a novel predictor of atrial fibrillation after coronary artery bypass surgery. Coron Artery Dis 1996;7(6):475–8.

54. Schulz R, Blau A, Borgel J, et al. Sleep apnoea in heart failure. Eur Respir J 2007;29(6):1201–5.

55. Javaheri S, Parker TJ, Liming JD, et al. Sleep apnea in 81 ambulatory male patients with stable heart failure. Types and their prevalences, consequences, and presentations. Circulation 1998;97(21):2154–9.

56. Sin DD, Fitzgerald F, Parker JD, et al. Risk factors for central and obstructive sleep apnea in 450 men and women with congestive heart failure. Am J Respir Crit Care Med 1999;160(4):1101–6.

57. Ferrier K, Campbell A, Yee B, et al. Sleep-disordered breathing occurs frequently in stable outpatients with congestive heart failure. Chest 2005;128(2): 2116–22.

58. Tkacova R, Wang H, Bradley TD. Night-to-night alterations in sleep apnea type in patients with heart failure. J Sleep Res 2006;15(3):321–8.

59. Ryan CM, Bradley TD. Periodicity of obstructive sleep apnea in patients with and without heart failure. Chest 2005;127(2):536–42.

60. Bailey JJ, Berson AS, Garson A Jr, et al. Recommendations for standardization and specifications in automated electrocardiography: bandwidth and digital signal processing. A report for health professionals by an ad hoc writing group of the Committee

on Electrocardiography and Cardiac Electrophysiology of the Council on Clinical Cardiology, American Heart Association. Circulation 1990;81(2):730–9.

61. Poets CF, Stebbens VA, Alexander JR, et al. Breathing patterns and heart rates at ages 6 weeks and 2 years. Am J Dis Child 1991;145:1393–6.

62. Poets CF, Samuels MP, Noyes JP. Home event recordings of oxygenation, breathing movements, and heart rate and rhythm in infants with recurrent life-threatening events. J Pediatr 1992;123: 693–701.

63. Findley LJ, Blackburn MR, Goldberger AL, et al. Apneas and oscillation of cardiac ectopy in Cheyne-Stokes breathing during sleep. Am Rev Respir Dis 1984;130(5):937–9.

64. Anonymous. Scoring manual FAQs. Available at: http://www.aasmnet.org/Resources/PDF/FAQsScoring Manual.pdf. Accessed October 1, 2008.

Multiple Sleep Latency Test and Maintenance of Wakefulness Test

Douglas Kirsch, MD[a,b,*], Josna Adusumilli, MD[c]

KEYWORDS

- Sleepiness • Multiple sleep latency test
- Maintenance of wakefulness test • Evaluation

Sleep, O Sleep! Elixir of life, why have thou escaped me? The alarm rings, and millions of Americans wake up to face the prospect of daytime sleepiness. This sleepiness may demonstrate itself in mild ways, such as a young medical student falling asleep during lectures, a mother of four children who battles the weight of sleep on her eyelids throughout the day, hoping for a nap, and, as a recent case of a history professor, who frequently dozed while driving through heavy traffic. These cases illustrate how excessive daytime sleepiness may cause embarrassment, impairment of performance, or even life-threatening injuries in our round-the-clock society.

Excessive daytime sleepiness (EDS), which is defined as "the inability to stay awake and alert during the major waking episodes of the day, resulting in unintended lapses into drowsiness or sleep," must occur at least 3 months before diagnosis.[1] Degrees of EDS can be quantified by obtaining a comprehensive history in conjunction with various diagnostic studies, such as overnight polysomnography, multiple sleep latency test (MSLT), and the maintenance of wakefulness test (MWT).

CLINICAL HISTORY

The first step in the evaluation of EDS is to obtain a thorough sleep and general medical history. It is important to discern whether a patient is presenting with sleepiness or fatigue. Although these terms may be used interchangeably by patients, sleepiness and fatigue have different etiologies. Although the former term is associated with sleep disorders or insufficient sleep, the latter term may be more likely associated with underlying medical or psychological problems. In patients with fatigue (or tiredness), there is not a clearly increased physiologic drive for sleep; if they were to lie down to rest, they would not necessarily fall asleep. It is also important to review a patient's sleep-wake schedule to identify problems with insufficient sleep or circadian rhythm disorders. Assessment for signs of other sleep disorders, such as obstructive sleep apnea or periodic limb movements, may prove helpful. Contributions to sleepiness from a patient's medical history, medications, and substance use should be evaluated.

Questionnaires such as the Epworth Sleepiness Scale (ESS), Stanford Sleepiness Scale (SSS), and Functional Outcomes of Sleep Questionnaire (FOSQ) are useful to assess the patient's perception of sleepiness in a variety of daily circumstances (**Boxes 1–2**). These questionnaires can be used as screening tests or to track response to treatment. The ESS is the most widely used subjective assessment for sleepiness. Although it has been found to be reliable and internally consistent with testing and retesting of individuals,[2] the correlation between subjective Epworth scores and objective measurement of mean sleep latency on the MSLT remains controversial. Other disadvantages of the ESS include the fact that the questions may not be typical or pertinent to an individual's daily routine and may not take into

[a] Division of Sleep Medicine, Harvard Medical School, Boston, MA, USA
[b] Sleep Health*Centers*, 1505 Commonwealth Ave, 5th Floor, Brighton, MA, 02135 USA
[c] Brigham and Women's Hospital, Boston, MA, USA
* Corresponding author. Sleep Health*Centers*, 1505 Commonwealth Ave, 5th Floor, Brighton, MA, 02135
E-mail address: Doug_Kirsch@sleephealth.com (D. Kirsch).

Sleep Med Clin 4 (2009) 385–392
doi:10.1016/j.jsmc.2009.04.006
1556-407X/09/$ – see front matter © 2009 Elsevier Inc. All rights reserved.

Box 1
Epworth Sleepiness Scale

ESS questions are answered using numbers from 0 to 4 (see answer key below):
How likely are you to doze off or fall asleep in the following situations, in contrast to just feeling tired?

0 = would never doze

1 = slight chance of dozing

2 = moderate chance of dozing

3 = high chance of dozing

Situation

1. Watching TV
2. Sitting inactively in a public place (eg, a theater or a meeting)
3. Being a passenger in a car for about an hour without a break
4. Lying down to rest in the afternoon when circumstances permit
5. Sitting and talking to someone
6. Sitting quietly after a lunch without alcohol
7. Sitting in a car while stopped for a few minutes in traffic

ESS scores range from 0 to 24, with increasing scores indicating increased sleepiness.
From Johns MW. A new method for measuring daytime sleepiness: the Epworth sleepiness scale. Sleep 1991;14(6):540–45; with permission.

Box 2
The Stanford Sleepiness Scale

Please record the scale value that best describes your state of sleepiness:

1. Feeling active and vital; alert; wide awake
2. Functioning at a high level, but not at peak; able to concentrate
3. Relaxed; awake; not at full alertness; responsive
4. A little foggy; not at peak; let down
5. Fogginess; beginning to lose interest in remaining awake; slowed down
6. Sleepiness; prefer to be lying down; fighting sleep; woozy
7. Almost in reverie; sleep onset soon; lost struggle to remain awake

SSS scores range from 1 to 7, with increasing scores indicating increased sleepiness.
From Hoddes E, Dement WC, Zarcone V. The history and use of the Stanford Sleepiness Scale [abstract]. Psychophysiology 1972;9:150; with permission.

---

account variation of sleepiness at different time points during the day. The SSS is a single-question assessment that tests current levels of sleepiness; it is often used in research protocols. A potential advantage of the SSS is that it can be given at various time points throughout the day; however, these individual time points may not fully demonstrate the real world effect of the patient's chronic level of sleepiness. The FOSQ was the first questionnaire created to determine the repercussion of disorders of EDS on activities of daily living. The literature has demonstrated that the FOSQ is useful in assessing the impact of sleep disorders on an individual's routine activities and providing documentation of improvement in these activities once the sleep disorder has been treated.[3]

POLYSOMNOGRAPHY

An overnight polysomnogram is valuable in identifying possible root causes of EDS, such as obstructive sleep apnea, periodic leg movements during sleep, and other sleep disorders. Although not routinely used for direct measurement of daytime sleepiness, a decreased sleep latency

and increased sleep efficiency on the overnight polysomnogram is suggestive of EDS. Technical details of the polysomnogram itself are reviewed elsewhere in this issue.

MULTIPLE SLEEP LATENCY TEST

The MSLT remains the gold standard test for objective assessment of EDS. This test measures the physiologic tendency of a patient to fall asleep in a quiet environment. It was developed by Drs. William Dement and Mary Carskadon in the 1970s at Stanford University for objective measurement of sleepiness in clinical and research settings. The recommendations for the MSLT protocol are described in detail in the January 2005 practice parameters published by the American Academy of Sleep Medicine and are summarized below.[1]

Preparation is essential before undergoing the MSLT. It is recommended that the patient obtain 2 weeks of regular sleep before the test. Having the patient keep a sleep log for documentation of sleep-wake schedules may prove helpful when evaluating the results of the MSLT. Stimulants, stimulant-like medications, and rapid eye movement (REM)-suppressing medications should be discontinued, if safe to do so, at least 15 days or five half-lives before the patient undergoes testing. Urinary drug screening can be performed the morning of the MSLT to ensure that findings of the MSLT are not pharmacologically altered. Caffeine and alcohol may alter sleep time and sleep architecture and should not be used during the test. Withdrawal from these agents also may modify test results.[4]

The night before the MSLT, a polysomnogram should be performed to document quality and duration of sleep. It is recommended that at least 6 hours of documented sleep occur before the administration of the MSLT. Even 6 hours of sleep may be insufficient for some patients, especially "long sleepers"; this "sleep deprivation" may cause observable sleepiness during the MSLT. Patients who suffer from delayed sleep phase syndrome may require alteration in the MSLT protocol. Delay of the patient's wake time from the overnight study and initiating the MSLT 2 hours from the delayed wake time is one possible strategy if altering the patient's circadian rhythm is not possible.

A standard MSLT montage includes a referential electroencephalogram (EEG) from central and occipital locations, two electro-oculograms (left and right) at the outer canthi, a mental or submental electromyogram, and an electrocardiogram. Frontal EEG leads, although not mentioned in the MSLT practice parameter, also may be added on the basis of the recent update to the visual scoring rules.[5] These measures are necessary to determine sleep onset, stages of sleep, and the patient's heart rhythm. The nap attempts should take place in a bedroom that is dark, quiet, and at a comfortable temperature setting. Five nap opportunities begin 1.5 to 3 hours after the end of the polysomnogram and continue every 2 hours. No sleeping is allowed between the naps, nicotine use is avoided 30 minutes before each test, and vigorous activity is suspended 15 minutes before each trial. Prior to each attempt, the patient is told to "please lie quietly, assume a comfortable position, keep your eyes closed, and try to fall asleep."[1] The technician monitors the transition from wake (**Fig. 1**) to electrographic sleep onset, defined as the first epoch of any stage of sleep, including stage N1 (**Fig. 2**). If sleep occurs at any time during one of the 20-minute trials, 15 additional minutes of recording are allowed to see whether "sleep-onset" REM sleep occurs (**Figs. 3** and **4**). If sleep does not occur, a nap session is terminated and a sleep latency of 20 minutes is recorded. The arithmetic average of the sleep latencies from all 5 naps is calculated to determine the mean sleep latency. Although clinically the sleep onset is determined by the first 30-second epoch of scored sleep of any type, in some research studies, the first three consecutive epochs of N1 sleep have been used an as alternate definition.

The value of a normal sleep latency has not been fully established because it likely relates to age, gender, and other genetic and medical factors. In general, a mean sleep latency of less than 5 minutes in adults indicates sleepiness, whereas a mean of 15 minutes or longer suggests normal alertness.[6] In a recent study, the mean sleep latency of narcoleptics was 3.1 ± 2.9 minutes, and the mean sleep latency of patients with idiopathic hypersomnia was 6.2 ± 3.0 minutes.[1] A mean value of 8 minutes or less is used to diagnose disorders that cause EDS.[1] It is important to keep in mind that healthy individuals may have variable sleep latencies, including a mean sleep latency less than or equal to 8 minutes, especially if nocturnal sleep is not normalized before the MSLT.

Clinically, the MSLT is used to quantify EDS for the diagnosis of narcolepsy with and without cataplexy and is often used to distinguish idiopathic hypersomnia from narcolepsy. The presence of sleep-onset REM periods during the MSLT naps is more specific for narcolepsy than a decreased mean sleep latency. Circadian rhythm disorders and chronic REM sleep–disrupting disorders, such as obstructive sleep apnea, medications, and affective disorders, also can cause sleep-onset REM periods.[7] The MSLT is not routinely indicated in the assessment of patients with obstructive sleep apnea, circadian rhythm disorders, insomnia, or medical or neurologic causes of sleepiness. Individuals with known sleep-disordered breathing, periodic limb movement disorder, or mood disorders who have continued excessive sleepiness despite optimal treatment may require evaluation for disorders of primary sleep drive, however, which may include use the MSLT.[1]

Case Study: Use of the Multiple Sleep Latency Test

The patient is a 28-year-old woman who has had difficulty with severe daytime sleepiness since her teenage years. This sleepiness has occurred although she has averaged 8 to 9 hours of sleep per night. She has required frequent naps throughout the day to be functional. When she was in school, she was unable to stay awake for more than one class in a row, and when returning home after school, she would require a late afternoon nap. She also slept through concerts and lectures and would easily fall asleep with sedentary activities. She has limited her driving to short drives of 5 to 10 minutes secondary to concerns about drowsy driving. She also reports episodes of muscle weakness in association with laughing too hard, beginning at the age 17. These episodes would result in drooping of her face and occasional knee buckling, which would last for less than a few minutes, with quick return to functioning. She has occasional episodes of sleep

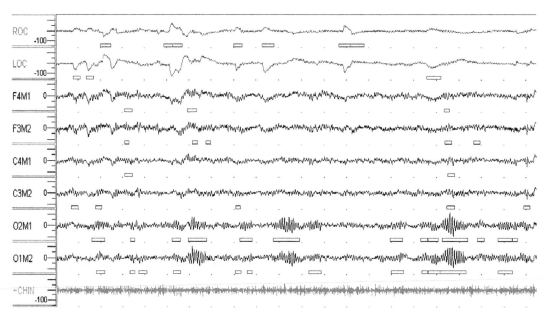

Fig. 1. Rapid eye movements and alpha frequency EEG activity during an epoch of wakefulness in the MSLT.

paralysis but denies any hypnogogic hallucinations. She states that her sleep is somewhat restless, but she denies any history of snoring, apneic spells, or leg jerking. She describes an uncle who has had similar levels of daytime sleepiness. Her physical examination did not demonstrate any abnormal findings. Her nocturnal polysomnogram demonstrated a sleep latency of 3 minutes, an REM sleep latency of 40 minutes, and a sleep efficiency of 87%. Her MSLT demonstrated a mean sleep latency of 2 minutes with four sleep-onset REM periods. She was given a diagnosis of narcolepsy and treated with gamma-hydroxybutyrate in two doses at night time with improvement in cataplexy and some improvement in EDS. Addition of daytime stimulant medication and scheduled napping further improved daytime functioning.

MAINTENANCE OF WAKEFULNESS TEST

The MWT is a validated measure of an individual's ability to remain awake during a period of time. Although the MSLT measures sleepiness, the MWT was developed by Dr. Merrill Mitler in 1982 to measure wakefulness, an alternative—but not necessarily opposite—phenomenon to sleepiness. Although one might predict that someone who is sleepy would not be able to keep himself or herself awake, the findings of the two tests do not correlate as well as might be expected. This fact suggests that the measurement of the ability to stay awake is at least partially independent of the ability to let oneself fall asleep. The measurement of wakefulness also has potential value in

an attempt to measure daytime alertness in a situation in which it may be difficult to maintain an alert state, however.

The recommendations for the MWT protocol are described in detail in the January 2005 practice parameters published by the American Academy of Sleep Medicine and are summarized in a later section.[1] Similar to the MSLT, the patient should avoid using caffeine, tobacco, and other stimulating medications before undergoing the MWT. Drug screening is often performed on the morning of the MWT to ensure the test results are not influenced by medications or other substance. This screening is particularly important for the MWT, because the patient may be tempted to pharmacologically improve test results in scenarios in which ability to return to work is being assessed.

It is usually recommended that the patient obtain a polysomnogram the night before having a MWT, which consists of four 20- to 40-minute sessions conducted at 2-hour intervals. The recording montage for a MWT is similar to that of a MSLT and consists of a referential EEG from central and occipital locations, two electro-oculograms (left and right) at the outer canthi, a mental or submental electromyogram, and an electrocardiogram. Before each attempt, the patient sits on a bed at room temperature and is told to "remain awake as long as possible." The patient should not use any stimulating measures, such as slapping the face or singing.[8] Bright light also can be stimulating, so it is recommended that a 0.10- to 1.13-lux light source be placed behind the patient's head, removed from his or her immediate

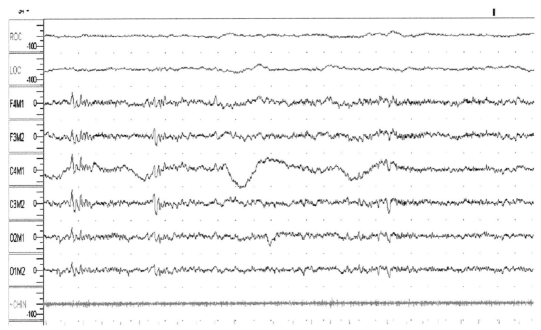

Fig. 2. A predominantly theta, mixed frequency EEG pattern with slow roving eye movements during an epoch of stage 1 sleep in the MSLT. Sleep onset during the MSLT is defined as the first epoch of any stage of sleep, including stage N1.

visual field. The technician subsequently monitors electrographic sleep onset, which is defined as the first epoch of any stage of sleep, including stage N1. The session terminates if three consecutive epochs of stage N1 sleep occur, if one epoch of stage N2, N3, or REM sleep occurs, or if no sleep occurs within 20 to 40 minutes.

Although normal values remain controversial, data were published by Doghramji and colleagues[8] for 20- and 40-minute nap lengths. The lower limit for normal sleep latency (first epoch of sleep scored) was considered two standard deviations below the mean. For a 20-minute MWT, the limit is 10.9 minutes (mean = 18.1 ± 3.6 min); for a 40-minute MWT, the lower limit is 12.9 minutes (mean 32.6 ± 9.9 min). Age and sex did not influence MWT sleep latency.[9] In general, mean sleep latencies less than 8 minutes are considered abnormal.[1] It has been suggested that patients should not be allowed to drive if their MWT sleep latency is less than 15 minutes, although a consensus has not yet been reached regarding MWT sleep latency for operators of any vehicle type.[10]

The MWT is most commonly used when an individual's ability to remain awake becomes a personal or professional safety issue. Patients with sleep disorders such as narcolepsy or obstructive sleep apnea who have been treated may need a MWT to document their ability to remain awake. The Federal Aviation Administration requires pilots with treated obstructive sleep apnea to undergo an MWT to assess alertness.[11] Compared with the MSLT, which measures the ability to fall asleep, the MWT assesses the ability to remain awake, which may be more relevant for daily functioning. The value of either test for predicting safety in real-world situations is unknown.

Case Study: Use of the Maintenance of Wakefulness Test

The patient is a 43-year-old male commercial airline pilot who presents to clinic with a history of snoring and occasional witnessed apneic spells. He describes worsening snoring in the setting of recent weight gain of approximately 20 pounds. He is unaware of any choking or gasping during the night but is aware of rare snort arousals during naps. He denies napping or having any significant daytime sleepiness while driving or flying. He obtains 7.5 hours of sleep per night, waking one time per night with nocturia. On examination, he is 5 ft 11 in tall and 235 lb (BMI of 32.8) with a Mallampati IV airway with an elongated soft palate, mildly enlarged uvula, and surgically removed tonsils. The patient underwent a split night polysomnogram with the finding of moderate obstructive sleep apnea (apnea-hypopnea index of 34 events/hour and a minimal oxygen saturation of 81%). Continuous positive airway pressure at

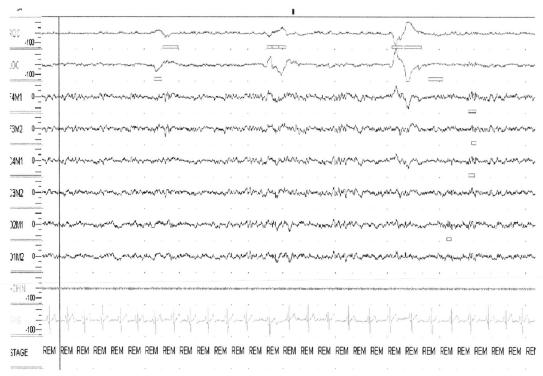

Fig. 3. A mixed frequency EEG (similar to stage N1), rapid eye movements, and muscle atonia during an epoch of REM sleep in the MSLT, indicating a sleep-onset REM period.

9 cm of water was recommended. The patient struggled with use of continuous positive airway pressure therapy initially, but after use of nasal steroids and a change of mask style to a full-face mask, he was able to use positive airway pressure therapy on a nightly basis. After 8 weeks, his continuous positive airway pressure data demonstrated 29/30 days of use with use on 25/30 days greater than 4 hours. To assess his response to therapy, he was scheduled for a repeat overnight sleep study on continuous positive airway pressure followed by a 40-minute MWT. His study did not indicate a need to change the continuous positive airway pressure, and the MWT did not demonstrate any significant sleepiness (MSL = 40 minutes over four naps). The patient was sent back to the company's physician for clearance to return to active flight duty.

POTENTIAL APPLICATIONS OF THE MULTIPLE SLEEP LATENCY TEST AND THE MAINTENANCE OF WAKEFULNESS TEST

Evaluation of daytime sleepiness can occur for several reasons, from attempting to objectively assess a patient complaining of a subjective symptom to attempting to assess fitness for jobs that require alertness. The current primary objective tests, the MSLT and MWT, do not evaluate the same symptom. Although the former tests a proclivity to sleepiness when patients allows themselves to sleep, the latter tests wakefulness in a setting in which they attempt to maintain alertness. Each of these tests should be applied to measure the specific symptom related to the patient's clinical scenario. Use of these tests primarily is indicated for clinical reasons, but research or legal grounds are alternate applications for these evaluations.

The MSLT was initially used to attempt to evaluate patients with narcolepsy and differentiate them from normal, nonsleepy patients. Its applications have broadened, however, as sleep medicine has advanced to dealing with many different patient scenarios. These scenarios may include assessment of narcolepsy or idiopathic hypersomnia, evaluation of patients complaining of a mix of fatigue or sleepiness, and objective assessment of symptomatic improvement of sleepiness after application of a form of treatment. In these cases, the MSLT is used to demonstrate the presence or degree of sleepiness. The test results can be skewed in several ways, most obviously by patients who attempt to avoid allowing themselves fall asleep. Although in some locations toxicology screens are routinely performed, many different

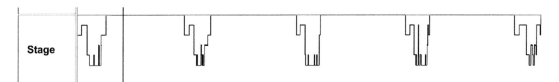

Fig. 4. Hypnogram of a five-nap MSLT. Each nap session demonstrates sleep. The mean sleep latency on this study was just over 5 minutes, and four of the five naps had at least some REM sleep. In the correct clinical context, this study could be consistent with narcolepsy.

pharmacologic interventions can alter test results. The MSLT may not be helpful in the assessment of future task performance, because the test was not designed with that need in mind. The MSLT has been used in tracking patient response to treatment, particularly after intervention of positive airway pressure therapy or alternate treatment of obstructive sleep apnea or use of medication in cases of idiopathic hypersomnia or narcolepsy. The absolute value of the mean sleep latency may be less useful than the patient's clinical description of symptoms, however. One example is the application of stimulant medications to narcolepsy; although the patient's clinical response in day-to-day life may be significantly improved, the mean sleep latency may be altered by only a few minutes.[12]

The MWT tests the ability to maintain the wake state, which is the converse to the sleepiness tested by the MSLT. This test is performed in low-light situations and tests a patient's ability to maintain the wake state in four 40-minute blocks over the course of the day. The application of this test primarily has been to assess work-related function or general alertness to a task, whether it be driving, piloting, or some function that requires consistent attention for safety. The Federal Aviation Administration has used this test to evaluate pilots for fitness for active duty, particularly after diagnosis and treatment of sleep-disordered breathing.[13] Other considerations for the use of this test could include commercial trucking, driving a bus, or jobs that require alertness for safety. The MWT, however, is a one-time test of an ability to remain awake and may not predict long-term performance. It also requires the cooperation of the patient, who must attempt to maintain alertness; a false-positive test result could occur from patients who allow themselves to doze or who used a medication that might induce sleepiness. The MWT is also difficult to interpret. Although a clearly negative test result with zero sleep is straightforward, even the normative values that are published may not help discriminate exactly how normal or abnormal the MSL is. Although the MWT is one of the most used measures of wakefulness, it may not reflect

adequately what many clinicians would prefer, that is, a replicable measure of task-specific alertness.

ALTERNATIVE TESTS OF SLEEPINESS

Other diagnostic studies to assess sleepiness include the Oxford Sleep Resistance Test (OSLER) test and pupillometry. These tests are uncommonly administered, and further research needs to be performed to assess their role. The OSLER test is a simpler, less laborious version of the MSLT, because sleep onset is measured behaviorally rather than by EEG staging. The patient sits in front of an LED screen and is told to push a button after seeing a light that flashes once every 3 seconds. If seven consecutive flashes (21 seconds) occur without a pushing of the button from the patient, then sleep onset is assumed.[14] Pupillometry was first used by the Mayo Clinic group in the 1960s. It involves measuring the pupil of the eye, because pupil stability and size are inversely proportional to the degree of an individual's sleepiness. One study showed that as SSS scores increased, pupillary fluctuations increased and pupil size decreased.[15] To administer this test, an individual is placed in a dark room for 15 minutes. Someone who is alert generally maintains a stable pupil size, whereas someone who is sleepy may have an increased number of pupillary fluctuations. This technique requires specialized equipment and has not been used widely.

MOVING FORWARD

Current assessments of sleepiness may not adequately fulfill the need for "real world" evaluations of daytime sleepiness. Unlike assessment of alcohol intoxication, which currently can be performed before starting a car, immediate estimation of sleepiness before driving or while operating a motor vehicle is not currently available for general use. Although the MSLT and MWT are laboratory-based assessments of sleepiness and wakefulness, respectively, the matter facing sleep specialists in the future will be how to better assess patient levels of sleepiness, particularly in settings that could cause danger to themselves and others. Some clinicians have suggested use of driving or flight simulators to more closely replicate the conditions in which sleepiness could occur. Critics suggest, however, that even these simulators may not simulate real life well enough, particularly when taking into account variability of sleep amounts on a daily basis. Future assessments of daytime sleepiness may be in vehicles or on the job, with remote or computerized assessment of ongoing sleepiness. This task may be done via monitoring of eyelid movement, pupil size, and motor activity or behavior. Further research is needed to elevate the evaluation of sleepiness from research models to a more practical level.

SUMMARY

EDS is a ubiquitous symptom seen by clinicians everywhere. With sharp clinical acumen and appropriately used diagnostic tools, physicians can diagnose and treat patients effectively. However, continued research and new tests may be needed to better address the concerns of task-specific sleepiness in the workplace and on the roads. Perhaps, in the future, even an alarm will become a pleasant sound!

REFERENCES

1. Littner MR, Kushida C, Wise M, et al. Practice parameters for clinical use of the multiple sleep latency test and the maintenance of wakefulness test. Sleep 2005;28(1):113–21.
2. Johns MW. Reliability and factor analysis of the Epworth Sleepiness Scale. Sleep 1992;15(4):376–81.
3. Weaver TE, Laizner AM, Evans LK, et al. An instrument to measure functional status outcomes for disorders of excessive sleepiness. Sleep 1997; 20(10):835–43.
4. Carskadon MA, Dement WC, Mitler MM, et al. Guidelines for the multiple sleep latency test (MSLT): a standard measure of sleepiness. Sleep 1986;9: 519–24.
5. Silber MH, Ancoli-Israel S, Bonnet MH, et al. The visual scoring of sleep in adults. J Clin Sleep Med 2007;3(2):121–31.
6. Thorpy M, Westbrook P, Ferber R, et al. The clinical use of the multiple sleep latency test. Sleep 1992;15: 268–76.
7. Chervin RD, Aldrich MS. Sleep onset REM periods during multiple sleep latency tests in patients evaluated for sleep apnea. Am J Respir Crit Care Med 2000;161(2 Pt 1):426–31.
8. Doghramji K, Mitler MM, Sangal RB, et al. A normative study of the maintenance of wakefulness test. Electroencephalogr Clin Neurophysiol 1997;103: 554–62.
9. Mitler MM, Doghramji K, Shapiro C. The maintenance of wakefulness test: normative data by age. J Psychosom Res 2000;49:363–5.
10. Poceta JS, Timms RM, Jeong DU, et al. Maintenance of wakefulness test in obstructive sleep apnea syndrome. Chest 1992;101:893–7.
11. Office of Aerospace Medicine. Guide for aviation medical examiners. Available at: http://www.faa. gov. Accessed Febrauary 1, 2009.
12. Wise MS, Arand DL, Auger RR, et al. Treatment of narcolepsy and other hypersomnias of central origin. Sleep 2007;30(12):1712–27.
13. Available at: http://www.faa.gov/about/office_org/ headquarters_offices/avs/offices/aam/ame/guide/ special_iss/all_classes/sleep_apnea. Accessed February 1, 2009.
14. Bennett LS, Stradling JR, Davies RJO. A behavioural test to assess daytime sleepiness in obstructive sleep apnea. J Sleep Res 1997;6:142–5.
15. Wilhelm B, Wilhelm H, Ludtke H, et al. Pupillometric assessment of sleepiness in sleep-deprived healthy subjects. Sleep 1998;21:258–65.

Pediatric Polysomnography

Suzanne E. Beck, MD, Carole L. Marcus, MBBCh*

KEYWORDS

- Obstructive sleep apnea • Scoring • Child
- Sleep-disordered breathing • Pediatric sleep laboratory

Pediatric polysomnography is the diagnostic study of choice to evaluate for obstructive sleep apnea in children, and to evaluate cardiorespiratory function in infants and children with chronic lung disease or neuromuscular disease when indicated.

INDICATIONS FOR PEDIATRIC POLYSOMNOGRAPHY
Obstructive Sleep Apnea Syndrome

Obstructive sleep apnea syndrome (OSAS) is the most common indication for polysomnography. OSAS is common in the pediatric age group, occurring in approximately 2% of young children.[1] The American Academy of Pediatrics recommends that all children be screened by history for snoring,[2] recognizing that OSAS is common and is frequently underdiagnosed. Whether or not primary snoring per se results in morbidity is controversial, and is beyond the scope of this article. It has been well established, however, that clinical history alone cannot distinguish primary snoring from OSAS in children.[2,3] Both the American Thoracic Society[4] and the American Academy of Pediatrics[2] recommend polysomnography as the diagnostic test of choice for children with suspected OSAS.

In most cases of pediatric OSAS, children present with signs or symptoms of obstructive breathing patterns during sleep, including snoring; labored breathing; witnessed apnea; gasping; mouth-breathing; or sleeping in unusual positions (eg, with the neck hyperextended). Failure to thrive or signs of right-sided heart failure may be present in severe cases. Associated daytime symptoms can be difficult to elicit. Unlike adults in whom excessive daytime sleepiness is often the presenting complaint, younger children tend to manifest daytime sleepiness as hyperactivity or inability to concentrate, leading to poor school performance or behavioral issues. Most children with obstructive sleep apnea have a normal physical examination. Physical findings, however, of retrognathia, oropharyngeal crowding, high arched palate, adenotonsillar hypertrophy, mouth breathing, or stertor at rest suggest the need for further evaluation for OSAS. Prematurity, hypotonia (eg, children with cerebral palsy or muscular dystrophy, Down syndrome), or craniofacial anomalies are risk factors for OSAS. Polysomnography is indicated in any child who snores and has labored breathing during sleep, and who has any predisposing physical examination findings or daytime symptoms. Polysomnography is the gold standard for the diagnosis of OSAS. Other diagnostic studies, such as nocturnal oximetry,[5] videotaping,[6] and nap studies,[7] may be helpful if positive, but underestimate the presence of OSAS,[2,3] in part because they may not capture rapid eye movement (REM) sleep, during which most obstructive events occur (**Fig. 1**).[8] Finally, direct observation of a sleeping child who is obstructing may be diagnostic of OSAS, but does not quantitate the severity of OSAS and cannot predict perioperative risk or the likelihood of persistent abnormalities postoperatively.

Central Apnea, Periodic Breathing, and Central Hypoventilation Syndromes

Pediatric polysomnography is indicated to evaluate infants and children with suspected

This research was supported by the National Institutes of Health grant R01 HL58585.

Sleep Center, Division of Pulmonary Medicine, Department of Pediatrics, The Children's Hospital of Philadelphia, University of Pennsylvania School of Medicine, Fifth Floor, Wood Center, 34th Street and Civic Center Boulevard, Philadelphia, PA 19104, USA

* Corresponding author.

E-mail address: marcus@email.chop.edu (C.L. Marcus).

Sleep Med Clin 4 (2009) 393–406

doi:10.1016/j.jsmc.2009.04.007

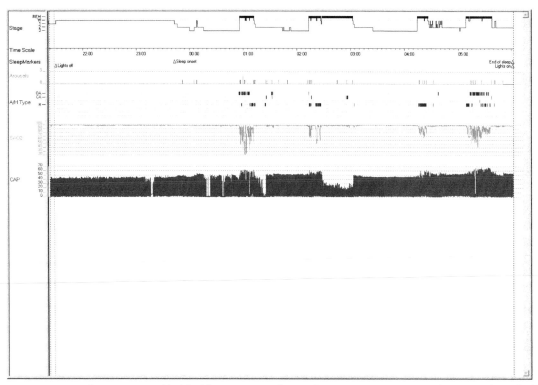

Fig.1. Hypnogram from a 4-year-old girl with OSAS. Note that pediatric OSAS occurs primarily in REM sleep (*bold bars*), with sleep architecture preserved. *Abbreviations:* A/H type, apnea/hypopnea type; CA, central apnea; CAP, capnography (mm Hg); H, hypopnea; MA, mixed apnea; OA, obstructive apnea; Sao$_2$, oxygen saturation (%). Stage: W, wake; 1, stage N1; 2, stage N2; 3, stage N3.

pathologic central apnea, periodic breathing, or central hypoventilation. These children may present with cyanosis, observed apnea during sleep, daytime symptoms, apparent life-threatening events, postanesthetic respiratory depression, or cor pulmonale. It is crucial to monitor end-tidal Pco$_2$ levels to evaluate for hypoventilation, which if not detected and treated promptly may lead to poor developmental outcomes.

Neuromuscular Disorders

Polysomnography is useful to evaluate underlying cardiorespiratory function in children with neuromuscular disorders. The timing of the study in the patient's clinical course is variable and is determined by their physician's interpretation of signs and symptoms.[9] In addition to evaluation of complaints of difficulty breathing during sleep, a polysomnogram is indicated to detect sleep-disordered breathing if there has been a change in growth velocity; developmental progress; daytime symptoms (eg, sleepiness, headache); pulmonary function;[10] development of daytime hypercapnia;[11] polycythemia; or heart failure.

Children with respiratory muscle weakness may not show signs of labored breathing during sleep and may not manifest airway obstruction by snoring. CO$_2$ monitoring is crucial during polysomnography in these patients to evaluate for sleep hypoventilation.

Chronic Lung Disease

Polysomnography can be used to evaluate for nocturnal hypoventilation and hypoxemia in infants and children with chronic lung disease, and to titrate supplemental oxygen. Children with chronic lung disease may have normal arterial oxygen saturation values during wakefulness, but desaturate during sleep.[12] In infants with bronchopulmonary dysplasia, maintaining arterial oxygen saturation levels greater than or equal to 93% during sleep results in improved growth.[13] Unattended overnight pulse oximetry monitoring can be used to assess oxygenation, but may be limited by motion artifact, and oxygen cannot be titrated during these studies; however, home oximetry studies have been proved to underestimate the degree of desaturation.[14]

Continuous Positive Airway Pressure Ventilator Titration Studies

Pediatric polysomnography is used to titrate continuous positive airway pressure (CPAP) and bilevel pressures, and home ventilators, in children. One of the main differences in pediatric CPAP titration studies compared with adults is that split night studies (diagnostic studies converted to titrations after demonstration of clinically significant OSAS) are not commonly performed, for several reasons. Often, the children referred to the sleep laboratory have complex medical issues, and the decision to initiate CPAP is multifaceted and is best done in an office setting. In addition, because adenotonsillectomy is the first line of treatment for childhood OSAS, CPAP is often not necessary. Most importantly, placing CPAP on a child for the first time in the middle of the night can be frightening and disturbing for the child. This can result in behavioral issues that unfavorably influence future CPAP adherence. A behavioral program with desensitization is preferable. For ventilator titration studies, the presence of a respiratory therapist during the study is advisable.

Tracheostomy Decannulation

Polysomnography is a useful tool to assess functional airway obstruction in children who are thought to be ready for tracheostomy decannulation. In pediatrics, tracheostomies are often placed temporarily (eg, in a neonate requiring prolonged ventilatory support, or while awaiting adequate airway growth for an infant to tolerate airway reconstruction). Children may breathe adequately when the tracheostomy tube is capped during wakefulness, but develop upper airway obstruction caused by hypotonia during sleep.[15] During these polysomnograms, the patient is monitored initially with the tracheostomy uncapped. The tracheostomy tube is then capped and airflow and end-tidal Pco_2 are monitored by the nose and mouth. It is necessary that oxygen, if required for chronic lung disease, be weaned to low flow so that it can be delivered through a nasal cannula. During the study, careful attention is paid to work of breathing and the presence of obstructive apneas or hypopneas. The laboratory staff must be trained in tracheostomy care, and should uncap the tracheostomy tube immediately if adverse events are noted. If there is concern that the child may not tolerate the procedure, the study can be done as a bedside study in the ICU. Tracheostomy tube capping studies should only be done in patients who have tolerated capping of the tracheostomy during wakefulness. Ideally, the tracheostomy tube should be downsized before the study.

Parasomnias

A common complaint evaluated in a pediatric sleep center is frequent night awakenings. In most cases, polysomnography is not indicated to evaluate this complaint. Rather, a good history helps determine if these night awakenings are caused by sleep terrors or confusional arousals versus behavioral insomnia of childhood or some other cause. There are uncommon cases where polysomnography is useful in determining whether there is a pathologic cause precipitating the night waking, however, such as gastroesophageal reflux or OSAS. In some unusual cases, polysomnography can be helpful in differentiating parasomnias from seizures; hysterical conversion reactions; or malingering (eg, for school avoidance). In these cases, videotaping and good documentation by the sleep technologist are essential. Examining the electroencephalogram (EEG) for epileptiform activity during unusual movements during sleep is useful in differentiating true seizure activity from other motor activity during sleep.

Restless Legs Syndrome and Periodic Limb Movement Disorder

It is the authors' practice to place limb leads on every infant and child having a polysomnogram. Polysomnography is useful to evaluate for periodic limb movement disorder in young children with symptoms suggestive of restless legs syndrome in whom a definitive history can be hard to elicit; however, it is not indicated in straightforward cases.

Excessive Daytime Sleepiness

In most cases of excessive daytime sleepiness, history, sleep diaries, or actigraphy reveal the cause (eg, insufficient sleep or poor sleep hygiene) and polysomnography is unnecessary. Polysomnography is indicated in the evaluation of excessive daytime sleepiness, however, if the history elicits suspicion of a pathologic cause, such as OSAS, narcolepsy, periodic limb movement disorder, or nocturnal seizures. If narcolepsy is suspected, a multiple sleep latency test is indicated. Normal, school-aged children are physiologically unlikely to fall asleep during the day, and age-appropriate normative data must be used to interpret the multiple sleep latency test. The tendency to fall asleep during the day increases with increasing pubertal Tanner stage.[16] Some investigators have recommended using multiple sleep latency tests with naps longer than

20 minutes when young children are studied for research purposes. The clinical use of this longer multiple sleep latency test protocol for the diagnosis of narcolepsy in children is unknown. Infants usually enter sleep by REM, but in older children, REM-onset naps are suggestive of narcolepsy. In children younger than 5 years of age, in who napping is commonplace, multiple sleep latency tests are hard to perform and normative data are unavailable.

Ambulatory and Unattended Polysomnography

There are no randomized, controlled trials and limited information on pediatric unattended home polysomnography. Jacob and colleagues[17] used a specialized, noncommercial polysomnography system in a carefully selected population in the home, and compared this with in-laboratory recordings. They reported adequate data, with a close correlation between home and laboratory values. In contrast, Poels and colleagues[18] studied children aged 2 to 7 years of age, using a commercial system, and found that only 29% of recordings were successful. Goodwin and colleagues[19] reported the feasibility of performing home unattended studies in selected patients as part of a research protocol that involved sending a team to the home to hookup the patient; the initial failure rate was 9%. Clearly, further studies are needed.

CREATING A CHILD-FRIENDLY LABORATORY

Polysomnography can be challenging in pediatrics because children have a limited ability to cooperate with the setup, and may have trouble sleeping in a strange environment. There are many things a sleep laboratory can do to ease the burden on the child, the family, and the technologists, and to improve the diagnostic quality of the polysomnogram (**Fig. 2**).

The authors' approach is to have a mindset of family-centered care, with the parent remaining with the child at all times and the least amount of trauma created for the child. The goal of the laboratory should be to put the needs of the child first and the needs of the laboratory and technicians second. The environment in the waiting room and in the "bedroom" should be child-friendly. In a combined adult-pediatric laboratory, consider a separate waiting area for children, because they may be intimidated by seeing older or ill-appearing adults just before bedtime. A parent should stay with the child, and there should be comfortable accommodations for the parent including a bed in the same room, and shower facilities. The patient bed should be age- and

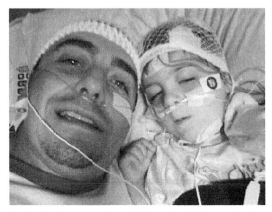

Fig. 2. Photograph of a child and his father just after hook up. Note that the father has engaged in playfully placing a nasal cannula and head wrap on himself as a distraction technique during the hook up. The father took this image with his cell phone at the start of the polysomnogram.

developmentally appropriate (eg, a crib for infants and toddlers, and side rails for the young or for children with special needs). The type of bed required should be known ahead of time so that the room is ready when the patient arrives.

Psychologic preparation should be offered to the child and parent before the sleep study. This often starts with the clinician who orders the study explaining the procedure and reason for the study in detail. The preparation is reinforced during the scheduling process, where parents are reminded of the procedure and allowed to ask questions. A visit to the sleep laboratory for a tour before the sleep study can be very helpful in easing anxiety associated with the study.

Staffing and laboratory hours might need to be extended for pediatric polysomnograms because children go to bed earlier than adults and need more sleep (eg, an 8 year old typically needs 10 hours for sleep a night). Ideally, there should be a 1:1 technologist/patient ratio during the patient hookup. Some laboratories have used swing shifts during the evening to accomplish this. The child should be allowed to sit on the parent's lap and should not be forced to lie down for the hookup. The technician should partner with the parent and the child during the setup and engage the child as much as possible, assigning roles, giving choices, and encouraging age- and developmentally appropriate coping strategies. Each step of the hookup should be explained in a child-friendly manner. Lots of praise and smiles should be given. A few laboratories have child life specialists present during the hookup. The laboratory should be equipped with a "distraction box" full of toys, such as soap bubble kits, stickers, and books to be used during the hookup.[20] Although watching television and other electronic screens before bedtime is not good sleep hygiene, making an exception (carefully explained to the parents as such) for polysomnography and having the child watch a video or play video games during hookup can be a powerful distraction. Instead of the hookup proceeding from head to toe, the technician should place the least invasive sensors on first (eg, leg leads) and save the more noxious ones (EEG, nasal cannula) for later. If necessary, the nasal cannula can be placed after the child falls asleep.

During the night, the technologist/patient ratio should be 1:1 or 1:2, depending on the type of study being performed. Children should be allowed to sleep in their usual position.

The reader is encouraged to consult other sources for a detailed description of making polysomnography more child-friendly.[20]

PEDIATRIC POLYSOMNOGRAPHIC TECHNIQUES

The new American Academy of Sleep Medicine (AASM) scoring manual[21] is the first to delineate pediatric scoring criteria clearly, and the AASM mandates the use of this manual in all accredited sleep laboratories. The physiologic parameters typically measured during pediatric polysomnography are similar to those measured during polysomnography in adults, with a few exceptions. Recommended sampling rates and filter settings for each channel can be found in the AASM manual.[21] The characteristic montage includes:

- EEG: AASM recommends F4-M1, C4-M1, and O2-M1; contralateral leads also are typically applied (F3-M2, C3-M2, and O1-M2)
- Electromyogram: submental and bilateral tibial
- Electro-oculogram (right and left)
- ECG
- Nasal pressure
- Oronasal airflow (thermistry)
- End-tidal P_{CO_2}
- Arterial oxygen saturation (Sp_{O_2}) with pulse waveform
- Chest and abdominal wall motion
- Body position monitor
- Snoring microphone (optional)
- Video

EEG Monitoring

Children have high-amplitude brain waves. EEG recordings may need a sensitivity of 10 to 15 $\mu V/mm$, compared with 5 $\mu V/mm$ in adults. Because infants and young children have smaller heads than adults, chin electromyogram electrodes may need to be placed 1 cm apart rather than 2 cm apart, and electro-oculographic leads may need to be placed 0.5 cm from the outer canthi. Because children frequently displace leads during the night, applying redundant leads (eg, the contralateral EEG leads, or several monitors of airflow) can obviate the need to awaken the child during the night to reattach leads. Extended EEG montages are used if nocturnal seizures are suspected. This procedure, however, extends the setup time. Furthermore, the more leads attached, the more difficulty a child may have falling asleep.

Airflow Monitoring

The use of multiple measures of airflow is highly recommended; signals are often lost because of moisture in the sensors, secretions, displacement of the sensor by the child, or sucking artifact. In particular, it is crucial to include a sensor for oral breathing, because many children with OSAS have an enlarged adenoid and breathe through their mouth. All of the sensors used have both advantages and disadvantages (**Table 1**). The authors' laboratory simultaneously measures oronasal thermistry (primarily to detect mouth-breathing); nasal pressure (primarily as a semi-quantitative assessment of airflow); end-tidal P_{CO_2} (primarily as a measure of hypercapnia); and respiratory inductance plethysmography (primarily to assess respiratory effort). They measure nasal pressure and end-tidal P_{CO_2} using a single nasal cannula with a distal Y-connection to a pressure manometer and a capnometer, and combine this with a very thin, flat thermistor. This system is tolerated by even very young children. For CPAP studies, they use the pneumotachometer within the CPAP circuit as the primary sensor of airflow.

Oximetry

Oximeter signal averaging time should be no more than 3 seconds.[21] Children tend to move frequently during sleep, so the monitoring of the pulse waveform in addition to the saturation value is helpful in distinguishing motion artifact from true desaturation. Most pulse oximeters provide an output for the plethysmographic pulse waveform. This output can also be used for more sophisticated analyses, such as the measurement of pulse transit time.[22] Oximeters with artifact-reduction algorithms can be very useful.[23]

Table 1
Airflow sensors used in pediatric polysomnography

Sensor	Methodology	Advantages	Disadvantages	Recommendation
Thermistor	Detects changes in temperature	Measures oral and nasal flow	Provides a qualitative rather than quantitative assessment of airflow	AASM recommends use for detection of apnea
Nasal pressure	Detects changes in nasal pressure	Provides a semiquantitative assessment of airflow	Poor signal in mouth-breathing patients; frequently obstructed by secretions and so forth	AASM recommends use for detection of hypopnea
End-tidal CO_2	Measures P_{CO_2}	Provides a quantitative assessment of the P_{CO_2}	Poor signal in mouth-breathing patients; frequently obstructed by secretions and so forth; may be oversensitive in detecting airflow	Use as a quantitative measure of P_{CO_2} rather than a primary measure of airflow
Respiratory inductance plethysmography sum signal	Derives tidal volume from changes in inductance of coils	Tolerated well because no sensors on face	Difficult to maintain calibrated; cannot distinguish between obstructive apnea and paradoxing from other causes (eg, in a young child or child with neuromuscular disease)	Useful for assessing respiratory effort in addition to airflow
Pneumotachometer	Measurement of airflow by measuring pressure differences across a known resistance	Quantitative assessment of airflow	Requires a snug-fitting face mask	Use in continuous positive airway pressure studies

Capnometry

Most adult sleep laboratories do not measure carbon dioxide (CO_2). CO_2 measurements are usually obtained in pediatric studies, however, and can be extremely useful in identifying obstructive hypoventilation (see Scoring section later). In addition, the measurement of CO_2 is useful in children with chronic lung disease or those receiving ventilatory support. It is especially important to measure CO_2 when supplemental oxygen is initiated in the sleep laboratory, because some patients may be dependent on their hypoxic drive to breathe. Adding oxygen without monitoring CO_2 may lead to worsening hypoventilation, and clinical deterioration of the patient.[24]

Measurements of CO_2 have been used in two contexts during polysomnography: as an indicator of airflow obstruction, and for quantitative measurement of hypoventilation. As a measure of airflow, end-tidal CO_2 is often oversensitive, and is not recommended other than as an adjunct signal. In pediatric laboratories, end-tidal P_{CO_2} is usually measured as an indicator of hypoventilation rather than obstruction. End-tidal P_{CO_2} can be measured directly from a tracheostomy or endotracheal tube, or as a side-stream measure from a nasal cannula. It is imperative that a good signal, consisting of a plateau during exhalation, be obtained (**Fig. 3**). If not, the measure can severely underestimate the actual P_{CO_2}. Furthermore, software should be used that provides the peak P_{CO_2} rather than random time points during a breath. To maintain a good signal, the technologist needs to be vigilant about clearing secretions and humidity from the line. In children who mouth-breathe, satisfactory signals can sometimes be obtained by placing the cannula over the mouth. It is common to see a single breath with an elevated end-tidal P_{CO_2} value, especially after sighs or body movements, when previously atelectatic alveoli re-expand. The percentage of total sleep time with hypercapnia is more important than the peak end-tidal P_{CO_2} value for the night. End-tidal P_{CO_2} values may be inaccurate in patients with obstructive lung disease with long time constants, such as patients with advanced cystic fibrosis.

An alternative measurement option for evaluating hypoventilation is transcutaneous P_{CO_2}. The transcutaneous electrode warms the skin, thereby

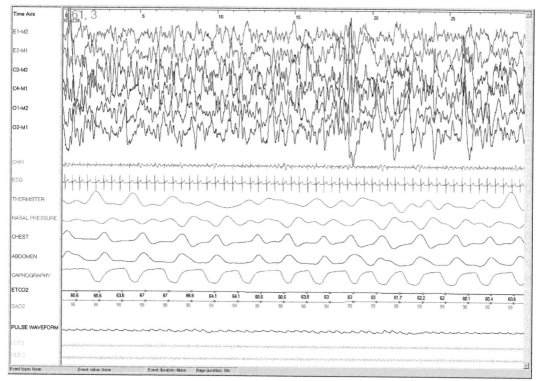

Fig. 3. A 30-second epoch from a polysomnography recording in a 7-month-old girl with meningomyelocele with Arnold-Chiari malformation and central hypoventilation. Note excellent CO_2 waveform and good expiratory plateau. *Abbreviations:* Chin, chin EMG; E1-M2, E2-M1, electro-oculogram; C3-M2, C4-M1, O1-M2, O2-M1, EEG; ETCO2, end tidal P_{CO_2} (mm Hg); Sao_2, arterial oxygen saturation (%).

arterializing the capillary blood flow. The sensor must be moved during the night to prevent skin burns. In contrast to end-tidal measurements, trans-cutaneous measurements can be slow-reacting, and provide a trend rather than a breath-by-breath measurement. Transcutaneous measurements may be preferable, however, to end-tidal measure-ments in children with advanced obstructive lung disease; infants with rapid respiratory rates; children who breathe through their mouth; and children receiving CPAP, in whom the CPAP airflow may interfere with end-tidal measurements.

Many children, particularly those less than 3 years of age, have a pattern of persistent, partial upper airway obstruction associated with hyper-capnia or hypoxemia, rather than cyclic discrete obstructive apneas. This has been termed "obstructive hypoventilation."[4] Most studies comparing end-tidal and transcutaneous P_{CO_2} with arterial samples have been performed in the ICU or during anesthesia, rather than in sleep labo-ratories. In general, these studies show a good correlation between the transcutaneous–end-tidal and arterial values, with a small bias evident in subjects without lung disease. In general, end-tidal values tended to underestimate arterial CO_2, with the largest discrepancies occurring in hypercapnic subjects or in subjects with respiratory disease. Transcutaneous values tended to have a smaller bias compared with arterial values than the end-tidal P_{CO_2} measurements, but tended to overesti-mate the P_{CO_2}.[25]

Respiratory Effort

Chest and abdominal wall motion can be measured in a number of ways. Respiratory induc-tance plethysmography is the preferred method, and is typically used in the uncalibrated mode in children, because calibration procedures need to be repeated after body movements. Other sensors that have been used include piezoelectric belts, which are provided with many commercial poly-somnography systems; intercostal EMG; and esophageal pressure monitoring. In one non-randomized study of normal children, paradoxical breathing was seen much more commonly with piezoelectric belts than with respiratory induc-tance plethysmography.[26] Esophageal pressure monitoring is rarely used because it is invasive, and the nasal pressure flow signal is often used as a surrogate when the upper airway resistance syndrome is suspected.

Body Position

Body position is frequently measured during poly-somnography, although the measurement of body position is less important in young children than in adults, because OSAS is less positional.[27,28]

Esophageal pH

Esophageal pH is occasionally measured to deter-mine whether gastroesophageal reflux is contrib-uting to night wakings, apnea, or desaturation. pH probe insertion is more invasive than the rest of the leads on a polysomnogram and takes specialized skill; placement must be confirmed by radiograph. The percentage of total sleep time with pH less than 4 and the number and length of pH drops less than 4 can be quantified and re-viewed for an association with respiratory disturbances.

Videotaping

Videotaping can be extremely helpful in the assessment of parasomnias, seizures, and unusual respiratory events. In rare cases, such as a very autistic child who refuses many of the monitoring leads, videotaping can be a valuable diagnostic tool. It may also be useful at times by revealing unusual parental interactions. In the authors' experience, videotapes and technolo-gist's observations have revealed cases where a lead radiology vest was used by parents to restrain a neurologically impaired child's nocturnal movements; a cardboard box over the child's head was substituted for an oxygen hood; a teen-ager complaining of daytime fatigue wrapped her entire face and body in a sheet cocoon, resulting in increased inspired and end-tidal P_{CO_2} levels; and an infant admitted with cyanotic spells had a bible placed over his face during sleep (**Fig. 4**).

PEDIATRIC POLYSOMNOGRAPHY SCORING

Pediatric scoring rules are detailed in the AASM manual.[21] This article highlights the differences between adult and pediatric scoring rules.

Sleep Architecture

The EEG changes considerably with age. The new AASM rules, with a few minor modifications, are applicable to pediatric patients older than 2 months postterm. In infants younger than 2 months of age, Anders criteria, which rely heavily on behavioral observations in addition to EEG, should be used.[29] Sleep spindles, K complexes, and slow wave activity are typically first noted at 2 to 3 months, 4 to 6 months, and 4 to 5 months postterm, respec-tively, and thereafter become more prominent. If these distinguishing EEG characteristics cannot be discerned after 2 months of age, sleep should be scored as stage N (non-REM) and R (REM).

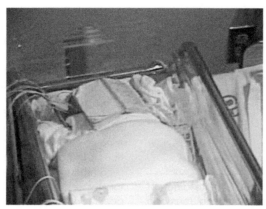

Fig. 4. Still image obtained from an overnight video recording of an 8-week-old infant whose parent placed a bible over the child's face in hopes of it benefiting the child, resulting in rebreathing of CO_2 without arousal.

By 6 months of age, most infant studies can be scored using the adult non-REM stages (ie, stages N1, N2, and N3). The EEG continues to show differences from the adult EEG, however, with higher amplitude and a slower dominant posterior rhythm than the alpha rhythm seen in adults.[30]

It should be recognized that the amount of REM and slow wave sleep changes dramatically during infancy, childhood, and adolescence. In infants, it is normal to enter sleep by REM. The amount of REM sleep as a percentage of total sleep time decreases during infancy and childhood. The

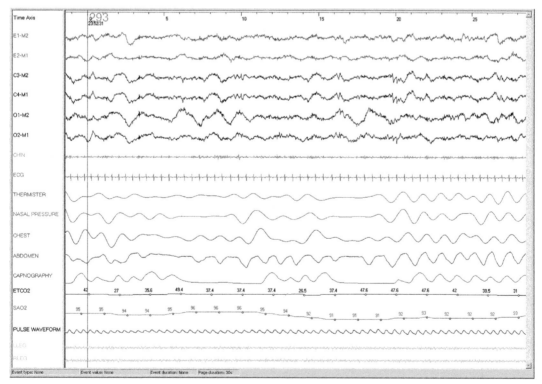

Fig. 5. A 30-second epoch from a polysomnography recording in a 4-month-old infant with OSAS. Note the short duration (4.5–5 seconds) of the obstructive apneas, associated with paradoxical chest and abdominal wall motion and desaturation but no arousal. Ander's sleep staging was used. *Abbreviations:* Chin, chin EMG; E1-M2, E2-M1, electro-oculogram; C3-M2, C4-M1, O1-M2, O2-M1, EEG; ETCO2, end tidal P_{CO_2} (mm Hg); Sao_2, arterial oxygen saturation (%).

amount of slow wave sleep also decreases during childhood, particularly during adolescence.

Arousals

Arousal scoring rules are the same for children as for adults. Children have a higher arousal threshold than adults, so it is common for them to have obstructive events that are not associated with EEG arousals.[31]

Respiratory

Respiratory scoring in children is quite different from that in adults. Pediatric scoring must be used for children less than or equal to 12 years of age. Because there is a paucity of data for adolescents, the use of pediatric scoring criteria for teenagers between 13 and 17 years of age is optional. Small studies that incorporated adolescents indicate that their breathing patterns during sleep are similar to that of younger children, and hence the use of pediatric scoring criteria is appropriate.[32–35] Adult criteria are used for patients greater than or equal to 18 years of age.

In adults, apneas and hypopneas are only scored if they are greater than or equal to 10 seconds duration. Children have a faster respiratory rate than adults, and a lower functional residual capacity. They are more likely to desaturate and suffer physiologic consequences from brief apneas. Because of this, obstructive apneas and hypopneas are scored if they are at least two breaths duration, even if they are less than 10 seconds duration (**Fig. 5**).[21] Hypopneas are defined as a 50% reduction in airflow associated with either arousal or greater than or equal to 3% desaturation.[21] In contrast to adults, the AASM does not recommend any alternative Medicare scoring rules for hypopneas. Obstructive events in children occur primarily during REM sleep.[8] If sufficient REM sleep is not obtained during a polysomnogram, the degree of OSAS is likely to be underestimated.

Some children, especially very young children, have a pattern of persistent partial upper airway obstruction associated with hypercapnia and desaturation, rather than discrete obstructive apneas or hypopneas. This pattern has been termed "obstructive hypoventilation" (**Fig. 6**).[4] Obstructive hypoventilation differs from hypopneas in that a reduction in airflow may not be detected using usual airflow sensors, and events may be very long (many

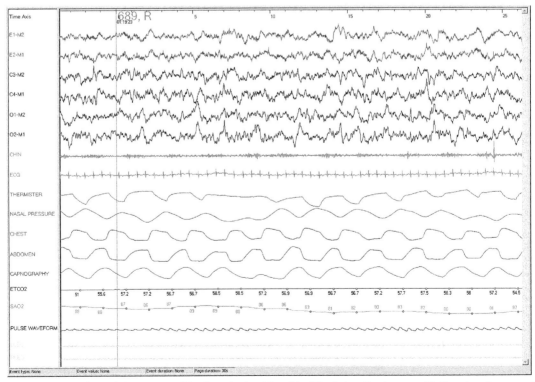

Fig. 6. A 30-second epoch in a 6-year-old otherwise healthy girl with obstructive hypoventilation showing overall preserved nasal airflow with prolonged paradoxical chest and abdominal wall motion, elevated end tidal CO_2, and prolonged desaturation. *Abbreviations:* Chin, chin EMG; E1-M2, E2-M1, electro-oculogram; C3-M2, C4-M1, O1-M2, O2-M1, EEG; ETCO2, end tidal P_{CO_2} (mm Hg); Sao_2, arterial oxygen saturation (%).

minutes). It can be differentiated from hypoventilation secondary to central nervous system abnormalities or pulmonary disease by the presence of snoring and paradoxical respiratory efforts. In addition, although hypoventilation from any cause is usually worse during sleep than wakefulness, in patients with obstructive hypoventilation the discrepancy between sleep and wakefulness is very large.

Respiratory effort–related arousals are not scored in all laboratories. Scoring details can be found in the AASM manual.[21] The prevalence of the upper airway resistance syndrome during childhood is not known, but many practitioners believe that it is rare, and that these children tend to exhibit mild forms of classic sleep-disordered breathing that can be detected using conventional polysomnographic acquisition and scoring techniques, including the monitoring of nasal pressure and end-tidal Pco_2.

Central apneas are common during sleep in children. Children have an active Hering-Breuer reflex (compensatory central respiratory pauses following the stimulation of pulmonary stretch receptors), and frequently have central apneas following sighs and movements, and during REM sleep. Central apneas or periodic breathing at sleep onset is relatively uncommon. Because long central apneas are frequently seen in normal children, central apneas are only scored if they are greater than or equal to 20 seconds duration or shorter, but associated with either arousal or greater than or equal to 3% desaturation.[21]

Periodic breathing occurs relatively frequently in premature infants or children at high altitude, and is occasionally seen in older children with central nervous system abnormalities, or as a brief normal phenomenon at sleep onset. Periodic breathing is defined as greater than three episodes of central apnea lasting greater than 3 seconds each, and separated by less than or equal to 20 seconds of normal breathing.[21] It is different from Cheyne-Stokes breathing in that it typically lacks a waxing and waning pattern (**Fig. 7**).

Central and obstructive apneas have very different pathophysiologic mechanisms and treatments. Hence, the obstructive and central event indices should be presented separately, rather than being combined as a respiratory disturbance index. Mixed apneas and hypopneas are included in the obstructive index.

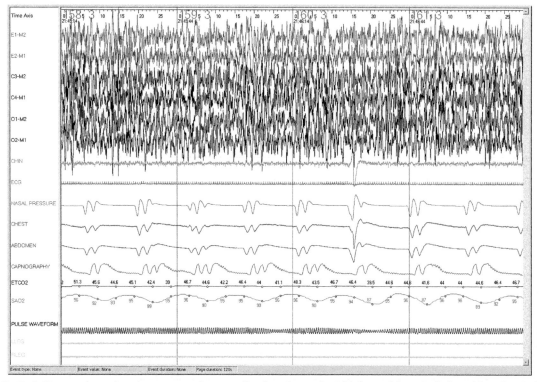

Fig. 7. A 60-second epoch polysomnography recording in a 4-month-old infant with periodic breathing showing pathologic periodic breathing, with characteristic repeated short central apneas and desaturations. Note also high-amplitude delta waves, typically seen in infants. *Abbreviations:* Chin, chin EMG; E1-M2, E2-M1, electro-oculogram; C3-M2, C4-M1, O1-M2, O2-M1, EEG; ETCO2, end tidal Pco_2 (mm Hg); Sao$_2$, arterial oxygen saturation (%).

Table 2
Typical sleep architecture values for normal children aged 1–18 years

Parameter	Usual Value	References
Sleep efficiency (%)	89%, large variability	26,41,42
Sleep latency (min)	23, large variability	26,41,42
REM latency (min)	87–155 (<10 years of age) 136–156 (>10 years of age)	41,42
Arousal index (N/h)	9–16	26,41,42
Stage N1 (% TST)	4–5	26,34,42
Stage N2 (% TST)	44–56	26,34,42
Stage N3 (% TST)	29–32 (<10 years of age) 20 (>10 years of age)	26,34,42
Stage R (% TST)	17–21 (can be higher in young children)	26,34,42

Data are approximated from mean and median values provided in references from large studies of normal children. Sleep stage distributions from Ref.[41] are not provided because data in that study are quoted as percent of total sleep period and not % TST.
   Abbreviation: TST, total sleep time.

REPRODUCIBILITY OF PEDIATRIC POLYSOMNOGRAPHIC RESULTS

Several studies have examined polysomnographic reproducibility. Infants do not display a first night effect.[36] When studied on two consecutive nights, older children have an increased sleep latency and decreased sleep efficiency on the first night, and may also show changes in REM sleep, consistent with a first night effect.[37,38] Differences in respiratory parameters from one night to another are minimal, however, and not clinically significant.[37,38] When polysomnography was repeated over several weeks, or even after a year in children with primary snoring, some very minor changes were noted in the apnea-hypopnea index, but not enough to be clinically important.[39,40] One night of polysomnography is adequate for clinical purposes, although several nights of recording may be needed to evaluate sleep architecture for research purposes.

CLINICAL IMPLICATIONS OF PEDIATRIC POLYSOMNOGRAPHIC SCORING

Tables 2 and **3**[41–43] show suggested normative data for the different polysomnographic variables. It should be emphasized that these are statistical norms rather than clinical criteria on which to base treatment decisions. There are very few studies assessing the polysomnographic predictors of morbidity in children, and these outcome studies need to be performed before clear clinical recommendations can be made. That being said,

Table 3
Recommended normative polysomnographic values for children aged 1–18 years

Parameter	Usual Value	Comments and References
Obstructive AHI (N/h)	≤1.4	26,33,41,43
Central apnea index (N/h)	≤0.4	[26]Only study using AASM criteria
Time with SpO_2 <90% (% TST)	0	41
SpO_2 nadir (%)	≥91	33,34 (Data from Ref.[26] were discrepant, with a value of 86%)
Time with peak Pco_2 ≥50 mm Hg (% TST)	>25	Data are from Ref.[41] Values from Ref.[34] were much lower than Refs.[33,41] are not consistent with the authors' personal experience; Ref.[33] did not use infrared capnometry and is not included.
Periodic limb movement index (N/h)	≤4.3	26,41

Recommended data derived from the mean ± 2 standard deviations based on the highest value from comparable values resulting from large studies. Discordant data are commented on separately. TST, total sleep time.

children do tend to have clinical complications of OSAS with a much lower apnea-hypopnea index than adults, and many centers treat children with an apnea-hypopnea index in the 2 to 5 per hour range. An apnea-hypopnea index of 10 per hour, which is considered mild in adults, is generally considered to be moderately severe in children.[39] A multicenter randomized trial (the Childhood Adenotonsillectomy Study), funded by the National Institutes of Health, is currently underway to evaluate neurocognitive morbidity associated with mild to moderate OSAS in children, and whether surgical intervention influences neurocognitive outcomes. More information should become available over the next few years.

SUMMARY

Pediatric polysomnography is the diagnostic study of choice to evaluate for obstructive sleep apnea in children, and to evaluate cardiorespiratory function in infants and children with chronic lung disease or neuromuscular disease when indicated. It is helpful to investigate atypical cases of parasomnias. It is important to understand that children are not just small adults when being studied in a sleep laboratory; they require a child friendly atmosphere and approach, need smaller and specialized equipment, and because of developmental and physiologic differences from adults, have age-adjusted rules for the scoring and interpretation of polysomnograms.

ACKNOWLEDGMENTS

The authors thank the patients and families in the Sleep Center who have given us the experience to become proficient in pediatric sleep medicine, the technicians in the sleep laboratory who make hooking a child up for a sleep study look fun and easy, and especially to Joe Traylor, RPSGT, for his expertise in preparing the figures for this article.

REFERENCES

1. Redline S, Tishler PV, Schluchter M, et al. Risk factors for sleep-disordered breathing in children: associations with obesity, race, and respiratory problems. Am J Respir Crit Care Med 1999;159: 1527–32.
2. American Academy of Pediatrics. Clinical practice guideline: diagnosis and management of childhood obstructive sleep apnea syndrome. Pediatrics 2002;109(4):704–12.
3. Schechter MS. Technical report: diagnosis and management of childhood obstructive sleep apnea syndrome. Pediatrics 2002;109(4):E69.
4. American Thoracic Society. Standards and indications for cardiopulmonary sleep studies in children. Am J Respir Crit Care Med 1996;153:866–78.
5. Brouillette RT, Morielli A, Leimanis A, et al. Nocturnal pulse oximetry as an abbreviated testing modality for pediatric obstructive sleep apnea. Pediatrics 2000;105(2):405–12.
6. Sivan Y, Kornecki A, Schonfeld T. Screening obstructive sleep apnoea syndrome by home videotape recording in children. Eur Respir J 1996;9(10): 2127–31.
7. Marcus CL, Keens TG, Ward SL. Comparison of nap and overnight polysomnography in children. Pediatr Pulmonol 1992;13(1):16–21.
8. Goh DYT, Galster P, Marcus CL. Sleep architecture and respiratory disturbances in children with obstructive sleep apnea. Am J Respir Crit Care Med 2000;162:682–6.
9. Finder JD, Birnkrant D, Carl J, et al. Respiratory care of the patient with Duchenne muscular dystrophy: ATS consensus statement. Am J Respir Crit Care Med 2004;170(4):456–65.
10. Toussaint M, Steens M, Soudon P. Lung function accurately predicts hypercapnia in patients with Duchenne muscular dystrophy. Chest 2007;131(2):368–75.
11. Hukins CA, Hillman DR. Daytime predictors of sleep hypoventilation in Duchenne muscular dystrophy. Am J Respir Crit Care Med 2000;161(1):166–70.
12. Moyer-Mileur LJ, Nielson DW, Pfeffer KD, et al. Eliminating sleep-associated hypxemia improves growth in infants with bronchopulmonary dysplasia. Pediatrics 1996;98:779–83.
13. Groothuis JR, Rosenberg AA. Home oxygen promotes weight gain in infants with bronchopulmonary dysplasia. Am J Dis Child 1987;141(9): 992–5.
14. Wiltshire N, Kendrick AH, Catterall JR. Home oximetry studies for diagnosis of sleep apnea/hypopnea syndrome: limitation of memory storage capabilities. Chest 2001;120(2):384–9.
15. Tunkel DE, McColley SA, Baroody FM, et al. Polysomnography in the evaluation of readiness for decannulation in children. Arch Otolaryngol Head Neck Surg 1996;122(7):721–4.
16. Carskadon MA, Harvey K, Duke P, et al. Pubertal changes in daytime sleepiness. Sleep 1980;2(4): 453–60.
17. Jacob SV, Morielli A, Mograss MA, et al. Home testing for pediatric obstructive sleep apnea syndrome secondary to adenotonsillar hypertrophy. Pediatr Pulmonol 1995;20(4):241–52.
18. Poels PJ, Schilder AG, van den BS, et al. Evaluation of a new device for home cardiorespiratory recording in children. Arch Otolaryngol Head Neck Surg 2003;129(12):1281–4.
19. Goodwin JL, Enright PL, Kaemingk KL, et al. Feasibility of using unattended polysomnography in

children for research: report of the Tucson Children's Assessment of Sleep Apnea study (TuCASA). Sleep 2001;24(8):937–44.

20. Zaremba EK, Barkey ME, Mesa C, et al. Making polysomnography more child friendly: a family-centered care approach. J Clin Sleep Med 2005; 1(2):189–98.

21. Iber C, editor. The AASM Manual for the Scoring of Sleep and Associated Events: rules, terminology and technical specification. Westchester (IL) American Academy of Sleep Medicine; 2007. p. 1–59.

22. Katz ES, Lutz J, Black C, et al. Pulse transit time as a measure of arousal and respiratory effort in children with sleep-disordered breathing. Pediatr Res 2003;53(4):580–8.

23. Brouillette RT, Lavergne J, Leimanis A, et al. Differences in pulse oximetry technology can affect detection of sleep-disordered breathing in children. Anesth Analg 2002;94(Suppl 1):S47–53.

24. Marcus CL, Carroll JL, Bamford O, et al. Supplemental oxygen during sleep in children with sleep-disordered breathing. Am J Respir Crit Care Med 1995;152(4 Pt 1):1297–301.

25. Redline S, Budhiraja R, Kapur V, et al. The scoring of respiratory events in sleep: reliability and validity. J Clin Sleep Med 2007;3(2):169–200.

26. Traeger N, Schultz B, Pollock AN, et al. Polysomnographic values in children 2-9 years old: additional data and review of the literature. Pediatr Pulmonol 2005;40(1):22–30.

27. Fernandes do Prado LB, Li X, Thompson R, et al. Body position and obstructive sleep apnea in children. Sleep 2002;25(1):66–71.

28. Dayyat E, Maarafeya MM, Capdevila OS, et al. Nocturnal body position in sleeping children with and without obstructive sleep apnea. Pediatr Pulmonol 2007;42(4):374–9.

29. Anders T, Emde R, Parmelee A, editors. A manual of standardized terminology, techniques and criteria for scoring of states of sleep and wakefulness in newborn infants. UCLA Brain Information Service, NINDS Neurological Information Network; 1971. Ref type: serial (book, monograph).

30. Grigg-Damberger M, Gozal D, Marcus CL, et al. The visual scoring of sleep and arousal in infants and children. J Clin Sleep Med 2007;3(2):201–40.

31. McNamara F, Issa FG, Sullivan CE. Arousal pattern following central and obstructive breathing abnormalities in infants and children. J Appl Physiol 1996;81:2651–7.

32. Acebo C, Millman RP, Rosenberg C, et al. Sleep, breathing, and cephalometrics in older children and young adults. Chest 1996;109:664–72.

33. Marcus CL, Omlin KJ, Basinki DJ, et al. Normal polysomnographic values for children and adolescents. Am Rev Respir Dis 1992;146(5 Pt 1):1235–9.

34. Uliel S, Tauman R, Greenfeld M, et al. Normal polysomnographic respiratory values in children and adolescents. Chest 2004;125(3):872–8.

35. Tapia IE, Karamessinis L, Bandla P, et al. Polysomnographic values in children undergoing puberty: pediatric vs. adult respiratory rules in adolescents. Sleep 2008;31(12):1737–44.

36. Rebuffat E, Groswasser J, Kelmanson I, et al. Polygraphic evaluation of night-to-night variability in sleep characteristics and apneas in infants. Sleep 1994;17(4):329–32.

37. Li AM, Wing YK, Cheung A, et al. Is a 2-night polysomnographic study necessary in childhood sleep-related disordered breathing? Chest 2004;126(5):1467–72.

38. Scholle S, Scholle HC, Kemper A, et al. First night effect in children and adolescents undergoing polysomnography for sleep-disordered breathing. Clin Neurophysiol 2003;114(11):2138–45.

39. Katz ES, Greene MG, Carson KA, et al. Night-to-night variability of polysomnography in children with suspected obstructive sleep apnea. J Pediatr 2002;140(5):589–94.

40. Marcus CL, Hamer A, Loughlin GM. Natural history of primary snoring in children. Pediatr Pulmonol 1998;26:6–11.

41. Montgomery-Downs HE, O'Brien LM, Gulliver TE, et al. Polysomnographic characteristics in normal preschool and early school-aged children. Pediatrics 2006;117(3):741–53.

42. Mason TB, Teoh L, Calabro K, et al. Rapid eye movement latency in children and adolescents. Pediatr Neurol 2008;39(3):162–9.

43. Witmans MB, Keens TG, Davidson Ward SL, et al. Obstructive hypopneas in children and adolescents: normal values. Am J Respir Crit Care Med 2003; 168(12):1540.

Polysomnographic Features of Medical and Psychiatric Disorders and Their Treatments

David T. Plante, MD[a], John W. Winkelman, MD, PhD[b,c],*

KEYWORDS
- Polysomnography • Sleep architecture
- Pharmacology • Rapid eye movement
- Slow-wave sleep

It is not surprising that psychiatric, neurologic, and medical illnesses, and their pharmacologic treatments affect the polysomnographic manifestations of sleep. As many of the patients who have sleep studies have multiple medical problems and often are taking many medications, it is crucial that those interpreting sleep studies have an understanding of these effects. In this way, all the potential contributors to the polysomnographic findings can be addressed adequately. This article serves as a primer on changes in polysomnography (PSG) caused by commonly encountered disease states and their pharmacologic treatments.

Because so many illnesses and medications can affect PSG, this article focuses primarily on their effects on the electroencephalogram (EEG), electrooculogram (EOG), and electromyogram (EMG), and their related effects on sleep architecture. Effects on the EEG not typically used in standard diagnostic PSG (eg, spectral analysis) are considered beyond the scope of this article. In addition, this article focuses primarily on disorders affecting the central nervous system (CNS), as sleep is generated in the brain, and the effects of CNS-related illnesses and treatments on PSG have been studied most widely. For organizational purposes, psychotropic medications commonly used to treat specific illnesses are reviewed, along with illness-related polysomnographic findings, with the caveat that drugs from a particular class may be used to treat various illnesses, and that the discussion of medications with certain illnesses does not equate with specific treatment recommendations by the authors. A summary of polysomnographic effects of medications is found in **Table 1**.

Interpretation of effects of a particular drug on PSG often is complicated by the fact that medications most commonly are studied in the disorder they are designed to treat, rather than healthy subjects. This methodological issue will be handled primarily here by presenting data in healthy subjects when available, with supplemental data in patient populations when such information is not available.

In addition to disorders of the CNS, this article also covers the polysomnographic effects of

[a] Department of Medicine, Brigham and Women's Hospital, Harvard Medical School, 75 Francis Street, Boston, MA 02115, USA
[b] Department of Medicine, Divisions of Sleep Medicine and Psychiatry, Brigham & Women's Hospital, Harvard Medical School, Boston, MA 02115, USA
[c] Sleep Health Center®, Affiliated with Brigham & Women's Hospital, 1505 Commonwealth Avenue, Brighton, MA 02459, USA
* Corresponding author. Sleep Health Centers, 1505 Commonwealth Avenue, Brighton, MA 02459.
E-mail address: jwwinkelman@partners.org (J. Winkelman).

Sleep Med Clin 4 (2009) 407–419
doi:10.1016/j.jsmc.2009.04.008
1556-407X/09/$ – see front matter © 2009 Elsevier Inc. All rights reserved.

Table 1
Summary of the drug effects on sleep architecture

Drug	Sleep Onset Latency	Sleep Efficiency	Slow Wave Sleep	Rapid Eye Movement Sleep
Antidepressants				
Selective serotonin reuptake inhibitors	↑	↓	-	↓
Serotonin and norepinephrine reuptake inhibitors	↑	↓	-	↓
Tricyclic antidepressants	↓/↑	↑/↓	-	↓
Monamine oxidase inhibitors	↑	↓	-	↓
Bupropion	↑	-	↑/-	-
Mirtazapine	↓	↑	↑	-
Trazodone	↓	↑	↑	↓/↑
Nefazodone	↓	↑	-	↑
Mood stabilizers				
Lithium	-/↓	↓	↑	↓
Anxiolytics				
Benzodiazepines	↓	↑	↓	↓
Buspirone	-	-	-	↓
Antipsychotics				
Typical Antipsychotics	↓	↑	-	-/↓
Clozapine	↓	↑	↓	-
Risperidone	↓	↑	-	↓
Olanzapine	↓	↑	↑	↓/↑
Quetiapine	↓	↑	-	-/↓
Ziprasidone	↓	↑	↑	↓
Older antiepileptic drugs (AEDs)				
Barbiturates	↓	-	-	↓
Carbamazepine	↑	↑	↑	↓
Phenytoin	↓	-	↓	↓
Valproic acid	-	↑/-	-/↑	-
Newer AEDs				
Gabapentin	-	-	↑	-/↑
Lamotrigine	-	-	↓	-
Levetiracetam	-	-/↑	-/↑	-/↓
Pregablin	↓	↑	↑	↓
Tiagabine	-	↑	↑	↓
Anti-Parkinson				
Levodopa	-	↓	-/↑	↓/↑
Ropinirole	↓	-/↑	-	-
Cognitive enhancers				
Acetylcholinesterase inhibitors	↓	-/↑	-	↑
Cardiovascular				
Beta-blockers	↑	-/↓	-	↑
Angiotensin-converting enzyme inhibitors	-	-	-	-
Clonidine	-/↓	↑	↑/↓	↓
Prazosin	-/↓	↑	-	↑
Statins	-/↑	-	-	-

(continued on next page)

Table 1
(continued)

Drug	Sleep Onset Latency	Sleep Efficiency	Slow Wave Sleep	Rapid Eye Movement Sleep
Gastrointestinal				
H2-antagonists	-	-	-/↑	-
Rheumatologic				
Corticosteroids	-/↑	-/↓	↓/↑	↓
Other				
Acetaminophen	-	-	-	-
Aspirin	-	↓	↓	-
Ibuprofen	-	-/↓	-	-
Opiates	-/↓	↓	↓	↓
H1-antagonists	-/↓	-/↑	↑	↓

- Indicates no effect; ↓ indicates decreases; ↑ indicates increases.
Abbreviation: AED, antiepileptic drugs

several important medical conditions and medications used to treat them. It does not focus on primary sleep disorders (eg, obstructive sleep apnea, restless legs syndrome [RLS], narcolepsy, and insomnia) or their treatments, as their effects on the polysomnogram are documented elsewhere. There likely will be overlap regarding the pharmacologic treatment of sleep disorders, however, as several medications used to treat sleep disorders first were developed for use in other psychiatric, neurologic, and medical illnesses.

PSYCHIATRIC DISORDERS

Patients who suffer from mental illness likely have the most disrupted sleep and greatest proportion of sleep-related complaints outside of the sleep clinic. According to the *Diagnostic and Statistical Manual of Mental Disorders, Fourth Edition (DSM-IV)*, sleep disturbance is often a diagnostic criterion for the diagnosis of a several psychiatric maladies.[1] Because the pathophysiology of most psychiatric disorders remains to be elucidated, many of these disorders have been studied using a multitude of diagnostic modalities, including PSG.

MOOD DISORDERS

The two broadest categories of mood (affective) disorders are major (unipolar) depression and bipolar disorder, the latter a disorder characterized by both depressive and manic states. Depression was one of the first psychiatric illnesses to be investigated thoroughly using PSG, and most depressed patients exhibit polysomnographic abnormalities.[2] In particular, patients who have depression may exhibit alterations in rapid eye movement (REM) sleep, slow-wave sleep (SWS), and sleep continuity.[3] Decreased REM latency is the most commonly reported polysomnographic finding in depression, and a prolonged first REM period, increased REM density (eg, increased number of eye movements per time in REM), and increased amount of REM as a percentage of total sleep time (TST) also can occur.[3] Decreased REM latency in depression is typically less than 60 minutes, but may even be so short as to cause sleep onset REM periods (SOREMPs; REM latency less than 10 minutes).[4,5] Often, extremely short REM latency occurs in severe, psychotic, or geriatric depression.[5] Additionally, depressed individuals may have a decrement in SWS, and the greatest amount of SWS may move to the second sleep cycle, when in healthy individuals, it tends to be greatest during the first cycle.[6] Depressed persons also exhibit increased sleep fragmentation or decreased sleep efficiency with increased sleep onset latency (SOL), increased awakenings and wake after sleep onset (WASO), and early morning awakenings.

Initially, there was hope in the psychiatric community that objective changes in PSG (particularly alterations in REM sleep) were a specific marker for depression. Studies using PSG in several other mental illnesses, however, have demonstrated these findings are not specific to depression and can be seen across the spectrum of psychiatric illness.[2,7] For example, the depressive phase of bipolar disorder exhibits similar polysomnographic findings to unipolar depression in regards to changes in REM and SWS variables compared with healthy controls.[8] In fact, the manic phase of bipolar disorder, characterized by a decreased need for sleep, is marked by decreased REM latency, increased REM density, and sleep continuity disturbances, similar to unipolar depression.[9,10]

There are several antidepressant medications used to treat depressive illness, all of which can affect the polysomnogram. The most commonly prescribed antidepressants are selective serotonin reuptake inhibitors (SSRIs), which notably are considered first-line for several psychiatric illnesses besides unipolar depression. Additionally, serotonin and norepinephrine reuptake inhibitors (SNRIs) (eg, venlafaxine and duloxetine), have similar effects on PSG as SSRIs. SSRIs and SNRIs decrease amount of REM sleep and can increase REM latency significantly in depressed and healthy subjects.[11] These antidepressants also increase periodic limb movements of sleep (PLMS) and can increase EMG activity during REM sleep, occasionally inducing REM sleep behavior disorder (RBD).[12–14] The effects of SSRIs and SNRIs on sleep initiation and maintenance are more variable, but they tend to increase latency to sleep onset, increase WASO, and worsen sleep efficiency, while having minimal effects on SWS in both subjects with depression and healthy volunteers.[11] In addition, SSRIs increase eye movements in non-REM (NREM) sleep that may persist months after drug discontinuation.[15] Although this effect is not documented for SNRIs, it is likely that NREM eye movements may be observed with these agents as well.

Older antidepressants including tricyclic antidepressants (TCAs) and monoamine oxidase inhibitors (MAOIs) also have pronounced polysomnographic effects. Most TCAs are sedating and increase sleep continuity, while prolonging REM latency and decreasing total REM sleep.[11] Some secondary amines (eg, protriptyline and desipramine), however, can be alerting, and be more disruptive to sleep onset and maintenance, with resultant increase in SOL and WASO. Also, unlike most TCAs, trimipramine has not been shown to decrease REM, and in fact, may increase REM sleep.[16] Like SSRIs, TCAs seem to have minimal effect on SWS.[11] MAOIs often cause significant insomnia with disruptions in sleep onset and maintenance, in addition to suppression of REM sleep with little effect on SWS.[17] These agents are used less commonly given their risk of hypertensive crisis with consumption of tyramine, but they still are used to treat refractory cases of depression.

There are other commonly encountered antidepressants that may have unique mechanisms of action and different effects on PSG than those previously mentioned. Bupropion, a norepinephrine and dopamine reuptake inhibitor (NDRI), may increase SWS and decrease stage 2 sleep in depressed people.[18,19] Reported effects on REM sleep in depressed subjects vary between studies. Increased, decreased, and unchanged REM latency, and decreased or unchanged total REM have been reported in depressed subjects.[18–21] These differing effects on REM in depressed subjects may be related to antidepressant response rather than a direct medication effect on PSG.[18,19] Bupropion, unlike SSRIs/SNRIs, does not induce PLMS and in fact may reduce them.[13,21] Mirtazapine, an antidepressant with alpha-2, 5-HT2A, 5-HT2C, 5-HT3, and histamine antagonist properties, when tested in healthy volunteers, increased SWS and sleep efficiency (SE), decreased stage 1 sleep and awakenings, and had no significant effect on REM sleep.[22] It also can produce RBD in patients who have Parkinson's disease.[23] Trazodone, which has alpha-1, 5-HT2A, 5-HT2C, and histamine antagonist properties, and is used commonly as an off-label sedative hypnotic, increases SWS while decreasing stage 1 and 2 sleep. It has inconsistent effects on REM sleep, however.[24,25] Nefazodone, a potent 5-HT2A receptor antagonist, was used more as a hypnotic in the past; however, it is seen less frequently clinically because of the risk of hepatotoxicity. Still, it increases sleep continuity, REM sleep, and REM latency, with minimal effects on SWS.[26–29]

The use and efficacy of antidepressants in bipolar disorder are somewhat controversial; however, mood stabilizers are considered standard treatments for managing the disorder.[30] Lithium is the most extensively studied mood stabilizer; however, given its potential for detrimental effects on numerous organ systems, there are few studies of its effects on PSG in healthy subjects. One small study in healthy volunteers demonstrated lithium decreased sleep efficiency and REM sleep, while increasing SWS and WASO.[31] There are myriad other medications used as mood stabilizers; however, most were developed as antiepileptic medications, and thus they will be discussed later.

ANXIETY DISORDERS

Anxiety disorders are related closely to mood disorders, and they are often comorbid with affective illness. Subjective sleep disturbance is often a component of this group of disorders, and it often is considered a criterion for diagnosis.[1] Generalized anxiety disorder (GAD) is characterized by chronic worry and frequently by sleep disturbance. Unlike affective disorders, GAD typically is not characterized by changes in REM sleep; however, increased SOL and sleep fragmentation and decreased SWS are common polysomnographic findings.[32–34] Panic disorder, characterized by sudden onset of episodes of intense anxiety with associated autonomic symptoms (eg, tachycardia, diaphoresis), often is associated with insomnia, with most studies showing polysomnographic evidence of increased SOL and difficulties with sleep maintenance.[35] Posttraumatic stress disorder (PTSD), characterized by re-experiencing, avoidance, and hypervigilance after a traumatic event, often manifests with impaired sleep and nightmares. Studies using PSG to assess sleep initiation and maintenance in PTSD have been mixed.[36] Several studies, however, have demonstrated increased phasic motor activity during REM, increased REM density, and arousals during REM in PTSD.[37–40]

Other anxiety disorders have not shown alterations consistently on PSG, although they typically have been studied less frequently than the aforementioned disorders. Specific phobias, characterized by fear and avoidance of specific situations or entities, typically are not associated with alteration of the PSG.[41] Similarly, PSG findings in obsessive–compulsive disorder (OCD) have not been consistent, with most studies showing no significant PSG effects of the disorder.[42,43] One small study, however, demonstrated SOREMPs occurring in some patients who had OCD without comorbid depression, although this finding has not been replicated.[44]

Although antidepressants such as SSRIs often are considered first-line agents for many anxiety disorders, benzodiazepines are used commonly as anxiolytics or sedative hypnotics. Their effects on the polysomnogram are well documented, with decreased SOL and increased TST, decreased stage 1 and SWS, and increased stage 2 sleep with a marked increase in sleep spindles.[45] Buspirone, a selective 5HT-1A agonist, unlike traditional benzodiazepines, is less apt to cause daytime sedation, and has no significant effects on most polysomnographic variables except for increasing REM latency and decreasing REM.[46,47]

PSYCHOTIC DISORDERS

The most commonly encountered psychotic disorder is schizophrenia, a mental illness characterized by a marked decline in functioning with positive (eg, hallucinations, delusions) and negative (affective flattening, alogia, avolition) symptoms.[1] The most consistently replicated polysomnographic finding is prolonged SOL in schizophrenic patients.[48] Although alterations in REM and SWS variables have been observed in individual studies,

large meta-analyses have failed to demonstrate consistent PSG effects on these measures.[2,49] This may be because of medication effects, methodological differences between studies, or it may reflect heterogeneity of schizophrenia spectrum disorders.[48]

Antipsychotic (neuroleptic) medications are the most commonly used medications for managing schizophrenia. Typical antipsychotics (eg, haloperidol, chlorpromazine) were the first neuroleptic medications available, and were so named because their potency paralleled their propensity to cause extrapyramidal symptoms (EPS) because of D2 receptor blockade, their primary mechanism of action. Typical antipsychotics produce decreased SOL and increased TST; however, their effects on REM and SWS variables are inconsistent between studies, although they may have a tendency to increase REM latency.[17,50] Atypical antipsychotics are less likely to cause EPS, and, in addition to dopaminergic antagonism, produce 5HT-2 receptor antagonism. Each of the atypical antipsychotics (clozapine, risperidone, olanzapine, quetiapine, ziprasidone, and aripiprazole) has different receptor binding profiles and also has varied polysomnographic findings.[51]

Clozapine was the first atypical antipsychotic, and it still is used commonly in treatment refractory psychosis. The authors, however, know of no PSG studies of clozapine in healthy volunteers, likely because of the potentially fatal adverse effect of agranylocytosis that can occur with this medication. In schizophrenic patients, clozapine decreases SOL and WASO, increases TST and stage 2 sleep, decreases SWS, and has minimal effects on REM sleep.[52,53] In healthy subjects, risperidone decreases WASO and REM sleep, increases stage 2 sleep, and has minimal effect on SWS.[50,54] Interestingly, patients with schizophrenia have shown increases in SWS on risperidone.[55] In a study of olanzapine in healthy subjects at 5 and 10 mg doses, findings included increased TST, SE, and a dramatic elevations in SWS, and decreased WASO.[56] In the authors' experience, patients taking olanzapine can have SWS percentages of over 50%. Effects on REM sleep caused by olanzapine in healthy subjects are inconsistent, with both increased and decreased REM reported in the literature.[50,56] In healthy volunteers, quetiapine in low dose (25 mg) decreased SOL and WASO, increased TST and stage 2 sleep, and had minimal effects on SWS and REM sleep.[57] At doses of 100 mg, however, quetiapine decreased REM sleep and increased the frequency of PLMS.[57] From clinical experience, an increase in PLMS also may occur with other antipsychotics. Ziprasidone increases

TST, SE, stage 2 sleep, REM latency, and SWS, while decreasing arousals and percentage of REM.[58] The authors are not aware of any studies examining the effects of aripiprazole on sleep architecture.

NEUROLOGIC DISORDERS
Seizure Disorders

It long has been known that sleep and epilepsy have a complex inter-relationship. Sleep deprivation may influence seizure frequency, and specific seizures may arise during particular sleep stages. Specific EEG changes seen in epilepsy syndromes during sleep are beyond the scope of this article, but are detailed elsewhere.[59] In general, interictal epileptiform discharges (ie, spikes, sharp waves, spike-wave complexes) are more common in NREM than REM sleep, and in many epilepsy syndromes, seizures occur primarily during NREM sleep.[59]

There are several pharmacologic agents (antiepileptic drugs, AEDs) used in the treatment of seizures, with variable mechanisms of action and effects on the CNS. Similar to polysomnographic studies that assess the role of medication on sleep architecture in other forms of neuropsychiatric illness (eg, psychiatric disease), studies that examine the effects of AEDs on sleep have been conducted predominantly in patients who have epilepsy, particularly studies of older agents with high adverse effect burden.[60] Interpretation of the literature documenting polysomnographic effects of AEDs is particularly complicated, because (1) seizures themselves may affect sleep architecture, (2) patients may be on multiple AEDs when studied, (3) there are often significant methodological differences across studies (eg, dose, duration).[61,62]

Most older AEDs and their effects on the polysomnogram have been studied primarily in patients who have epilepsy. Barbiturates, in healthy volunteers, may decrease SOL and REM sleep, increase stage 2 sleep, and have minimal effects on SWS.[63] In patients who have epilepsy, phenytoin decreases SOL, SWS, and REM sleep, and increases arousals and stage 1 sleep.[64,65] Carbamazepine, when examined in healthy volunteers, has shown variable effects on sleep architecture, with increases in SE, SOL, and SWS, and decreases in arousals and REM sleep reported.[66,67] Interestingly, a recent study showed no significant effects caused by carbamazepine treatment on sleep architecture in patients with epilepsy admitted for long-term monitoring.[65] Valproate, in patients who have epilepsy, increases stage 1 sleep, although it does not affect REM or SWS significantly.[65] Valproate in non-epileptic populations, however, increases SE and SWS, decreases stage 1 sleep and PLMS, with no significant effect on REM sleep.[68]

The effects of newer AEDs on PSG have been studied more frequently than their older counterparts. Gabapentin increases SWS in healthy volunteers, with no significant effects on other polysomnographic variables.[69,70] The authors know of no studies of lamotrigine in healthy volunteers, but when used as an add-on medication in patients who have epilepsy on phenytoin or carbamazepine, lamotrigine increases stage 2 sleep and decreases SWS, with no other significant effects on polysomnographic variables.[71] Pregabalin, when compared with placebo, produces modest reductions in SOL, increases SWS, decreases REM sleep, and decreases awakenings.[72] Reports regarding the effects of levetiracetam on sleep architecture in healthy volunteers have been conflicting, with one study demonstrating increased stage 2 and REM latency, one study demonstrating only an increase in awakenings, and another study demonstrating increased TST, SE, SWS, and WASO.[73–75] Tiagabine in healthy older adults increases SE and SWS.[76] Tiagabine also has been studied in subjects with primary insomnia, demonstrating increased SWS and decreased REM sleep, with minimal effects on SOL, TST, or WASO.[77,78]

There are several AEDs that are used commonly but, to the best of the authors' knowledge, they have not been evaluated systematically for their effects on PSG. These include: topiramate, zonisamide, felbamate, vigabatrin, and oxcarbazepine.

Parkinson's Disease and Related Disorders

The synucleinopathies comprise a set of heterogenous neurodegenerative disorders characterized by progressive decline in motor, cognitive, autonomic, and behavioral functioning, and include Parkinson's disease (PD), dementia with Lewy bodies (DLB), and multiple system atrophy (MSA). Sleep architecture frequently is disturbed in these disorders, with increases in WASO and arousals from sleep, and decreases in SE and SWS.[79–83] The diffuse slow-wave activity observed at times in sleep in PD, however, can produce difficulties distinguishing different NREM stages from each other, making the results of some studies difficult to interpret.[84] Effects on REM sleep are less consistent among studies, although REM sleep may be decreased in unmedicated patients, and increased by treatment with levodopa.[79,80] There are also reports, however, of decreases in REM sleep with levodopa administration in patients who have PD and other neuropsychiatric disorders.[85,86]

In addition, the nocturnal EMG frequently is altered in these patients, with PD patients exhibiting an increased number of PLMS compared with healthy controls.[83] Furthermore, there is a clear connection between synucleinopathies and the development of RBD, characterized by an absence of atonia during REM sleep.[87] In some instances, the finding of REM sleep without atonia may precede the clinical symptoms of PD and related disorders; however, REM sleep without atonia also can be induced by pharmacologic agents such as antidepressants, making this finding nonspecific. In addition, 20% to 50% of patients who have PD have obstructive sleep apnea that often is not correlated clearly with body weight.[88]

Because patients who have PD exhibit an array of sleep disturbances, the effects of pharmacologic treatments for PD on PSG are difficult to interpret, and there are few studies of anti-Parkinsonian drugs in healthy volunteers. Nearly all of the dopaminergic agents used in PD have been associated with diurnal sleep attacks; however, it is not clear if this occurs in healthy subjects.[89] Ropinirole has minimal effects on nocturnal PSG in healthy volunteers, but decreases SOL during naps on the multiple sleep latency test (MSLT), without causing SOREMPs.[90] The dopamine agonists ropinirole and pramipexole also dramatically decrease PLMS and modestly improve sleep architecture in patients who have RLS.[91,92]

Dementias and Other Neurodegenerative Disorders

The most common dementia is Alzheimer's disease (AD), which is characterized by progressive loss of memory and cognitive function, with the pathologic finding of neurofibrillary tangles and amyloid plaques. Sleep disturbance in this population is a significant problem, and may lead to increased caregiver burnout and nursing home placement. Polysomnographic findings in AD include an increased number of awakenings and WASO, with decreased SWS and REM.[93,94] In addition, characteristic features of stage 2 sleep (K-complexes and sleep spindles) often diminish significantly, leading to an increase in stage 1 sleep and a diminution of stage 2 sleep.[95]

The most broadly used class of medications used in the treatment of AD are acetylcholinesterase inhibitors (AChEIs). The AChEI donepezil, when used in healthy volunteers, increased total REM, but did not significantly alter other measures of sleep architecture.[96] Rivastigmine also decreases REM latency and increases the duration of the first REM period in healthy subjects.[97] In patients who have AD, donepezil increases REM and overall sleep efficiency, while shortening SOL.[98] The increases in REM sleep caused by AChEIs appear to be a class effect, although there may be subtle differences in other sleep-related variables, such as increased stage 2 compared with stage 1 sleep with donepezil compared with rivastigmine or galantamine.[99]

Progressive supranuclear palsy (PSP) is a tauopathy that typically presents in the sixth decade of life with supranuclear gaze dysfunction, cognitive dysfunction, and extrapyramidal symptoms. PSG in these patients shows decreased TST, SE, sleep spindles, K complexes, and REM sleep, with increased awakenings and SOL.[100,101] PSP, like PD, also is associated with REM sleep without atonia and RBD.[102] Huntington's disease, a choreiform disorder caused by a trinucleotide repeat in the Huntington gene, which causes progressive motor, cognitive, and psychiatric disturbance, also has been studied using PSG. Patients who have Huntington's chorea demonstrate decreased SWS and SE, with increased SOL, awakenings, and spindle density on PSG.[103,104]

MEDICAL DISORDERS
Cardiovascular Disease

Diseases of the cardiovascular system, particularly congestive heart failure, and their effects on sleep architecture through sleep-disordered (eg, Cheyne-Stokes) breathing are beyond the scope of this article, but can be found in detail elsewhere.[105] There are several commonly encountered medications, however, used to manage cardiovascular disease, whose effects on PSG merit further discussion.

Beta-blockers, as a class, have a tendency to disrupt sleep, with increases in SOL and nighttime awakenings, and can increase REM.[106] The effect on SOL seems in part a function of their lipophilicity and thus, their tendency to cross the blood–brain barrier. Clonidine, a centrally acting alpha-2 agonist that is used as an antihypertensive agent and to manage some psychiatric disorders, has shown variable effects on sleep architecture across several studies.[107–110] Clonidine decreases REM and increases REM latency, with variable effects on SWS, and increases stage 2 sleep and TST. Some of the REM-suppressing effects of clonidine appear to be dose- dependent.[107] The alpha antagonist prazosin increases TST and REM, and decreases REM latency in patients who have PTSD; however, the overall effects in healthy subjects is less clear.[111] Angiotensin-converting enzyme inhibitors (ACE-Is) do not alter the PSG significantly.[112,113] The authors know of no data that systematically evaluate polysomnographic effects of calcium channel blockers on sleep architecture.

Statins are among the most widely prescribed classes of agents in the United States, and are taken commonly by patients undergoing PSG. Statin drugs, however, regardless of their hydrophilicity, seem to have minimal effects on PSG, although they may be subjectively associated with insomnia in some instances.[114,115]

Renal Disease

Patients who have end-stage renal disease (ESRD) undergoing hemodialysis (HD) frequently have multiple sleep disturbances. Polysomnographic findings in patients undergoing HD include decreased TST, SE, and REM sleep, with corresponding increases in SOL, REM latency, and arousals.[116] Also, patients who have ESRD have a significantly higher prevalence of RLS and PLMS than the general population. The PLM index in ESRD-related RLS is often very high (50 to 100/h), and may predict mortality in ESRD.[117,118] These sleep-related motor manifestations are not improved with traditional treatments (eg, HD) but do improve after renal transplantation.[119,120] Furthermore, approximately 60% of patients who have ESRD have sleep apnea, which is improved by transplantation or nightly HD, but not with traditional HD regimens.[121,122]

Gastrointestinal Disorders

Gastroesophageal reflux disease (GERD) is a very common disorder, and can lead to increased arousals during PSG.[123] H2-antagonists used to treat GERD typically do not cross the blood–brain barrier and thus have minimal effects on sleep architecture. The exception is cimetidine, which may increase SWS.[124,125] There are no known effects of proton pump inhibitors (PPIs) directly on the PSG independent of their effects on GERD.

Irritable bowel syndrome (IBS) has been associated with increased stage 1/2 sleep and frequency of arousals, with decreased TST, SE, and SWS; however, effects on REM sleep have been inconsistent across studies.[126] Inflammatory bowel diseases (Crohn's disease or ulcerative colitis) have been studied only minimally using PSG, with minimal significant alterations in sleep architecture found.[127]

Rheumatologic Illness

Rheumatologic diseases frequently are associated with sleep disturbance. Patients who have rheumatoid arthritis (RA) demonstrate variable changes on PSG, including increased SOL, awakenings, WASO, and PLMS, with decreased SE, but relatively unchanged REM and SWS.[128,129] Patients who have systemic lupus erythematosus (SLE) exhibit increased PLMS, stage 1 sleep, and arousals; decreased SWS and SE; and no significant alteration in REM sleep.[130,131] Patients who have Sjögren's syndrome exhibit increased awakenings from sleep and WASO, with subsequent decreases in SE.[132] Patients who have fibromyalgia classically note subjective nonrestorative sleep, and objectively have increased frequency of arousal and stage 1 sleep, with diminished SWS.[133] In addition, the nonspecific sleep EEG finding of alpha-intrusion is found commonly in fibromyalgia patients. This can take the form of phasic alpha sleep (alpha intrusion into SWS) or tonic alpha sleep (alpha intrusion into all stages of NREM sleep).[134]

Although not exclusively used to treat rheumatologic illness, corticosteroids have been shown to decrease REM, with variable effects on SWS and stage 2 sleep.[135,136]

Other Common Medications

Patients undergoing PSG are often on analgesic medication. Nonsteroidal anti-inflammatory drugs (NSAIDS) have somewhat variable effects on PSG. Acetaminophen does not affect PSG variables significantly.[137] Ibuprofen decreases SE in some studies, while having no significant effect on sleep architecture in others.[137,138] Aspirin decreases SE and SWS and increases stage 2 sleep and awakenings, although these findings are not consistent across studies.[137,139]

Opiates are also commonly encountered medications in the sleep laboratory. The effect of opioid medications on sleep architecture depends largely on the duration of treatment. In the acute phase, opiates tend to decrease REM, SWS, TST, and SE, while increasing stage 2 sleep and WASO.[140] With protracted use, sleep architecture tends to normalize.[140] In addition, up to 50% of those who use opiates on a chronic basis develop central sleep apnea, which is in part, dose-dependent.[141]

Other commonly encountered medications include over-the-counter (OTC) antihistamines. Older H1-antagonists (eg, diphenhydramine) are more likely to cross the blood–brain barrier, and thus are more likely to affect sleep architecture (and produce sedation), while newer

H1-antagonists are more hydrophilic and have less effect on sleep. H1-antagonists (primarily examining older agents) increase SWS and stage 2 sleep, while decreasing REM.[125]

SUMMARY

Myriad psychiatric, neurologic, and medical disorders, and their treatments, can affect PSG. A working knowledge of common disorders and medications used to treat them is critically important for those interpreting PSG. Several psychiatric disorders disrupt sleep continuity and affect sleep architecture. Depression classically demonstrates decreased REM latency, and antidepressants typically increase REM latency and suppress REM. Benzodiazepines flatten the PSG, with significant decreases in SWS and increases in stage 2 sleep. Antipsychotics may improve sleep continuity, and in some instances, increase SWS. Antiepileptic medications have differing effects on PSG, reflecting a diversity of mechanisms of action within the CNS. PD and related disorders are associated with several sleep disturbances, including increased PLMS and REM sleep without atonia. Other neurodegenerative disorders demonstrate a breakdown of sleep architecture, often with decreases in REM and SWS. Several medical disorders and nonpsychotropic medications also affect PSG. In particular, renal failure is associated with increased PLMS. Fibromyalgia often is associated with alpha intrusion into the sleep EEG. Pain medications have variable effects on PSG, with chronic opiate use frequently causing central sleep apnea.

REFERENCES

1. American Psychiatric Association. Diagnostic and statistical manual of mental disorders, fourth edition, text revision. Washington: American Psychiatric Association; 2000.
2. Benca RM, Obermeyer WH, Thisted RA, et al. Sleep and psychiatric disorders. A meta-analysis. Arch Gen Psychiatry 1992;49:651–68 [discussion: 669–70].
3. Peterson MJ, Benca RM. Sleep in mood disorders. Sleep Med Clin 2008;3:231–49.
4. Coble PA, Kupfer DJ, Shaw DH. Distribution of REM latency in depression. Biol Psychiatry 1981;16: 453–66.
5. Kupfer DJ, Reynolds CF III, Grochocinski VJ, et al. Aspects of short REM latency in affective states: a revisit. Psychiatry Res 1986;17:49–59.
6. Kupfer DJ, Reynolds CF III, Ulrich RF, et al. Comparison of automated REM and slow-wave sleep analysis in young and middle-aged depressed subjects. Biol Psychiatry 1986;21: 189–200.
7. Kupfer DJ, Foster FG. Interval between onset of sleep and rapid eye movement sleep as an indicator of depression. Lancet 1972;2:684–6.
8. Riemann D, Voderholzer U, Berger M. Sleep and sleep–wake manipulations in bipolar depression. Neuropsychobiology 2002;45(Suppl 1):7–12.
9. Hudson JI, Lipinski JF, Frankenburg FR, et al. Electroencephalographic sleep in mania. Arch Gen Psychiatry 1988;45:267–73.
10. Hudson JI, Lipinski JF, Keck PE Jr, et al. Polysomnographic characteristics of young manic patients. comparison with unipolar depressed patients and normal control subjects. Arch Gen Psychiatry 1992;49:378–83.
11. Gursky JT, Krahn LE. The effects of antidepressants on sleep: a review. Harv Rev Psychiatry 2000;8:298–306.
12. Winkelman JW, James L. Serotonergic antidepressants are associated with REM sleep without atonia. Sleep 2004;27:317–21.
13. Yang C, White DP, Winkelman JW. Antidepressants and periodic leg movements of sleep. Biol Psychiatry 2005;58:510–4.
14. Ebrahim IO, Peacock KW. REM sleep behavior disorder–psychiatric presentations: a case series from the United Kingdom. J Clin Sleep Med 2005; 1:43–7.
15. Schenck CH, Mahowald MW, Kim SW, et al. Prominent eye movements during NREM sleep and REM sleep behavior disorder associated with fluoxetine treatment of depression and obsessive–compulsive disorder. Sleep 1992;15:226–35.
16. Wiegand M, Berger M, Zulley J, et al. The effect of trimipramine on sleep in patients with major depressive disorder. Pharmacopsychiatry 1986; 19:198–9.
17. Yang CK, Winkelman JW. Antidepressant and antipsychotic drugs and sleep. In: Kilduff TS, Armitage R, Marcus CL, editors. SRS basics of sleep guide. 1st edition. Westchester (IL): Sleep Research Society; 2005. p. 167–73.
18. Ott GE, Rao U, Nuccio I, et al. Effect of bupropion-SR on REM sleep: Relationship to antidepressant response. Psychopharmacology (Berl) 2002;165: 29–36.
19. Ott GE, Rao U, Lin KM, et al. Effect of treatment with bupropion on EEG sleep: relationship to antidepressant response. Int J Neuropsychopharmacol 2004;7:275–81.
20. Nofzinger EA, Reynolds CF III, Thase ME, et al. REM sleep enhancement by bupropion in depressed men. Am J Psychiatry 1995;152:274–6.
21. Nofzinger EA, Fasiczka A, Berman S, et al. Bupropion SR reduces periodic limb movements associated with arousals from sleep in depressed

patients with periodic limb movement disorder. J Clin Psychiatry 2000;61:858–62.

22. Aslan S, Isik E, Cosar B. The effects of mirtazapine on sleep: a placebo-controlled, double-blind study in young healthy volunteers. Sleep 2002;25:677–9.

23. Onofrj M, Luciano AL, Thomas A, et al. Mirtazapine induces REM sleep behavior disorder (RBD) in parkinsonism. Neurology 2003;60:113–5.

24. Yamadera H, Nakamura S, Suzuki H, et al. Effects of trazodone hydrochloride and imipramine on polysomnography in healthy subjects. Psychiatry Clin Neurosci 1998;52:439–43.

25. Yamadera H, Suzuki H, Nakamura S, et al. Effects of trazodone on polysomnography, blood concentration and core body temperature in healthy volunteers. Psychiatry Clin Neurosci 1999;53:189–91.

26. Vogal G, Cohen J, Mullis D, et al. Nefazodone and REM sleep: How do antidepressant drugs decrease REM sleep? Sleep 1998;21:70–7.

27. Sharpley AL, Walsh AE, Cowen PJ. Nefazodone— a novel antidepressant—may increase REM sleep. Biol Psychiatry 1992;31:1070–3.

28. Sharpley AL, Williamson DJ, Attenburrow ME, et al. The effects of paroxetine and nefazodone on sleep: a placebo-controlled trial. Psychopharmacology (Berl) 1996;126:50–4.

29. Ware JC, Rose FV, McBrayer RH. The acute effects of nefazodone, trazodone and buspirone on sleep and sleep-related penile tumescence in normal subjects. Sleep 1994;17:544–50.

30. Sachs GS, Nierenberg AA, Calabrese JR, et al. Effectiveness of adjunctive antidepressant treatment for bipolar depression. N Engl J Med 2007; 356:1711–22.

31. Friston KJ, Sharpley AL, Solomon RA, et al. Lithium increases slow wave sleep: possible mediation by brain 5-HT2 receptors? Psychopharmacology (Berl) 1989;98:139–40.

32. Saletu-Zyhlarz G, Saletu B, Anderer P, et al. Nonorganic insomnia in generalized anxiety disorder. Controlled studies on sleep, awakening, and daytime vigilance utilizing polysomnography and EEG mapping. Neuropsychobiology 1997;36: 117–29.

33. Arriaga F, Paiva T. Clinical and EEG sleep changes in primary dysthymia and generalized anxiety: a comparison with normal controls. Neuropsychobiology 1990;24:109–14.

34. Papadimitriou GN, Kerkhofs M, Kempenaers C, et al. EEG sleep studies in patients with generalized anxiety disorder. Psychiatry Res 1988;26:183–90.

35. Mellman TA. Sleep and anxiety disorders. Sleep Med Clin 2008;3:261–8.

36. Lavie P. Sleep disturbances in the wake of traumatic events. N Engl J Med 2001;345:1825–32.

37. Mellman TA, Nolan B, Hebding J, et al. A polysomnographic comparison of veterans with combat-related PTSD, depressed men, and nonill controls. Sleep 1997;20:46–51.

38. Ross RJ, Ball WA, Dinges DF, et al. Motor dysfunction during sleep in posttraumatic stress disorder. Sleep 1994;17:723–32.

39. Ross RJ, Ball WA, Dinges DF, et al. Rapid eye movement sleep disturbance in post-traumatic stress disorder. Biol Psychiatry 1994;35:195–202.

40. Breslau N, Roth T, Burduvali E, et al. Sleep in lifetime posttraumatic stress disorder: a community-based polysomnographic study. Arch Gen Psychiatry 2004;61:508–16.

41. Brown TM, Black B, Uhde TW. The sleep architecture of social phobia. Biol Psychiatry 1994;35: 420–1.

42. Robinson D, Walsleben J, Pollack S, et al. Nocturnal polysomnography in obsessive–compulsive disorder. Psychiatry Res 1998;80:257–63.

43. Hohagen F, Lis S, Krieger S, et al. Sleep EEG of patients with obsessive-compulsive disorder. Eur Arch Psychiatry Clin Neurosci 1994;243:273–8.

44. Kluge M, Schussler P, Dresler M, et al. Sleep onset REM periods in obsessive compulsive disorder. Psychiatry Res 2007;152:29–35.

45. Lancel M. Role of GABAA receptors in the regulation of sleep: initial sleep responses to peripherally administered modulators and agonists. Sleep 1999;22:33–42.

46. Rao U, Lutchmansingh P, Poland RE. Contribution of development to buspirone effects on REM sleep: a preliminary report. Neuropsychopharmacology 2000;22:440–6.

47. Seidel WF, Cohen SA, Bliwise NG, et al. Buspirone: an anxiolytic without sedative effect. Psychopharmacology (Berl) 1985;87:371–3.

48. Benson KL. Sleep in schizophrenia. Sleep Medicine Clinics 2008;3:251–60.

49. Chouinard S, Poulin J, Stip E, et al. Sleep in untreated patients with schizophrenia: a meta-analysis. Schizophr Bull 2004;30:957–67.

50. Gimenez S, Clos S, Romero S, et al. Effects of olanzapine, risperidone and haloperidol on sleep after a single oral morning dose in healthy volunteers. Psychopharmacology (Berl) 2007;190:507–16.

51. Cohrs S. Sleep disturbances in patients with schizophrenia: impact and effect of antipsychotics. CNS Drugs 2008;22:939–62.

52. Wetter TC, Lauer CJ, Gillich G, et al. The electroencephalographic sleep pattern in schizophrenic patients treated with clozapine or classical antipsychotic drugs. J Psychiatr Res 1996;30:411–9.

53. Hinze-Selch D, Mullington J, Orth A, et al. Effects of clozapine on sleep: a longitudinal study. Biol Psychiatry 1997;42:260–6.

54. Sharpley AL, Bhagwagar Z, Hafizi S, et al. Risperidone augmentation decreases rapid eye movement sleep and decreases wake in

treatment-resistant depressed patients. J Clin Psychiatry 2003;64:192–6.

55. Yamashita H, Morinobu S, Yamawaki S, et al. Effect of risperidone on sleep in schizophrenia: a comparison with haloperidol. Psychiatry Res 2002;109:137–42.

56. Sharpley AL, Vassallo CM, Cowen PJ. Olanzapine increases slow-wave sleep: evidence for blockade of central 5-HT(2C) receptors in vivo. Biol Psychiatry 2000;47:468–70.

57. Cohrs S, Rodenbeck A, Guan Z, et al. Sleep-promoting properties of quetiapine in healthy subjects. Psychopharmacology (Berl) 2004;174: 421–9.

58. Cohrs S, Meier A, Neumann AC, et al. Improved sleep continuity and increased slow-wave sleep and REM latency during ziprasidone treatment: a randomized, controlled, crossover trial of 12 healthy male subjects. J Clin Psychiatry 2005;66: 989–96.

59. Malow BA. Sleep and epilepsy. Neurol Clin 2005; 23:1127–47.

60. Sammaritano M, Sherwin A. Effect of anticonvulsants on sleep. Neurology 2000;54:S16–24.

61. Bazil CW. Effects of antiepileptic drugs on sleep structure: are all drugs equal? CNS Drugs 2003; 17:719–28.

62. Foldvary-Schaefer N. Sleep complaints and epilepsy: the role of seizures, antiepileptic drugs, and sleep disorders. J Clin Neurophysiol 2002;19:514–21.

63. Karacan I, Orr W, Roth T, et al. Dose-related effects of phenobarbitone on human sleep–waking patterns. Br J Clin Pharmacol 1981;12:303–13.

64. Roder-Wanner UU, Noachtar S, Wolf P. Response of polygraphic sleep to phenytoin treatment for epilepsy. A longitudinal study of immediate, short- and long-term effects. Acta Neurol Scand 1987; 76:157–67.

65. Legros B, Bazil CW. Effects of antiepileptic drugs on sleep architecture: a pilot study. Sleep Med 2003;4:51–5.

66. Yang JD, Elphick M, Sharpley AL, et al. Effects of carbamazepine on sleep in healthy volunteers. Biol Psychiatry 1989;26:324–8.

67. Gann H, Riemann D, Hohagen F, et al. The influence of carbamazepine on sleep-EEG and the clonidine test in healthy subjects: results of a preliminary study. Biol Psychiatry 1994;35:893–6.

68. Ehrenberg BL, Eisensehr I, Corbett KE, et al. Valproate for sleep consolidation in periodic limb movement disorder. J Clin Psychopharmacol 2000;20:574–8.

69. Rao ML, Clarenbach P, Vahlensieck M, et al. Gabapentin augments whole blood serotonin in healthy young men. J Neural Transm 1988;73:129–34.

70. Foldvary-Schaefer N, De Leon Sanchez I, Karafa M, et al. Gabapentin increases slow-wave sleep in normal adults. Epilepsia 2002;43:1493–7.

71. Foldvary N, Perry M, Lee J, et al. The effects of lamotrigine on sleep in patients with epilepsy. Epilepsia 2001;42:1569–73.

72. Hindmarch I, Dawson J, Stanley N. A double-blind study in healthy volunteers to assess the effects on sleep of pregabalin compared with alprazolam and placebo. Sleep 2005;28:187–93.

73. Bell C, Vanderlinden H, Hiersemenzel R, et al. The effects of levetiracetam on objective and subjective sleep parameters in healthy volunteers and patients with partial epilepsy. J Sleep Res 2002;11:255–63.

74. Bazil CW, Battista J, Basner RC. Effects of levetiracetam on sleep in normal volunteers. Epilepsy Behav 2005;7:539–42.

75. Cicolin A, Magliola U, Giordano A, et al. Effects of levetiracetam on nocturnal sleep and daytime vigilance in healthy volunteers. Epilepsia 2006; 47:82–5.

76. Mathias S, Wetter TC, Steiger A, et al. The GABA uptake inhibitor tiagabine promotes slow-wave sleep in normal elderly subjects. Neurobiol Aging 2001;22:247–53.

77. Walsh JK, Zammit G, Schweitzer PK, et al. Tiagabine enhances slow-wave sleep and sleep maintenance in primary insomnia. Sleep Med 2006;7: 155–61.

78. Roth T, Wright KP Jr, Walsh J. Effect of tiagabine on sleep in elderly subjects with primary insomnia: a randomized, double-blind, placebo-controlled study. Sleep 2006;29:335–41.

79. Kales A, Ansel RD, Markham CH, et al. Sleep in patients with Parkinson's disease and normal subjects prior to and following levodopa administration. Clin Pharmacol Ther 1971;12:397–406.

80. Bergonzi P, Chiurulla C, Gambi D, et al. L-dopa plus dopa-decarboxylase inhibitor. Sleep organization in Parkinson's syndrome before and after treatment. Acta Neurol Belg 1975;75:5–10.

81. Neil JF, Holzer BC, Spiker DG, et al. EEG sleep alterations in olivopontocerebellar degeneration. Neurology 1980;30:660–2.

82. Manni R, Morini R, Martignoni E, et al. Nocturnal sleep in multisystem atrophy with autonomic failure: polygraphic findings in ten patients. J Neurol 1993; 240:249–50.

83. Wetter TC, Collado-Seidel V, Pollmacher T, et al. Sleep and periodic leg movement patterns in drug-free patients with Parkinson's disease and multiple system atrophy. Sleep 2000;23:361–7.

84. Bliwise DL, Willians ML, Irbe D, et al. Inter-rater reliability for identification of REM sleep in parkinson's disease. Sleep 2000;23:671–6.

85. Wyatt RJ, Chase TN, Scott J, et al. Effect of L-dopa on the sleep of man. Nature 1970;228:999–1001.

86. Gillin JC, Post RM, Wyatt RJ, et al. REM inhibitory effect of L-DOPA infusion during human sleep. Electroencephalogr Clin Neurophysiol 1973;35:181–6.

87. Gagnon JF, Postuma RB, Mazza S, et al. Rapid-eye-movement sleep behaviour disorder and neurodegenerative diseases. Lancet Neurol 2006; 5:424–32.

88. Comella CL. Sleep disorders in Parkinson's disease: an overview. Mov Disord 2007;22(Suppl 17):S367–73.

89. Ferreira JJ, Galitzky M, Montastruc JL, et al. Sleep attacks and Parkinson's disease treatment. Lancet 2000;355:1333–4.

90. Ferreira JJ, Galitzky M, Thalamas C, et al. Effect of ropinirole on sleep onset: a randomized, placebo-controlled study in healthy volunteers. Neurology 2002;58:460–2.

91. Saletu M, Anderer P, Saletu-Zyhlarz G, et al. Acute placebo-controlled sleep laboratory studies and clinical follow-up with pramipexole in restless legs syndrome. Eur Arch Psychiatry Clin Neurosci 2002;252:185–94.

92. Allen R, Becker PM, Bogan R, et al. Ropinirole decreases periodic leg movements and improves sleep parameters in patients with restless legs syndrome. Sleep 2004;27:907–14.

93. Prinz PN, Peskind ER, Vitaliano PP, et al. Changes in the sleep and waking EEGs of nondemented and demented elderly subjects. J Am Geriatr Soc 1982;30:86–93.

94. Prinz PN, Vitaliano PP, Vitiello MV, et al. Sleep, EEG and mental function changes in senile dementia of the Alzheimer's type. Neurobiol Aging 1982;3: 361–70.

95. Petit D, Gagnon JF, Fantini ML, et al. Sleep and quantitative EEG in neurodegenerative disorders. J Psychosom Res 2004;56:487–96.

96. Kanbayashi T, Sugiyama T, Aizawa R, et al. Effects of donepezil (aricept) on the rapid eye movement sleep of normal subjects. Psychiatry Clin Neurosci 2002;56:307–8.

97. Schredl M, Weber B, Braus D, et al. The effect of rivastigmine on sleep in elderly healthy subjects. Exp Gerontol 2000;35:243–9.

98. Mizuno S, Kameda A, Inagaki T, et al. Effects of donepezil on Alzheimer's disease: the relationship between cognitive function and rapid eye movement sleep. Psychiatry Clin Neurosci 2004;58:660–5.

99. Cooke JR, Loredo JS, Liu L, et al. Acetylcholinesterase inhibitors and sleep architecture in patients with Alzheimer's disease. Drugs Aging 2006;23: 503–11.

100. Aldrich MS, Foster NL, White RF, et al. Sleep abnormalities in progressive supranuclear palsy. Ann Neurol 1989;25:577–81.

101. Montplaisir J, Petit D, Decary A, et al. Sleep and quantitative EEG in patients with progressive supranuclear palsy. Neurology 1997;49:999–1003.

102. Arnulf I, Merino-Andreu M, Bloch F, et al. REM sleep behavior disorder and REM sleep without atonia in patients with progressive supranuclear palsy. Sleep 2005;28:349–54.

103. Hansotia P, Wall R, Berendes J. Sleep disturbances and severity of Huntington's disease. Neurology 1985;35:1672–4.

104. Wiegand M, Moller AA, Lauer CJ, et al. Nocturnal sleep in Huntington's disease. J Neurol 1991;238: 203–8.

105. Garcia-Touchard A, Somers VK, Olson LJ, et al. Central sleep apnea: implications for congestive heart failure. Chest 2008;133:1495–504.

106. McAinsh J, Cruickshank JM. Beta-blockers and central nervous system side effects. Pharmacol Ther 1990;46:163–97.

107. Miyazaki S, Uchida S, Mukai J, et al. Clonidine effects on all-night human sleep: opposite action of low- and medium-dose clonidine on human NREM-REM sleep proportion. Psychiatry Clin Neurosci 2004;58:138–44.

108. Gentili A, Godschalk MF, Gheorghiu D, et al. Effect of clonidine and yohimbine on sleep in healthy men: a double-blind, randomized, controlled trial. Eur J Clin Pharmacol 1996;50:463–5.

109. Nicholson AN, Pascoe PA. Presynaptic alpha 2-adrenoceptor function and sleep in man: studies with clonidine and idazoxan. Neuropharmacology 1991;30:367–72.

110. Autret A, Minz M, Beillevaire T, et al. Effect of clonidine on sleep patterns in man. Eur J Clin Pharmacol 1977;12:319–22.

111. Taylor FB, Martin P, Thompson C, et al. Prazosin effects on objective sleep measures and clinical symptoms in civilian trauma posttraumatic stress disorder: a placebo-controlled study. Biol Psychiatry 2008;63:629–32.

112. Dietrich B, Herrmann WM. Influence of cilazapril on memory functions and sleep behaviour in comparison with metoprolol and placebo in healthy subjects. Br J Clin Pharmacol 1989;27(Suppl 2): 249S–61S.

113. Peter JH, Gassel W, Mayer J, et al. Effects of cilazapril on hypertension, sleep, and apnea. Am J Med 1989;87:72S–8S.

114. Kostis JB, Rosen RC, Wilson AC. Central nervous system effects of HMG CoA reductase inhibitors: lovastatin and pravastatin on sleep and cognitive performance in patients with hypercholesterolemia. J Clin Pharmacol 1994;34:989–96.

115. Eckernas SA, Roos BE, Kvidal P, et al. The effects of simvastatin and pravastatin on objective and subjective measures of nocturnal sleep: a comparison of two structurally different HMG CoA reductase inhibitors in patients with primary moderate hypercholesterolaemia. Br J Clin Pharmacol 1993; 35:284–9.

116. Parker KP, Bliwise DL, Bailey JL, et al. Polysomnographic measures of nocturnal sleep in patients on

chronic, intermittent daytime haemodialysis vs those with chronic kidney disease. Nephrol Dial Transplant 2005;20:1422–8.

117. Wetter TC, Stiasny K, Kohnen R, et al. Polysomnographic sleep measures in patients with uremic and idiopathic restless legs syndrome. Mov Disord 1998;13:820–4.

118. Benz RL, Pressman MR, Hovick ET, et al. Potential novel predictors of mortality in end-stage renal disease patients with sleep disorders. Am J Kidney Dis 2000;35:1052–60.

119. Perl J, Unruh ML, Chan CT. Sleep disorders in end-stage renal disease: "markers of inadequate dialysis"? Kidney Int 2006;70:1687–93.

120. Beecroft JM, Zaltzman J, Prasad GV, et al. Improvement of periodic limb movements following kidney transplantation. Nephron Clin Pract 2008; 109:c133–9.

121. Kraus MA, Hamburger RJ. Sleep apnea in renal failure. Adv Perit Dial 1997;13:88–92.

122. Hanly PJ, Pierratos A. Improvement of sleep apnea in patients with chronic renal failure who undergo nocturnal hemodialysis. N Engl J Med 2001;344: 102–7.

123. Dickman R, Green C, Fass SS, et al. Relationships between sleep quality and pH monitoring findings in persons with gastroesophageal reflux disease. J Clin Sleep Med 2007;3:505–13.

124. Idzikowski C, Shapiro CM. ABC of sleep disorders. non-psychotropic drugs and sleep. BMJ 1993;306: 1118–21.

125. Qureshi A, Lee-Chiong T Jr. Medications and their effects on sleep. Med Clin North Am 2004;88:751–66x.

126. Rotem AY, Sperber AD, Krugliak P, et al. Polysomnographic and actigraphic evidence of sleep fragmentation in patients with irritable bowel syndrome. Sleep 2003;26:747–52.

127. Keefer L, Stepanski EJ, Ranjbaran Z, et al. An initial report of sleep disturbance in inactive inflammatory bowel disease. J Clin Sleep Med 2006;2:409–16.

128. Hirsch M, Carlander B, Verge M, et al. Objective and subjective sleep disturbances in patients with rheumatoid arthritis. A reappraisal. Arthritis Rheum 1994;37:41–9.

129. Drewes AM, Svendsen L, Taagholt SJ, et al. Sleep in rheumatoid arthritis: a comparison with healthy subjects and studies of sleep/wake interactions. Br J Rheumatol 1998;37:71–81.

130. Valencia-Flores M, Resendiz M, Castano VA, et al. Objective and subjective sleep disturbances in patients with systemic lupus erythematosus. Arthritis Rheum 1999;42:2189–93.

131. Iaboni A, Ibanez D, Gladman DD, et al. Fatigue in systemic lupus erythematosus: contributions of disordered sleep, sleepiness, and depression. J Rheumatol 2006;33:2453–7.

132. Gudbjornsson B, Broman JE, Hetta J, et al. Sleep disturbances in patients with primary Sjogren's syndrome. Br J Rheumatol 1993;32:1072–6.

133. Harding SM. Sleep in fibromyalgia patients: subjective and objective findings. Am J Med Sci 1998;315:367–76.

134. Roizenblatt S, Moldofsky H, Benedito-Silva AA, et al. Alpha sleep characteristics in fibromyalgia. Arthritis Rheum 2001;44:222–30.

135. Born J, Zwick A, Roth G, et al. Differential effects of hydrocortisone, fluocortolone, and aldosterone on nocturnal sleep in humans. Acta Endocrinol (Copenh) 1987;116:129–37.

136. Obermeyer WH, Benca RM. Effects of drugs on sleep. Neurol Clin 1996;14:827–40.

137. Murphy PJ, Badia P, Myers BL, et al. Nonsteroidal anti-inflammatory drugs affect normal sleep patterns in humans. Physiol Behav 1994;55: 1063–6.

138. Gengo F. Effects of ibuprofen on sleep quality as measured using polysomnography and subjective measures in healthy adults. Clin Ther 2006;28: 1820–6.

139. Horne JA, Percival JE, Traynor JR. Aspirin and human sleep. Electroencephalogr Clin Neurophysiol 1980;49:409–13.

140. Wang D, Teichtahl H. Opioids, sleep architecture and sleep-disordered breathing. Sleep Med Rev 2007;11:35–46.

141. Eckert DJ, Jordan AS, Merchia P, et al. Central sleep apnea: pathophysiology and treatment. Chest 2007;131:595–607.

Artifacts and Troubleshooting

Elise Maher, MA, RPSGT[a],*, Lawrence J. Epstein, MD[b,c]

KEYWORDS

- Polysomnography • Artifact • Troubleshooting
- Filters • Electrode

Recordings are made of the physiologic events during sleep to understand the mechanisms of sleep and wakefulness, identify sleep disorders, determine appropriate therapies, and monitor response to treatment. It is essential that the recorded signals accurately represent what is occurring. Correct interpretation depends on producing high-quality, artifact-free recordings. An artifact in a sleep recording is the presence of an undesirable signal, whether physiologic or environmental. By the nature of recording the input from multiple simultaneous sensors over 6 to 8 hours, chances are high of extraneous or undesirable signals arising that could have an impact on the ability to read and interpret the recording. The objectives of this article are to illustrate common artifacts in polysomnographic recordings, to show how to differentiate between physiologic and nonphysiologic artifacts, to describe the known causes of artifacts, to learn to identify the source of artifacts, and to explain how to optimize the postrecording signals.

IDENTIFYING ARTIFACT FROM FACT

Tracing the pathway from the signal source to the recording can be helpful in identifying and understanding some common artifacts. **Fig. 1** depicts the pathway from the patient, where the physiologic signals are generated, to the computer screen, where the signals can be observed. The physiologic signals are detected by sensors and then pass through electrical conducting wires to the junction box, also called a headbox, where they are bundled as separate channels to keep them organized and the patient mobile. The signals are then run through amplifiers, which process the signals for display and may be part of the junction box or separate components. An electric cable connects the junction box to the computer, and the signals are displayed on the computer screen.

Knowing the normal ranges and patterns of each channel is the foundation for detecting most artifacts. For most channels, this means simply knowing the frequencies of the wave patterns being recorded. For example, brain waves during sleep are produced mostly in the theta (4–8 Hz) and delta (0.5–2 Hz) frequencies, with the exception of sporadic brief configurations of known morphology and frequency. Stage N1 theta may be interrupted by faster vertex waves, stage N2 theta by spindles and K-complexes, stage N3 theta by delta waves, and rapid eye movement (REM) theta by sawtooth waves. When anything too fast or too slow (<0.5 Hz and >8 Hz) is seen in the electroencephalogram (EEG) and does not resemble any known pattern, a question should be raised about the true source of the signal. The same goes for respiratory and other sleep-related channels. For instance, a patient simply cannot breathe in sleep as rapidly as what is seen with a cardiogenic pulse.

Another important skill is to scan all other channels for a pattern similar to what is intruding in the channel in question. An undulation in an EEG channel that resembles the respiratory signal might indicate that a wire is lying under the ribcage and is getting tugged with each breath. Careful note taking on the part of the night technologist can help to identify unclear

[a] Sleep Health*Centers,* Medford, 200 Boston Avenue, Medford, MA 02155, USA
[b] Sleep Health*Centers,* 1505 Commonwealth Avenue, Brighton, MA 02135, USA
[c] Division of Sleep Medicine, Brigham and Women's Hospital, Harvard Medical School, 75 Francis Street, Boston, MA 02115, USA
* Corresponding author.
E-mail address: elise_maher@sleephealth.com (E. Maher).

Sleep Med Clin 4 (2009) 421–434
doi:10.1016/j.jsmc.2009.04.010

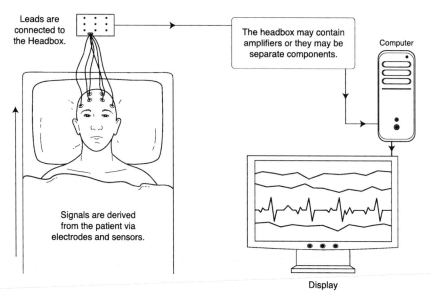

Leads are connected to the Headbox.

The headbox may contain amplifiers or they may be separate components.

Computer

Signals are derived from the patient via electrodes and sensors.

Display

The signal is processed by a computer system and displayed.

Fig. 1. The patient-to-computer circuit.

patterns and should be encouraged with feedback. Videotape playback can also be revealing. Sometimes the best detective work and research simply cannot uncover the unusual circumstances and behaviors causing artifact. Reviewing machine calibration (a test of the amplifier and filters) and bio-calibration (ie, when the patient goes through maneuvers to check proper detection of the signal) can verify the integrity of the recording and give a baseline of normal signals to compare suspected abnormalities against.

The two main categories of artifact in a sleep recording are unwanted environmental input and real physiologic input that obscures data in other channels. Other problems to be identified when reviewing a sleep study are real physiologic abnormalities that appear as artifact, absent data, and false data.

NONPHYSIOLOGIC ARTIFACT

The foundation of a good-quality recording in alternating current (AC) channels is low imped-ance, which is low resistance to the flow of electri-cal current. Low impedance is achieved by using electrodes with low electrical resistance, preparing the skin properly to remove dead skin, and creating secure and conductive contact between the electrode and patient.

Artifact at 60 Hz

Many polysomnographic channels detect electri-cal impulses that are conducted from the patient using an electrode connected to an amplifier. The amplification of this physiologic input makes the circuit susceptible to allowing environmental electricity from the testing suite into the recording. The frequency of electrical outlets in the United States is 60 Hz (50 Hz in Europe). This frequency can intrude and be displayed on the polysomno-gram (PSG) when there is a continuity or grounding problem anywhere in the patient circuit (**Fig. 2**). Causes of 60 Hz artifact include a bad ground (which can affect all AC channels), a broken or disconnected wire, poor electrode contact, external equipment interference (eg, adjustable bed motor, digital video disk player, laptop computer, medical equipment), and high or unbal-anced electrode impedance levels. Differential amplifiers used in referenced electrode channels, such as in an EEG, amplify differences between the exploring electrode and the reference. If either or both electrodes in the pair have a significantly high impedance, electrical noise becomes amplified.

Electromagnetic Interference

The use of cell phones or pagers in the testing suite can cause a pulse-like artifact to run through referential channels on the PSG. This can occur even if the ringer is off and calls are coming in unanswered. The technologist should ask that telephones be turned off before the study starts.

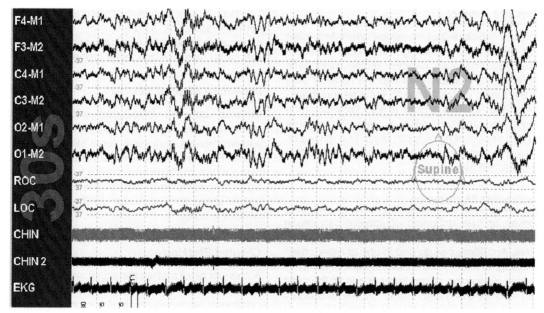

Fig. 2. A 60-Hz artifact is seen in EEG sites referenced to M2 (right mastoid) and also in both chin electromyelogram channels and the electrocardiogram. Impedance levels at these sites were all extremely high (>20 kohms).

Electrode Popping

Electrode popping is caused when conduction is temporarily or continuously interrupted in the patient circuit. In the EEG, electro-oculogram (EOG), and electrocardiogram (ECG), electrode pop displays as a sharp positive or negative deflection, although it often looks like a high-amplitude slow wave but with blocking (usually at the top and bottom of the wave, as seen in **Fig. 3**). Popping is often seen when the patient is moving, causing the electrode to be pulled away from the skin. Popping can occur if the conductive substance is drying, if the electrode is dirty, or when there is a minor break in the wire so that continuity is lost intermittently.

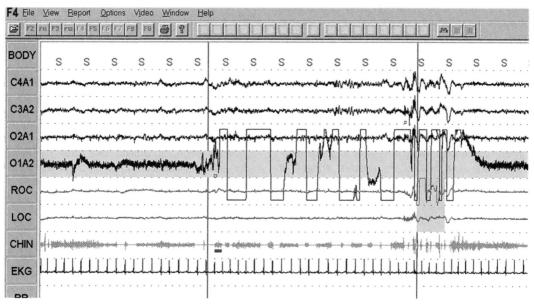

Fig. 3. Electrode popping. Electrode popping artifact is seen in O1. There is also 60-Hz artifact before and after the popping, indicating poor attachment to the patient, a bad electrode, or impedance mismatch in the electrode pair.

Moisture Artifact

Ambient moisture can introduce unwanted noise into the breathing tracing from nasal pressure channels. This can happen during diagnostic recordings if moisture gets into the cannula itself or the tubing connecting it to the pressure transducer (**Fig. 4**). This artifact is also fairly common during continuous positive airway pressure (CPAP) titration if there is too much of a mismatch between room temperature and the humidification of the CPAP circuit.

Equipment Malfunction

Broken or malfunctioning equipment can cause the system to display 60-Hz or other electronic noise. Amplifiers can go bad in one or more channels (**Fig. 5**) and should be tested against a known voltage during the calibration periods at the start and end of the sleep study. To the unstudied eye, electrodes connected to the headbox and amplifier but not to the patient can pick up mixed-frequency electronic noise that looks similar to EEG frequencies.

The integrity of recorded pulse oximetry values (oxygen saturation of arterial blood [Sao_2]) is critical for diagnosis and treatment of nocturnal disorders. The main oximetry artifact that occurs during a PSG is attributable to movement that dislodges the probe. This can cause an obvious dropout of the signal to a blank or zero value (**Fig. 6**). This signals the technologist to go in the room and re-attach the probe. A small slip of the probe can easily go undetected, however, and cause Sao_2 values to read significantly lower than the true signal. The technologist should beware of a sustained drop in saturation after any patient movement or sustained desaturation that occurs in the absence of concurrent position or sleep state change (**Fig. 7**). Falsely low readings can also occur when the patient places the probe under his or her body, or when dark nail polish interferes with the sensor. Low saturations should always be verified with a portable oximeter if it is not clear whether the low reading represents artifact or a true drop in saturation.

False readings can also present as higher than normal values. A saturation of 100% is not common in adults and can indicate an improperly calibrated oximeter or a faulty probe.

Implanted Medical Devices

Artifacts can be introduced into the sleep recording when implanted medical devices, such as pacemakers and vagal nerve stimulators, are active. Pacing spikes can be constant or intermittent and can cause an abnormally fast spike in the ECG and sometimes also in the EEG. A vagal nerve stimulator obscures all head channels when it is firing.

Channel Blocking

A channel blocks when the signal input is larger in amplitude than channel parameters allow. This commonly occurs in respiratory channels (**Fig. 8**). Sensitivity or gain controls can sometimes dampen down the signal so that the full waveform can be viewed. Pressure transducers (a separate piece of equipment from the amplifier) sometimes need to be adjusted during the recording, however. This type of artifact cannot be adjusted from within the system after the test. Likewise, if respiratory effort belts are overtightened, they can cause a blocked signal that cannot be filtered. Conversely, belts that are overly loose may only be minimally improved by changing settings after the test. The technologist needs to stay alert to respiratory signals so that subtle changes, particularly in airflow, can be viewed.

PHYSIOLOGIC ARTIFACTS

A signal recorded primarily in one channel of a PSG can also frequently appear in a physiologically related channel. In the case of sweat artifact, a physiologic response that is unwanted information in any channel type gets recorded. The following sections outline the most commonly seen artifacts that are normal biopotentials picked up in channels in which they do not originate.

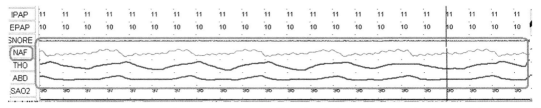

Fig. 4. Moisture artifact. Water in the nasal pressure airflow (NAF) channel causes the fast undulating signal artifact.

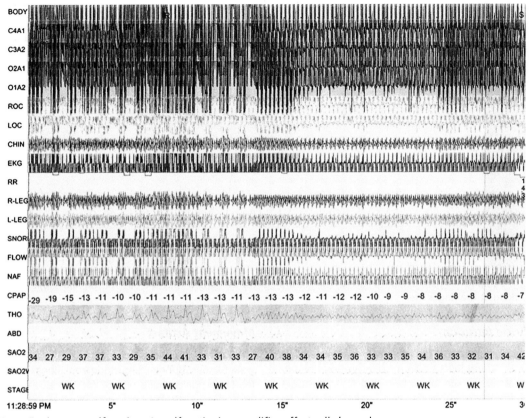

Fig. 5. Equipment malfunction. A malfunctioning amplifier affects all channels.

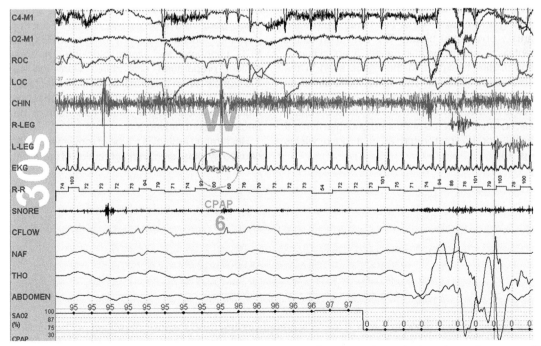

Fig. 6. Equipment malfunction: oximetry. The signal drops out of the Sao$_2$ channel when the probe comes off after patient movement.

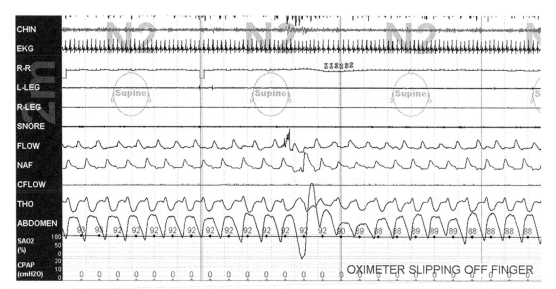

Fig. 7. Equipment malfunction: oximetry. The technologist documented that the Sao_2 probe had slipped after checking at the finger site.

Muscle Intrusion

Fast frequency (10–70 Hz) activity can intrude into the EEG and ECG when muscle groups beneath the electrode site are active (**Fig. 9**). In the EEG, the frontalis, temporalis, and occipitalis muscles are the source of "muscle tension." This generally subsides at sleep onset. Similarly, a fast, low-voltage, shivering artifact can be seen in the ECG when the room is too cool.

A patient who is snoring loudly may also be opening and closing his or her mouth with each partially obstructed breath. The activation of the mentalis muscle in the chin causes a signal fluctuation in direct relation to the signal seen in the snore sensor channel. This is not considered an artifact in the chin electromyogram (EMG) channel. Muscle activity can also intrude into the EEG channels, however, which is undesired because it might obscure or be interpreted as fast brain waves (**Fig. 10**).

Movement Artifact

The sleeping person moves during periods of wakefulness; during sleep stage transitions; during the hyperpneic phase of a respiratory event; and with sleep disturbances, such as periodic limb movements of sleep, parasomnias, seizures, or the arousal at the end of an apnea episode. Artifact caused by patient movement can obscure data in one or more channels. A major body movement can usually be seen in every channel. The artifacts from body movement can include electrode popping, muscle frequency activity in EEG and ECG channels, and signal blocking.[1] If proper patient preparation procedures were followed, the signals return to normal when the patient stops moving. Body position sensors, videotape recordings, and technologist notes can confirm suspected patient movement.

Respiration artifact is a type of movement artifact caused by expansion and contraction of the ribcage

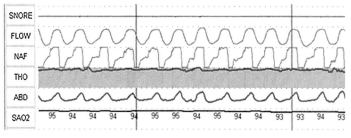

Fig. 8. Signal blocking. Blocking is seen in the nasal pressure airflow (NAF) channel. The output on the transducer needs to be reduced. The gain is set too high on the thorax belt channel, but the signal is still inadequate. The belt needs to be tightened to get a better signal. The gain can then be reduced, allowing the baseline to return to the center of the channel.

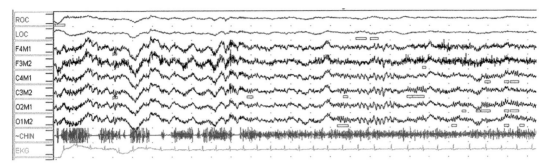

Fig. 9. Muscle tension. After arousal from sleep, muscle tension in the EEG persists most prominently in F4M1.

with respiratory effort. This artifact typically occurs when wires do not have enough slack and are lying close to the patient. The slow undulations in EEG, EOG, and ECG baselines can be differentiated from sweat sway artifact when they fluctuate synchronous with the respiratory channels (**Fig. 11**).

Sleep-related movement disorders can cause artifacts that make sleep staging difficult, including rhythmic movement disorder, bruxism, and REM behavior disorder. In rhythmic movement disorder, the movements have a frequency range of 0.5 to 2 Hz.[2] Bruxism can be phasic or sustained and has a duration range of 0.25 to 2 seconds; when recurrent, it commonly occurs at a 1-Hz frequency (**Fig. 12**).[3] Other medical conditions, such as seizures or Parkinson's disease, may cause movement artifact that can obscure the recording. Again, technologist documentation of patient behaviors and medical history should be reviewed.

Chewing causes a repetitive, fast, high-amplitude muscle artifact in multiple channels, including the EEG, EOG and ECG channels (**Fig. 13**). This resembles the patient response during biocalibrations to "grit your teeth." Respiratory channels may also reflect interruptions in regular breathing. Sucking and swallowing can elicit a glossokinetic artifact that resembles a slow wave because the tongue, like the eyeball, has a positive component and a negative component. As the negative tip of the tongue moves, the electrical field surrounding the head electrodes changes and is picked up in EEG electrode sites.

Electrocardiogram Artifact

The waveforms of heart conduction (particularly the R wave) can intrude into all physiologic channels, particularly AC channels, such as those of

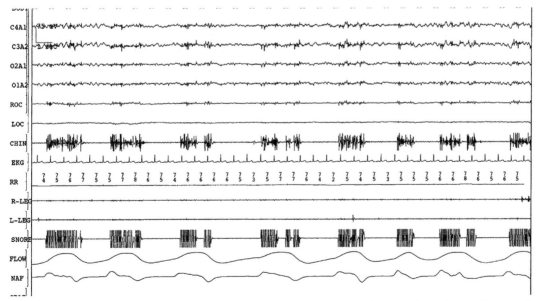

Fig. 10. Muscle tension. Snore-related activity is appropriate in the chin EMG, but muscle tension artifact can also be seen in the EEG and right EOG.

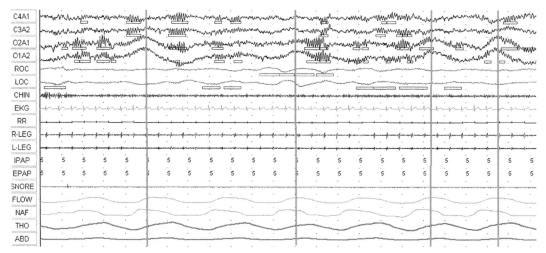

Fig. 11. Respiration movement artifact. Note that the baseline sway in occipital EEG channels lines up with respiration, as indicated by the red vertical bars.

the EEG, EOG, and chin and leg EMG. Referential derivations, in particular, are inadvertently placed in locations likely to capture the cardiac depolarization vectors. Imbalanced impedance values, fatty deposits over the mastoid reference site, or a short and thick neck can increase the potential of ECG intrusion, whereas linking references can help to eliminate it. Spacing bipolar EMG electrodes too far apart or placing them diagonally or horizontally instead of vertically also allows more ECG artifact, especially with imbalanced

impedances. The spike of an R wave appearing in the EEG should not be confused with abnormal EEG activity, and a quick scan to see if the timing lines up with the heart rhythm can help to confirm a cardiac source (**Fig. 14**).

A pulsatile artifact can be seen in the EEG when electrodes are placed over a pulsating blood vessel. There is a slight delay from the QRS complex to the appearance of the triangular slow artifact, which is caused by the pulse moving the electrode.[4] This most often occurs

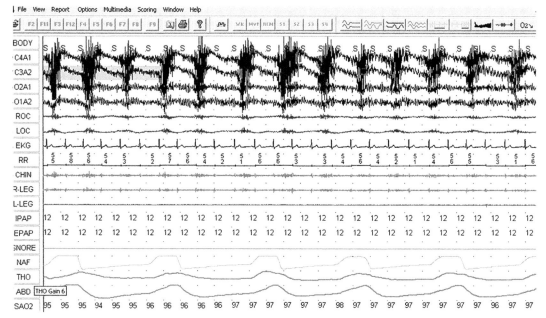

Fig. 12. Bruxism artifact. Rhythmic movement artifact is seen throughout the EEG and EOG channels and is attributable to teeth grinding.

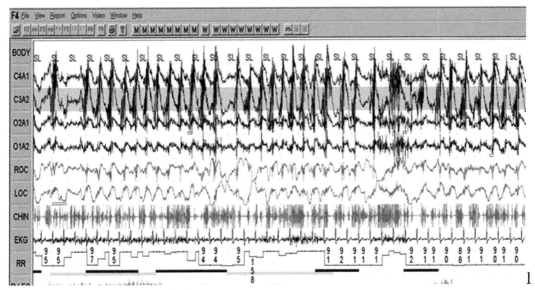

Fig.13. Chewing artifact. Rhythmic movement artifact from chewing is seen in the EEG, EOG, and ECG channels in addition to partial signal dropout in the chin EMG from agitation of the electrodes.

at the mastoid site of reference when the electrode is placed too low on the mastoid, a site at which there are more surface vessels, and when impedance is high. The movement of the body with each heartbeat, called cardioballistic motion, can cause an artifact that can also be picked up in effort channels, particularly during central events (**Fig. 15**).

Eye Movement Artifact

The eye creates a large potential field in the front of the head because the eyeball is positive in the front and negative in the back (the corneoretinal potential).[1] When the eye moves, this electrical change is picked up in EEG electrode sites close to the eyes, particularly frontal and central sites (**Fig. 16**). Likewise, high-voltage EEG waves can be displayed in the EOG channels (**Fig. 17**). Both share the same recommended low- and high-frequency settings of 0.3 and 35 Hz.[2]

The EOG channel detects little if any movement from a glass eye because there is no polarity change with movement. Some patients also have muscle or nerve damage that causes the eye not to move. A bad eye electrode may appear flat

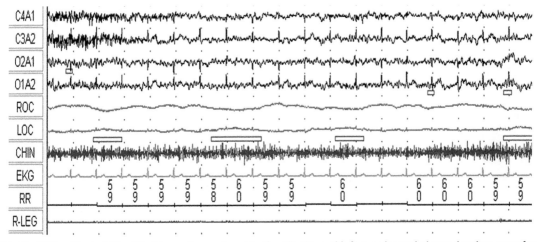

Fig.14. ECG artifact. ECG artifact is most prominent in the C3, O1, and left eye channel electrodes that are referenced to the right side, but it is also present in C4 and O2.

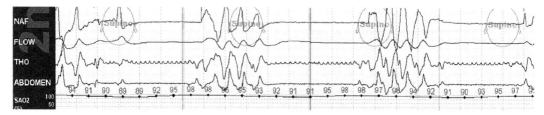

Fig. 15. Cardioballistic (cardiogenic) artifact. This artifact, with the same frequency as the heart rate, is seen in the thorax (THO) effort channel.

and not reflect eye movements seen in the other eye channel, or it may pick up EEG waves.

Sweat Sway

Sweat sway is a slow-frequency artifact that can affect all AC channels (EEG, EOG, ECG, and EMG), especially those that allow slower frequencies. This electrodermal artifact is caused when the patient sweats at the electrode site. The excretion and reabsorption or evaporation of sweat cause a direct current that alters the signal baseline. Causes include warm stagnant ambient room temperature, heavy bedclothes or bedding, and endogenous medical conditions that cause sweating (eg, diabetic reaction, respiratory exertion, chronic heart failure, hot flashes, medication side effects, fever).

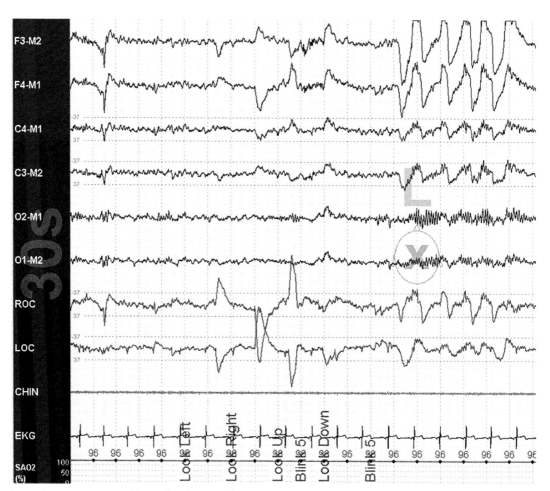

Fig. 16. Eye movement artifact. The electrical field change caused by eye movement during biocalibration is detected in the frontal and central electrode sites.

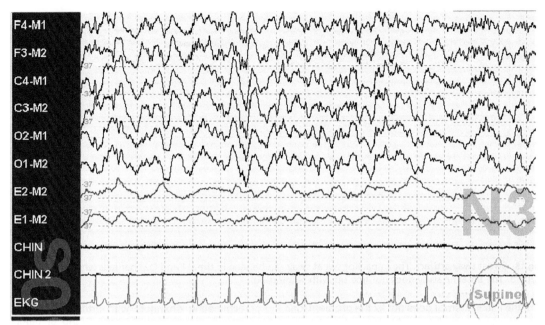

Fig. 17. Artifact in the EOG channels. High-voltage EEG waves are picked up in the EOG channels, particularly in E2, which is placed above the right outer canthus, compared with E1, which is placed below the left outer canthus.

The EEG, EOG, and ECG channels tend to be most affected, although not necessarily equally or concurrently. Low-frequency filters (LFFs) for EMG channels eliminate any slow activity regardless of whether the patient is sweating or not. Sweat sway can be a problem if it distends the true underlying physiologic waveforms. A sweat sway wave can look like a large delta wave, with a frequency less than 2 Hz. It is often more pronounced in occipital leads when the patient is supine and the back of the head is buried in the pillow (**Fig. 18**). This artifact disappears in REM sleep, when there is no thermoregulatory response. The technologist must assess and detect the site and cause and then try to remedy the cause, such as changing room temperature or patient position. Sometimes troubleshooting cannot improve the intrusion and changing the LFF (or "high-pass" filter) from 0.3 to 1.0 is necessary to determine sleep staging. Sweat sway may cause slow wave sleep (SWS, or N3) to be underestimated because some of the delta wave amplitude is attenuated.

TROUBLESHOOTING

The best way to avoid the disruption caused by artifacts is to prevent them from happening. Obtaining a clean record requires careful preparation of the patient and equipment, knowledge of the proper functioning of the equipment, following of established protocols, and familiarity with the proper appearance of the signals.

Once the technologist has recognized that a signal is an artifact rather than a true signal, the next step is to identify the source of the artifact and fix it. This process is called troubleshooting. Troubleshooting requires a thorough grounding in the fundamentals of signal generation, knowledge of the equipment, and an understanding of how artifacts occur. The key to successful troubleshooting is the development of a systematic approach to identification of the source of artifacts. The authors present an approach that, when used, allows one to find the source of artifact and correct it.

The premise for this approach is that the cause of any problem can be identified by systematically examining the potential sources of artifact starting from the patient and working back through each connection, the patient-to-computer circuit described in **Fig. 1**. Any connection site or mechanical device is a potential source of artifact and must be examined. Eventually, the source is uncovered.

First, if you can recognize the type of artifact, go to the most likely source. For example, if you notice respiratory artifact in the EEG channels, first check to see that the EEG wires are not lying close to the patient and moving with the patient's breathing movements.

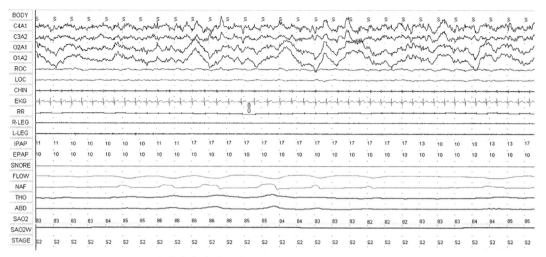

Fig. 18. Sweat sway artifact. The impact of sweat sway can be seen in the O1 and O2 channels while this patient is supine. The baseline sway does not line up with respiration.

If the initial attempt does not fix the problem, or if you do not recognize the type of artifact, begin a systematic evaluation of all possible sources of artifact from patient to computer. The authors have developed a pneumonic to help remember the possible sources to check: location, application, connection, equipment, settings (© 2008 Sleep Health*Centers* LLC).

Start with the location of the electrode. Is it placed in the appropriate place to get the correct signal? For instance, if the chin lead is not properly located over the mentalis muscle, it is difficult to detect changes in muscle tone associated with the changes in sleep stages. Then, check the application of the electrode to see if it is still well attached to the skin. Electrode pop often occurs when the electrode is coming off the skin. Does the electrode need to be reapplied? Next, check all the connections: electrode to wire, wire to jack box, jack box to amplifier, and, finally, to the computer. A loose connection can lead to extraneous signals or allow electrical interference from other sources. After that, check all your equipment to make sure it is turned on and in good working order. A broken wire, cracked amplifier, or malfunctioning oximeter can give spurious signals. Finally, check that your settings are correct. Are the filters, sensitivity, and gain set correctly, and do the tracings show the correct polarity? Following the systematic LACES approach ensures that you evaluate all possible sources of artifact. Once the source is identified, the artifact can be eliminated.

OPTIMIZING ANALYSIS

The interpreting physician needs to learn to maximize the display of the PSG recording by reducing or eliminating channels with artifact, amplifying critical signals, or viewing the study at varying time frames to suit each channel.

Filters and Sensitivity

Most systems have the ability to change filter and sensitivity settings during and after the recording. It is helpful to apply a variety of filter and sensitivity settings to a real recording to see the changes in signal response. The 60-Hz notch filter can be applied to one or all channels to reduce or eliminate electrical noise coming from the environment. The LFF can be changed from 0.3 to 1.0 to attenuate the slower sweat sway frequency, although SWS may then be underestimated. Sensitivity has an inverse relation to signal size (known as pen deflection in the days of analog PSGs). A seizure montage that adds extra leads to assist localization of abnormalities may best be viewed at a 7-μV/mm sensitivity setting, whereas a normal sleep montage has room to view the EEG at 5 μV/mm. Respiratory channels may need to be amplified by decreasing sensitivity to see any signal at all. Obstructive apneas can mistakenly be classified as central apneas if this is not tested (**Fig. 19**).

Electrode Selector Feature

The ability to re-reference electrodes can be invaluable in identifying and ameliorating a questionable signal. If, after re-referencing, an artifact appears in another channel, the amplifier was not the problem. If an amplifier channel does go bad, the input can be moved to a spare channel.

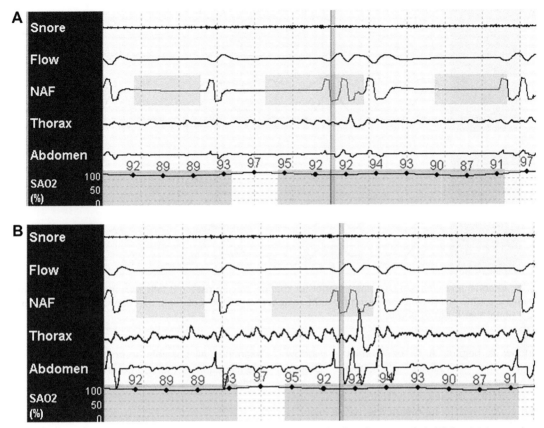

Fig. 19. Adjusting sensitivity. (*A*) Abdomen and thorax tracings are displayed as recorded. (*B*) Sensitivity was lowered, revealing the respiratory effort and showing this to be an obstructive event.

If a mastoid reference goes bad on one side, all electrodes can be re-referenced to the ipsilateral rather than contralateral side. Three chin electrodes are routinely applied, such that changing the pairs can eliminate the signal from a bad electrode.

Channel Inversion

When negative inputs are placed in the positive ports of the headbox, the signal is displayed but is inverted. This happens frequently in the ECG, although it is not always noticed by the acquiring technologist. There is usually a channel inversion software control in the digital system. Respiratory channels may also need to be inverted if the input is not correct (**Fig. 20**). Although out-of-phase signals can occur in upper and lower respiratory effort belts during obstructions, airflow signals measured by thermistor and nasal pressure should always fluctuate in phase with each other (even when at different amplitudes).

Montage Display

The montage can be crowded with all 20 American Academy of Sleep Medicine (AASM) recommended channels for PSGs; thus, it may be desirable to turn off channels that are not required. The backup EEG and chin EMG channels can be turned off if unneeded to allow more viewing space for the remaining channels. Bad channels can stand out and be distracting; thus, when artifact does emerge, it may be best to remove that channel during review if the data are not valuable (eg, 60 Hz).

Interpretation can be aided by visualizing channel waveforms at different time scales. EEGs and ECGs are normally viewed in 30-second epochs, but zooming in can allow precise scrutiny of waveform timing and morphology. In respiratory channels, a 60-second or 2-minute window allows long events or a series of events to be viewed in their entirety. To assess whether recurrent leg movements occur in a series of four 90-second intervals, which defines the maximum periodic limb movements of sleep frequency, a 5-minute

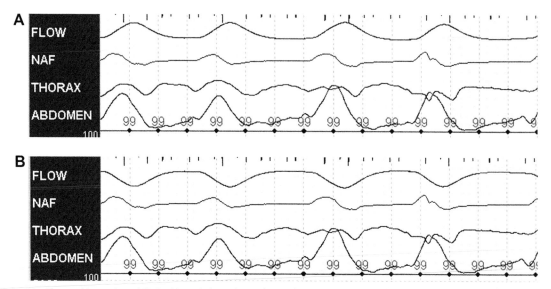

Fig. 20. Channel inversion. (*A*) Oral/nasal thermistor channel tracing rises and falls with the three other respiratory signals. (*B*) In the thermistor tracing from the same section of the recording, the channel is inverted, displaying a signal that is out of phase.

window is helpful. A 5- or 10-minute window shows the periodicity of Cheyne Stokes respiration.

The graphic display, or histogram, of all channels condensed to represent the whole night is a useful tool to demonstrate how the recorded parameters affect each other concurrently, as with sleep stage, patient position, and respiratory events. This graphic can also be a useful educational tool to show the patient what happens when he or she sleeps.

SUMMARY

Correct analysis and interpretation of a PSG requires that the recorded signals accurately represent what is happening in the body. Artifacts can lead to inaccurate interpretation. The most common categories of artifacts are unwanted environmental input and real physiologic input that obscures data in other channels. Using a systematic troubleshooting approach that

examines all possible sources of artifact allows identification of the source and correction of the artifact.

REFERENCES

1. Butkov N, Lee-Chiong T. Fundamentals of sleep technology. Philadelphia: Lippincott Williams & Wilkins; 2007. p. 362, 257.
2. Iber C, Ancoli-Israel S, Chesson A, et al. The AASM manual for the scoring of sleep and associated events: rules, terminology and technical specifications. 1st edition. Westchester (IL): American Academy of Sleep Medicine; 2007.
3. American Academy of Sleep Medicine, editors. International classification of sleep disorders diagnostic and coding manual, 2nd edition, Westchester (IL): American Academy of Sleep Medicine; 2005. p. 190.
4. Tyner FS, Knott JR, Mayer WB. Fundamentals of EEG technology, vol.1. Basic concepts and methods. New York: Raven Press; 1983. p. 88.

Portable Monitoring

Nancy A. Collop, MD

KEYWORDS
- Portable monitor • Oximetry • Polysomnography
- Obstructive sleep apnea • Sleep disordered breathing

Polysomnography (PSG) long has been considered the gold standard for diagnosing sleep-disordered breathing syndromes including obstructive sleep apnea (OSA). PSGs are the backbone of sleep centers and require trained technologists to perform and score the tests, and specialized physicians to professionally interpret the results. Because of the equipment and personnel costs, PSG is relatively expensive and often is considered inconvenient for the patient, who has to travel to the center and spend a night away from home. It has been argued that many patients who have sleep-disordered breathing in the form of OSA do not require such a comprehensive procedure to obtain an accurate diagnosis.

Because of this perception, various devices have been developed to test for sleep apnea outside the usual environment of a sleep center. These devices are hence more portable and allow studies to be done in the patient's home. Portable monitoring therefore in this context means technology that can be performed outside a sleep center and often is unattended. Such devices may be as simple as overnight oximetry or include all the same leads as performed with standard PSG.

PORTABLE MONITORING TIMELINE

In 1994, the American Sleep Disorders Association (now know as the American Academy of Sleep Medicine, AASM) published its first review on the use of PM devices.[1] In this review, PM devices were categorized into type 1, 2, 3, and 4 (**Table 1**). At that time, the authors noted that the available PM devices had insufficient reliability to allow for widespread usage.

Over the next decade, the number and types of PMs multiplied dramatically. This technology expansion was followed by numerous studies comparing the effectiveness of PM with PSG. Most studies were performed with the PM device on the patient during their PSG study, and analysis examined sensitivity and specificity.

In 2000, the Agency for Healthcare Research and Quality commissioned a meta-analysis examining PM.[2] As was observed in the 1994 American Sleep Disorders Association article, it concluded that PMs did not have sufficient sensitivity or specificity to replace PSG. Subsequent to this, a tri-society taskforce of the AASM, the American College of Chest Physicians and the American Thoracic Society was assembled to perform an evidence review specifically comparing PM to PSG.[3,4] This review looked at type 2, type 3 and type 4 studies. Studies only were included if they examined adults, if the PM was compared directly with PSG, and if the study had a minimum of 10 patients. Fifty-one studies between 1990 and 2001 met the inclusion criteria (35 studies on type 4, 12 studies on type 3, and 4 studies on type 2). A practice parameter subsequently was published using the information from the evidence review. Those recommendations stated that type 3 PMs were acceptable, but only when attended and with certain limitations, including a required review of raw data, the absence of comorbidities, and the need for a definitive evaluation if the study is nondiagnostic. Use of type 2 and type 4 devices was discouraged because of a lack of high-quality evidence. Once again, broad use of unattended PM was discouraged.

In 2005 and 2007, a different type of study emerged. These studies examined outcomes with PM compared with standard PSG. Both of those studies suggested that in highly selected populations, the outcomes with regards to the use of continuous positive airway pressure (CPAP) were at least equivalent with PM compared with

Division of Pulmonary and Critical Care Medicine, Department of Medicine, Johns Hopkins University, 1830 East Monument Street, Suite 555, Baltimore, MD 21205, USA
E-mail address: ncollop@jhmi.edu

Sleep Med Clin 4 (2009) 435–442
doi:10.1016/j.jsmc.2009.04.011

Table 1
ASDA portable monitoring types

	Type 1	Type 2	Type 3	Type 4
Number of leads	≥7	≥7	≥4	1–2
Type of leads	EEG, EOG, EMG, ECG, airflow, effort, oximetry	EEG, EOG, EMG, ECG, airflow, effort, oximetry	Airflow, effort, oximetry, ECG	Oximetry + other (usually airflow)
Setting	Attended usually in a sleep center	Unattended	Unattended	Unattended

Abbreviations: EEG, electroencephalogram; EMG, electromyogram; EOG, electro-oculogram.
Data from Ferber R, Millman R, Coppola M, et al. Portable recording in the assessment of obstructive sleep apnea. Sleep 1994;17:378.

PSG.[5,6] The diagnostic differences between PM and PSG did not appear to affect short-term outcomes, which examined CPAP acceptance and adherence.

In 2007, the Centers for Medicare and Medicaid Services (CMS) initiated another review of PM and commissioned two studies to examine the issue. These two papers were used to assist in their ultimate decision to allow reimbursement for CPAP based on PM studies. The titles of these papers were: "Home Diagnosis of Obstructive Sleep Apnea-Hypopnea Syndrome"[7] and "Obstructive Sleep Apnea-Hypopnea Syndrome: Modeling different diagnostic strategies.[8]" Later that year, another paper was published by the AASM, which set forth some clinical guidelines for use of PM.[9] Finally, PM appeared to have broken through many of the barriers that were preventing it from more widespread usage.

DIAGNOSTIC ACCURACY OF PORTABLE MONITORS

The physiologic variables measured and the information derived from portable monitoring depend upon the type of PM device that is used and the quality of the signals that are recorded. Some of the leads used may have the ability to derive more than one signal (eg, a pulse oximeter in addition to oxygen saturation also can provide a heart rate). Similarly from some airflow leads, one can derive a snoring signal. Therefore, the American Sleep Disorders Association system of types 1 through 4 may not actually correlate with the number of channels of information that might be available. In the AASM Clinical Guidelines paper, the technology was divided into different parameters, which may be a more useful way to approach PM types (**Table 2**).[9]

Table 2
American Academy of Sleep Medicine clinical guidelines: parameters used for portable monitors

Parameter	Examples
Oximetry	
Respiratory monitoring	Effort Airflow Snoring End-tidal CO2 Esophageal pressure
Cardiac monitoring	Heart rate Heart rate variability Arterial tonometry
Measures of sleep/wake activity	Electroencephalography Actigraphy
Body position	
Other	

Data from Collop N, Anderson W, Boehlecke B, et al. Clinical guidelines for the use of unattended portable monitors in the diagnosis of obstructive sleep apnea in adult patients. J Clin Sleep Med 2007;3(7):381.

Unattended full PSG has been used in several large research studies including the Sleep Heart Health Study.[10] This use requires expert technical assistance to attach the leads correctly to the patient, therefore requiring a hands-on interaction between patient and technician. In the right hands, unattended full PSGs can be accomplished with a relatively low number of studies that need to be repeated based on lost data. From a cost savings and personnel perspective, however, these studies do not save much and are not anticipated to generate large clinical usage at this time. These types of studies might be best for institutionalized patients who would have trouble getting to a sleep center, or for hospitalized patients.

Type 3 devices typically do not record sleep stage variables, as they usually lack a method of differentiating wake and sleep. Recordings from a typical type 3 portable monitoring device are shown in **Figs. 1** and **2**. In these examples, respiratory effort is detected by a piezo–electric belt; airflow is detected by a nasal cannula pressure transducer, and arterial oxygen saturation is measured by a pulse oximeter. Heart rate also is derived from the pulse oximeter signal. The physiologic variables measured by type 3 devices are sufficient to detect most apneas (including obstructive, central, and mixed) and hypopneas, as seen in the figures, although there are important

limitations. Because type 3 devices typically do not monitor electroencephalography (EEG), they cannot detect arousals from sleep. As a result, hypopneas with arousals and/or respiratory effort-related arousals (RERAs) are not scored, which may lead to an underestimation of the degree of sleep-disordered breathing. The traditional PSG-derived apnea hypopnea index (AHI) is calculated by dividing the number of apneas and hypopneas by the duration of sleep in hours. If RERAs also are counted, the respiratory disturbance index is the number of apneas plus hypopneas plus RERAs divided by the number of hours of sleep. In contrast, the AHI that is derived from a type 3 device is calculated by dividing the number of apneas and hypopneas (only scored with desaturations) by the entire study duration. These calculation changes cause the AHI derived by a type 3 PM to be lower than that derived by PSG (**Fig. 3**). This decreases the diagnostic sensitivity of type 3 devices, compared with type 1 and 2 devices. Some type 3 devices add on actigraphy in an attempt to improve the detection of sleep; however, studies have not shown that this additional lead significantly improves accuracy.[11,12]

The information derived from type 4 devices is even more limited and again depends on the physiologic variables measured. Most commonly, pulse oximetry is combined with an airflow measure. The

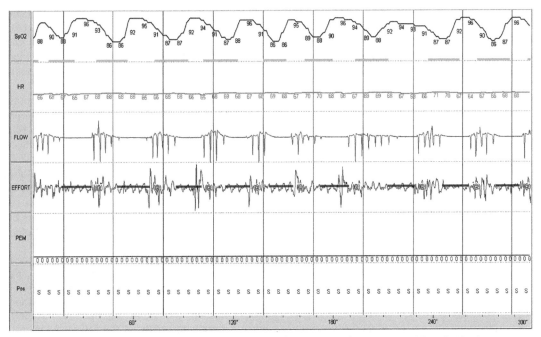

Fig. 1. This is an example of a 5-minute epoch from a portable monitor showing repetitive obstructive apneas as evidenced by periods of absent flow in the FLOW tracing and continued effort in the EFFORT tracing. The apneas are marked by a red line in the EFFORT tracing. Tracing labels: SpO₂, pulse oximetry; HR, heart rate derived from SpO₂; FLOW, airflow derived from nasal pressure; EFFORT, respiratory effort derived from piezoelectric belts; PEM, no signal; Pos, body position.

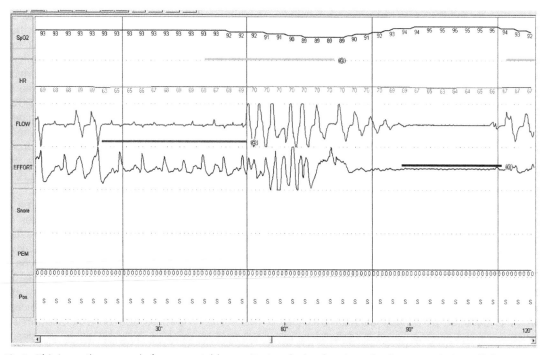

Fig. 2. This is another example from a portable monitoring device showing a 2-minute epoch. Two distinct events are seen here. The first event is hypopnea with a reduction in the FLOW and EFFORT tracing with an oxygen desaturation from 93% to 89%. The hypopnea is marked by a pink line. The second event is a central apnea showing absent FLOW and EFFORT, marked by a blue line. Tracing labels: SpO$_2$, pulse oximetry; HR, heart rate derived from SpO$_2$; FLOW, airflow derived from nasal pressure; EFFORT, respiratory effort derived from piezoelectric belts; PEM, no signal; Pos, body position.

information that can be collected from a type 4 device includes: frequency of apneas, frequency of hypopneas (with desaturation only), an AHI (as divided by total recording time), baseline arterial oxyhemoglobin saturation (SaO$_2$), mean SaO$_2$, frequency of desaturation, and nadirs of SaO$_2$. Therefore not only do all of the limitations of type 3 devices apply to type 4 devices, but type 4 devices also cannot differentiate between obstructive and central/mixed apneas.

Some other limitations should also be noted with regards to type 3 and 4 PMs. Unlike polysomnography, in which there are standardized rules for scoring events, there are no published standardized rules for PMs. Many devices use proprietary algorithms to score events, and the user cannot alter the scoring. SNAP (SNAP Laboratories, Glenview, Illinois) and Watch PAT (Itamar Medical LTD, Caesarea, Israel) are examples of devices with proprietary algorithms.[13,14] Such proprietary algorithms have been shown to decrease diagnostic accuracy.[11,15–18]

Similarly, the characteristics of overnight pulse oximetry depend upon the criteria used to define events. When using a quantitative measure such as a 4% desaturation, the sensitivity is relatively low for diagnosing OSA; however, the specificity is acceptable.[19–21] When using more qualitative criteria, however, such as analyzing the tracing for frequent desaturations often known as a sawtooth pattern, the sensitivity improves, but the specificity falls.[22] In fact, a more recent study

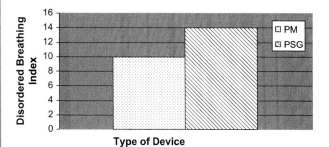

Fig. 3. In this graph, the disordered breathing indexes for a PSG-derived study and a PM-derived study are shown. The studies were done on the same night on the same patient. During the study, he had 70 disordered breathing events. In the PSG study, his total sleep time was 5 hours and, in the PM study, the total recording time was 7 hours.

showed poor consistency between pulmonary physicians interpreting overnight oximetry readings.[23] The low level of consistency suggests there are significant problems with either approach that will result in increased false-negative or -positive tests.

OUTCOME STUDIES USING PORTABLE MONITORS

Prior evidence reviews have suggested that PMs are not as accurate as polysomnography in diagnosing sleep apnea; however, in selected patient populations, PM has been shown to result in similar outcomes with regards to CPAP usage. Three studies have examined short-term outcomes in patients randomized to a diagnostic PM or PSG test.

In a study published in 2005, 288 patients referred by a family physician were randomized to either PSG or a SnoreSat (Saga Tech Electronics, Calgary, Alberta, Canada) followed by treatment with an auto-titrating CPAP.[5] After 4 weeks, a reassessment was done to determine their response to treatment. No difference was found between the two groups with regards to CPAP adherence or quality of life. Another study of 68 patients who were assigned randomly to PSG or PM (Remmers Sleep Recorder, Saga Tech Electronics, Calgary, Alberta, Canada) and re-evaluated after 3 months of CPAP usage again showed no differences with regards to CPAP adherence. In fact, the PM group actually demonstrated higher CPAP adherence.[6] It should be noted that in both of these studies, the patients were highly selected. All patients were referred for possible sleep apnea. There were relatively strict entry criteria that excluded patients who had comorbid disorders (like active heart disease, chronic lung disease, psychiatric disorders, and pregnancy), and all patients were evaluated in a sleep clinic. Therefore, the patients studied were chosen specifically to have a high pretest probability of having OSA.

A third study was published recently that examined another high-risk population, patients in a Veterans Administration medical center.[24] In this study, the patients were required to have an Epworth Sleepiness Scale score of greater than 11 and complain of two out of three of the following: loud habitual snoring, witnessed apneas, or hypertension. The patients were evaluated by a Watch PAT 100 PM; then they used an auto-CPAP for 2 to 3 nights with a switch to fixed CPAP. These patients were compared with the control group who underwent a typical split night study. One hundred and six patients were randomized, and 79 completed the trial. Ninety-three percent of the patients were found to have OSA

(AHI greater than 5), and after 6 weeks of CPAP use, there was again no difference between groups regarding CPAP adherence, change in Epworth scores, or CPAP satisfaction.

These studies demonstrate that with a clear-cut algorithmic approach that excludes patients who have comorbid diseases and includes patients at high risk for OSA, short-term outcomes are equivalent with PM and PSG. It should be noted that these studies were done by trained sleep specialists, and patients had several interactions with the health care teams to train and educate them on use of the PM and CPAP. Longer-term studies are needed to confirm these results.

CONSIDERATIONS FOR PORTABLE MONITORING USAGE

OSA occurs when there are repetitive narrowings or closures of the upper airway. These events are associated with oxygen desaturation; hypercapnia; changes in sympathetic tone, heart rate, and blood pressure; and sleep disruption. Measuring physiologic signals to capture these obstructive events is the goal of diagnostic testing. Therefore, the most common leads used to monitor for OSA include airflow, respiratory effort, and oxygen saturation. Other channels that also have been examined include but are not limited to: carbon dioxide monitors, peripheral arterial tonometry (which monitors sympathetic tone), heart rate, esophageal pressure, snore microphone with acoustic analysis, and actigraphy. Most sleep specialists agree that oximetry must be included for any PM; however, the number and type of other leads are not agreed upon fully. Clearly, a higher number of leads will increase the accuracy, but eventually the complexity of putting on multiple leads outweighs the diagnostic accuracy of the PM. In 2007, the AASM released the "Clinical Guidelines for the Use of Unattended Portable Monitors in the Diagnosis of Obstructive Sleep Apnea in Adult Patients.[8]" This paper was based on an evidence review and consensus; the recommendations suggested that a PM should record airflow, respiratory effort, and blood oxygenation. This statement was based on the review of accuracy of various polysomnography signals as outlined in the AASM scoring manual papers.[25] These signals were felt to have the most robust diagnostic accuracy. The most accurate airflow signals would include both a thermal-based sensor and a nasal pressure sensor, and the most accurate effort signals would use respiratory inductance plethysmography.

Another thing to consider when using a PM is the ease of conducting the study. Because these

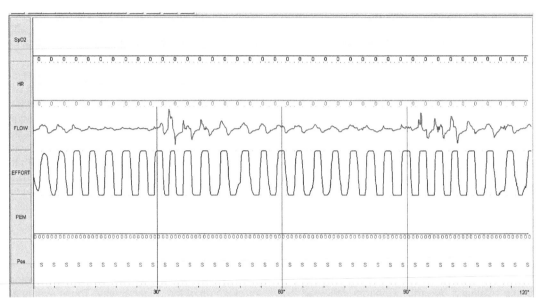

Fig. 4. This figure taken from a portable monitoring device demonstrates data loss. In this 2-minute epoch, the oximeter (SpO₂) is not working nor is the heart rate signal (HR), which is derived from the oximeter. Tracing labels: SpO₂, pulse oximetry; HR, heart rate derived from SpO₂; FLOW, airflow derived from nasal pressure; EFFORT, respiratory effort derived from piezoelectric belts; PEM, no signal; Pos, body position.

PMs are to be used in the home, ideally the patient should be able to put it on and take it off on his or her own. Thus, it must be relatively simple to use. Even if the patient is verbally instructed on the use of the PM including a demonstration on how to put on the device, he or she still must be able to do it at home. Additionally, the leads must remain on the patient throughout the night and therefore must

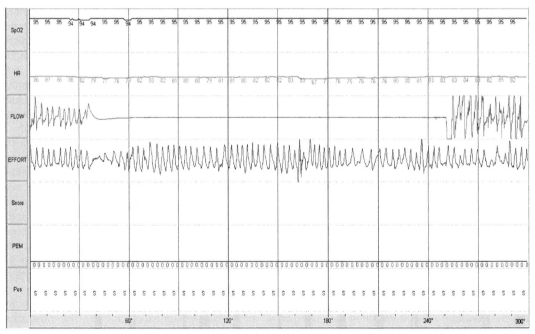

Fig. 5. This figure taken from a portable monitoring device also demonstrates data loss. In this 5-minute epoch, the FLOW signal flattens beginning shortly after the 30-second mark until just after the 240 -second mark. This can be identified as data loss, because if an event lasted that long, one would expect some change in oxygen saturation, heart rate, or effort, which is not observed. Tracing labels: SpO₂, pulse oximetry; HR, heart rate derived from SpO₂; FLOW, airflow derived from nasal pressure; EFFORT, respiratory effort derived from piezoelectric belts; PEM, no signal; Pos, body position.

be secured well. Duplication of leads to prevent data loss adds to complexity. In actuality, some degree of data loss must be assumed when considering use of PM; some minimal amount of data must be obtained to assure test validity. Studies of type 3 devices show anywhere between 2% and 18% data loss; for type 4 devices, data loss ranges from 7% to 10%.[4] **Figs. 4** and **5** show examples of data loss occurring during portable monitor acquisitions. Other issues typically not addressed in research studies include equipment breakage, sweat artifact, battery life, and use over extended periods of time by multiple patients. Clearly, durability is an important feature of any PM device.

This issue of cost savings from use of PM is not as well examined as one would think. Although studies that have estimated costs typically show substantial savings, many of them do not account for the costs associated with failure rates, nor do they compare with PSG using split night protocols. Other costs associated with PM include use of autotitrating CPAP devices, technician time to educate the patient about the PM, cost related to PM device depreciation or damage, and recurring supplies. Also, there are costs associated with getting the PM device to the patient, either the patient's or the courier's travel costs, or postage and shipping.

Choosing the appropriate population is extremely important when considering use of PM to diagnose OSA. As stated earlier, most of the studies showing positive outcomes with PM have been done on patients who had a high likelihood of having OSA. In addition, confounding disorders such as respiratory disease or cardiac disease are usually a reason to exclude patients for PM testing. All patients for whom PM is being considered should be evaluated by a health care professional trained in sleep medicine. Because of relatively high false-negative results with PM, careful assessment of pretest probability is necessary. The presence of other comorbid sleep disorders, such as insomnia, restless legs syndrome, or parasomnias are also likely to reduce the accuracy of PM, and their use should be avoided. In those patients in whom the risk appears high for OSA, and no significant comorbidities are present that might reduce the accuracy of the test, a PM test is a reasonable alternative.

SUMMARY

PM is a term that includes various monitoring devices typically used to diagnose obstructive sleep apnea. It is anticipated that use of PM in the United Stats will be expanding with the recent approval by CMS for use in patients with OSA who are eligible for treatment with CPAP. Three studies have shown equivalent short-term outcomes of treatment when using PM in patients undergoing CPAP therapy; these patient populations were highly selected for probable moderate-to-severe OSA. Practitioners contemplating use of PM in their practices must review the advantages and limitations of PMs systematically before embarking upon their usage.

REFERENCES

1. Ferber R, Millman R, Coppola M, et al. Portable recording in the assessment of obstructive sleep apnea. Sleep 1994;17:378–92.
2. Ross SD, Sheinhait IA, Harrison KJ, et al. Systematic review and meta-analysis of the literature regarding the diagnosis of sleep apnea. Sleep 2000;23:519–32.
3. Chesson AL Jr, Berry RB, Pack A. Practice parameters for the use of portable monitoring devices in the investigation of suspected obstructive sleep apnea in adults. Sleep 2003;26:907–13.
4. Flemons WW, Littner MR, Rowley JA, et al. Home diagnosis of sleep apnea: a systematic review of the literature. An evidence review cosponsored by the American Academy of Sleep Medicine, the American College of Chest Physicians, and the American Thoracic Society. Chest 2003;124(4):1543–79.
5. Whitelaw WA, Brant RF, Flemons WW. Clinical usefulness of home oximetry compared with polysomnography for assessment of sleep apnea. Am J Respir Crit Care Med 2005;171:188–93.
6. Mulgrew AT, Fox N, Ayas NT, et al. Diagnosis and initial management of obstructive sleep apnea without polysomnography: a randomized validation study. Ann Intern Med 2007;146:157–66.
7. Agency for Healthcare Research and Quality. Technology assessment: home diagnosis of obstructive sleep apnea–hypopnea syndrome. Available at: http://www.cms.hhs.gov/determinationprocess/downloads/id48TA.pdf. Accessed May 25, 2009.
8. Agency for Healthcare Research and Quality. Obstructive sleep apnea–hypopnea syndrome: modeling different diagnostic strategies. Available at: http://www.cms.hhs.gov/determinationprocess/downloads/id50TA.pdf. Accessed May 25, 2009.
9. Collop N, Anderson W, Boehlecke B, et al. Clinical guidelines for the use of unattended portable monitors in the diagnosis of obstructive sleep apnea in adult patients. J Clin Sleep Med 2007;3(7):737–47.
10. Iber C, Redline S, Kaplan Gilpin AM, et al. Polysomnography performed in the unattended home versus the attended laboratory setting—Sleep Heart Health Study methodology. Sleep 2004;27(3):536–40.
11. Overland B, Bruskeland G, Akre H, et al. Evaluation of a portable recording device (Reggie) with

actimeter and nasopharyngeal/esophagus catheter incorporated. Respiration 2005;72:600–5.

12. Penzel T, Kesper K, Pinnow I, et al. Peripheral arterial tonometry, oximetry, and actigraphy for ambulatory recording of sleep apnea. Physiol Meas 2004; 25:1025–36.

13. Liesching TN, Carlisle C, Marte A, et al. Evaluation of the accuracy of SNAP technology sleep sonography in detecting obstructive sleep apnea in adults compared to standard polysomnography. Chest 2004;125(3):886–91.

14. Bar A, Pillar G, Dvir I, et al. Evaluation of a portable device based on peripheral arterial tone for unattended home sleep studies. Chest 2003;123:695–703.

15. Dingli K, Coleman EL, Vennelle M, et al. Evaluation of a portable device for diagnosing the sleep apnoea/hypopnoea syndrome. Eur Respir J 2003;21:253–9.

16. Golpe R, Jimenez A, Carpizo R. Home sleep studies in the assessment of sleep apnea/hypopnea syndrome. Chest 2002;122:1156–61.

17. Reichert JA, Bloch DA, Cundiff E, et al. Comparison of the NovaSom QSG, a new sleep apnea home-diagnostic system, and polysomnography. Sleep Med 2003;4:213–8.

18. Esnaola S, Duran J, Infante-Rivard C, et al. Diagnostic accuracy of a portable recording device (MESAM IV) in suspected obstructive sleep apnoea. Eur Respir J 1996;9:2597–605.

19. Williams A, Yu G, Santiago S, et al. Screening of sleep apnea using pulse oximetry and a clinical score. Chest 1991;100:631–5.

20. Douglas N, Thomas S, Jan MA. Clinical value of polysomnography. Lancet 1992;339: 347–50.

21. Gyulay S, Olson LG, Hensley M, et al. A comparison of clinical assessment and home oximetry in the diagnosis of obstructive sleep apnea. Am Rev Respir Dis 1993;147:50–3.

22. Series F, Marc I, Cormier Y, et al. Utility of nocturnal home oximetry for case finding in patients with suspected sleep apnea hypopnea syndrome. Ann Intern Med 1993;119:449–53.

23. Ramsey R, Mehra R, Strohl KP. Variations in physician interpretation of overnight pulse oximetry monitoring. Chest 2007;132(3):852–9.

24. Berry RB, Hill G, Thompson L, et al. Portable monitoring and autotitration versus polysomnography for the diagnosis and treatment of sleep apnea. Sleep 2008;31(10):1423–31.

25. Redline S, Budhiraja R, Kapur R, et al. The scoring of respiratory events in sleep: reliability and validity. J Clin Sleep Med 2007;3(2):169–200.

Manual Titration of Positive Airway Pressure in Patients with Obstructive Sleep Apnea

Alejandro D. Chediak, MD, FAASM, FACP, FACCP[a,b,]*

KEYWORDS

- Positive airway pressure • Titration
- Continuous positive airway pressure
- Bilevel positive airway pressure
- Obstructive sleep apnea
- Sleep-related breathing disorder
- Sleep-disordered breathing

Obstructive sleep apnea (OSA), a sleep-related breathing disorder characterized by full or partial occlusion of the upper airway during sleep, is treated most often by positive airway pressure (PAP) therapy. Standard sleep medicine practice involves manual pressure adjustment by a sleep technologist during attended laboratory polysomnography (PSG) designed to eliminate obstructive respiratory-related events (apneas, hypopneas, respiratory effort-related arousals [RERAs], and snoring). The manual titration of PAP has been conducted for over 25 years,[1] yet no standardized protocols exist for this procedure.[2] A survey of accredited sleep centers reviewed titration protocols from 51 accredited centers and found that the procedures described for PAP titration varied widely among the centers. Twenty-two percent of these centers did not have a written protocol.[3] The lack of standardization results in clinicians and technologists from different sleep laboratories developing their own protocols[4] or relying on protocols obtained from industry or other sleep laboratories. When a standardized protocol is implemented, the optimal pressure for continuous positive airway pressure (CPAP) can be reproducible; one study revealed a Spearman correlation coefficient of 0.89 for the optimal pressure selected for two consecutive CPAP titration nights in 50 patients who had OSA.[5] Published PAP titration protocols are scarce, however, and there is a question as to what one would use or measure to advocate or support one particular protocol over another. Given this gap, an American Academy of Sleep Medicine (AASM) Task Force was charged with developing an evidence- and consensus-based standardized PAP titration protocol. The task force chose as its premise that a successful titration is one in which there is an optimized trade-off between increasing pressure to yield efficacy in elimination of respiratory events and decreasing pressure to minimize emergence of pressure-related adverse effects.[6] The guidelines for CPAP titration provided in this treatment on the topic are often duplicative of the recommendations made by the AASM CPAP Titration Task Force, and the reader is directed to that manuscript for details pertaining to the scientific basis for a specific recommendation.[7]

Several factors have been identified as potentially influencing optimal pressure, such as rapid eye movement (REM) sleep amounts,[8] the length of the soft palate, and the degree of respiratory

a University of Miami at Mount Sinai Medical Center, 4300 Alton Road, Miami Beach, FL 33140, USA
b Miami Sleep Disorders Center, 7029 SW 61st Avenue, South Miami, FL 33143, USA
* School of Medicine, University of Miami at Mount Sinai, FL.
E-mail address: miamisleep@bellsouth.net

Sleep Med Clin 4 (2009) 443–453
doi:10.1016/j.jsmc.2009.04.012
1556-407X/09/$ – see front matter © 2009 Elsevier Inc. All rights reserved.

effort.[9] Although there are some studies demonstrating reasonable correlation between the level of optimal CPAP and the apnea–hypopnea index (AHI)[10,11] or obesity,[11] a significant correlation for optimal CPAP and AHI has been observed only in patients whose apneas depend on body position.[12] Mathematical equations incorporating measures of OSA severity (AHI) and obesity (ie, body mass index [BMI] and neck circumference) developed to predict the optimal level of CPAP[11,13] have proven inaccurate in predicting the optimal CPAP level.[14,15] Hence, manual titration of PAP in the sleep laboratory remains the standard of care.

PAP delivery systems consist of three main components: a PAP device (a turbine- or fan-driven air pump), an interface (ie, nasal mask, nasal pillows, full-face mask) used to connect the subjects natural airway to the PAP device output, and a flexible hose that connects the PAP device to the interface. PAP devices are divided into four basic types depending on their pressure delivery system:

1. CPAP, which delivers a single, fixed pressure throughout the respiratory cycle

2. Bilevel positive airway pressure (BPAP), which delivers a higher PAP with inspiration (IPAP) than with expiration (EPAP)
3. Auto-titrating positive airway pressure (APAP), which, using a manufacturer specific paradigm, automatically alters CPAP or BPAP (IPAP/EPAP) intending to maintain airway patency
4. Adaptive servo-ventilation (ASV), which uses a servo-controller that automatically adjusts pressure to maintain steady minute ventilation

APAP device prescriptions account for only 4% of PAP devices prescribed, and in 2004, 30% of board-certified sleep physicians reported having never prescribed APAP devices.[16] Two types of PAP devices, CPAP and BPAP, will be discussed. As described in this article, BPAP refers to a BPAP device set in spontaneous mode unless otherwise specified. Data regarding usefulness of other PAP device types or device features including ASV will not be discussed. Unless specified otherwise, the information in this article pertains only to nighttime PAP titration studies. Manual titration of CPAP or BPAP is currently the gold standard for selecting the optimal (effective) pressure for CPAP and BPAP,

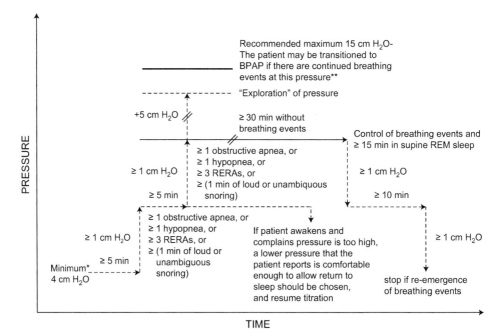

Fig. 1. Continuous positive airway pressure (CPAP) titration algorithm for patients younger than 12 years during full- or split-night titration studies. Note, upward titration at greater than or equal to 1 cm increments over greater than or equal to 5-minute periods is continued according to the breathing events observed until at least 30 minutes without breathing events is achieved. A higher starting CPAP may be selected for patients who have an elevated body mass index and for retitration studies (*). The patient also should be tried on bilevel positive airway pressure if he or she is uncomfortable or intolerant of high CPAP (**). (*From* Kushida CA, Chediak A, Berry R, et al. Clinical guidelines for the manual titration of positive airway pressure in patients with obstructive sleep apnea. J Clin Sleep Med 2008;4:157–71; with permission.)

and this article is limited to reflect current knowledge and practice of this procedure.

This article uses the following terminology. Unless stated otherwise, OSA is used synonymously with obstructive sleep apnea syndrome, obstructive sleep apnea–hypopnea syndrome, and obstructive forms of either sleep-disordered breathing or sleep-related breathing disorder. The scope of this work is restricted to adult (at least 12 years) and pediatric (younger than 12 years) patients who have OSA and does not apply to patients who have conditions such as neuromuscular disease or intrinsic lung disease. The respiratory disturbance index (RDI) refers to the total of apneas, hypopneas, and RERAs per hour of sleep, and for this article, this term is not synonymous with the AHI, which refers to the total of apneas and hypopneas per hour of sleep. Mild, moderate, and severe OSAs are defined according to following criteria in adults: mild, $5 \leq RDI \leq 15$; moderate, $15 \leq RDI \leq 30$; and severe, $RDI > 30$.[17] In children younger than 12 years of age, the criteria are as follows: mild, $1 \leq RDI < 5$; moderate, $5 < RDI < 10$; and severe, $RDI > 10$.[18,19]

GENERAL RECOMMENDATIONS FOR ADULT AND PEDIATRIC POSITIVE AIRWAY PRESSURE TITRATIONS

All potential PAP titration candidates (including those candidates where a split-night study is a possibility) should receive adequate PAP education, hands-on demonstration, careful mask fitting, and acclimatization before titration. Specific recommendations include:

- The indications, rationale for use, and adverse effects of PAP should be discussed in detail with the patient or caregiver *before* the PAP titration study.
- The patient should be fitted carefully for the interface with intent of maximizing comfort, compensating for significant nasal obstruction, and minimizing leak before the PAP titration.
- The patient should be acclimated to the PAP equipment (ie, wearing the interface with the pressure on) before lights off.[20,21]
- There should be several different types of PAP interfaces (ie, nasal mask, nasal pillows, full-face/oronasal mask) and

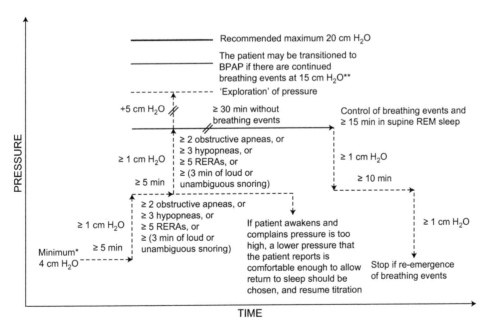

Fig. 2. Continuous positive airway pressure (CPAP) titration algorithm for patients greater than or equal to 12 years during full- or split-night titration studies. Note, upward titration at agreater than or equal to1-cm increments over greater than or equal to 5-minute periods is continued according to the breathing events observed until at least 30 minutes without breathing events are achieved. A higher starting CPAP may be selected for patients who have an elevated BMI and for retitration studies (*). The patient also should be tried on bilevel positive airway pressure if he or she is uncomfortable or intolerant of high CPAP (**). (*From* Kushida CA, Chediak A, Berry R, et al. Clinical guidelines for the manual titration of positive airway pressure in patients with obstructive sleep apnea. J Clin Sleep Med 2008;4:157–71; with permission.)

Box 1
Specific continuous positive airway pressure titration guidelines

The minimum starting CPAP should be 4 cm H_2O in pediatric and adult patients. A priori determination of CPAP cannot be supported by evidence. Nonetheless, a higher starting CPAP is sensible in retitration studies, in those who have very high BMI, and in cases where patients experience air hunger on lower doses of CPAP during the pretitration acclimation to CPAP.

The maximum CPAP should be 15 cm H_2O for patients younger than 12 years.

The maximum CPAP should be 20 cm H_2O for patients 12 years of age or older.

If there are continued obstructive respiratory events at 15 cm H_2O of CPAP for either adult or pediatric patients during the titration study, the patient may be switched to BPAP titration.

CPAP should be increased by at least 1 cm H_2O with an interval no shorter than 5 minutes, with the goal of eliminating obstructive respiratory events.

In patients younger than 12 years of age, increase CPAP as stipulated if:

At least one obstructive apnea is observed

At least one hypopnea is observed

At least three RERAs are observed

In patients 12 years of age or older, increase CPAP as stipulated if:

At least two obstructive apneas are observed

At least three hypopneas are observed

At least five RERAs are observed

CPAP may be increased by at least 1 cm H_2O with an interval no shorter than 5 minutes, with the goal of eliminating loud or unambiguous snoring after.

At least 1 minute of loud or unambiguous snoring in patients younger than 12 years

At least 3 minutes of loud or unambiguous snoring in patients 12 years of age or older

Exploration of CPAP pressure above the pressure at which control of obstructive respiratory events is achieved should not exceed 5 cm H_2O.

Elevated upper airway resistance with sleep disruption may persist despite selection of a pressure that eliminates apneas and hypopneas.[24,25]

A reduction in respiratory oscillations of esophageal pressure or resolution of inspiratory flattening on a flow–time curve in response to exploration with higher CPAP pressure may serve as surrogate markers of decreasing upper airway resistance. In this regard, CPAP exploration can have utility by increasing pressure by 2 cm H_2O but no higher than by 5 cm H_2O.[26]

Upward titration of the CPAP level to correct inspiratory flow limitation may be 2 to 5 cm H_2O higher than the level at which it reappears during downward titration, a phenomena explained by upper airway hysteresis.[26] Decreasing CPAP after controlling respiratory events (apneas, hypopneas, RERAs, and snoring) or up–down titration is an acceptable strategy employed to take advantage of upper airway hysteresis and allow for selection of a lower effective CPAP dose. Alternatively, an up-down-up CPAP titration paradigm, where pressure is increased in a stepwise fashion until respiratory events disappear then systematically decreased until respiratory abnormalities reappear (**Fig. 3**) followed by a reincrease in CPAP pressure to renormalize respiration, has been used to exploit the hysteresis effect.[27] If an up–down or up-down-up titration strategy is implemented:

At least one titration cycle (up–down or up-down-up) should be conducted.

At least 30 minutes without obstructive respiratory events should have passed before starting the titration cycle.

CPAP should be decreased by more than 1 cm H_2O with an interval no shorter than 10 minutes, until there is reemergence of obstructive respiratory events.

In up-down-up titration cycles, after completing the previously described CPAP reduction, CPAP pressure once again is increased in increments of 1 cm H_2O until respiratory events are corrected.

Complaints of excess pressure during the course of CPAP titration may be addressed by resuming the CPAP titration at a pressure at or just below that which the patient reports as uncomfortable.

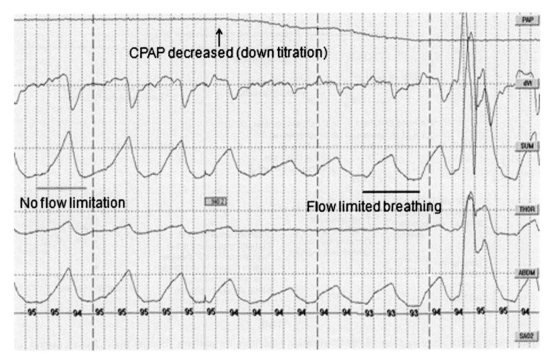

Fig. 3. Down titration phase of an up–down continuous positive airway pressure (CPAP) titration cycle. Note how flow becomes limited, and breath volume diminishes on abrupt reduction in CPAP pressure output, indicating insufficient treatment pressure at the lower CPAP pressure output. *Abbreviations:* ABDOM, abdominal contribution to breathing by respiratory inductive plethysmography (RIP); dVt, airflow derived by the instantaneous derivative of the tracing SUM (breath volume-time); PAP, positive airway pressure output; SAO$_2$, oxyhemoglobin saturation by pulse oximetry; SUM, breath volume derived by RIP; THOR, thoracic contribution to breathing by RIP.

accessories (chinstrap, heated humidifier) available if the patient encounters problems (eg, mouth leak, nasal congestion, or oronasal dryness) during the night.

- In patients who have combined insomnia and sleep apnea, a combination of daytime psychological and physiologic treatments before overnight PAP titration can facilitate acceptance of PAP titration[21]
- Because children have more problems adjusting to PAP than adults, additional steps may be required. Pediatric size interfaces should be available,[22] and behavioral modification techniques may be implemented to increase the tolerability and potential adherence to PAP equipment.[16,23]
- PAP assembly, optional equipment, importance of daily/nightly use, adherence issues, necessity of cleaning the equipment, and implications of the purchase/ rental of the equipment (when applicable) should be discussed in detail with the patient or caregiver, preferably following the PAP titration study.

GUIDELINES FOR CONTINUOUS POSITIVE AIRWAY PRESSURE TITRATION

In full-night CPAP titration PSG and split-night PSG when CPAP is used in the titration arm of the study, CPAP should be increased until obstructive respiratory events are eliminated (apneas, hypopneas, RERAs, and snoring) or a recommended maximum CPAP is reached. Oxyhemoglobin desaturation–resaturation events occurring without associated obstructive respiratory events should not be considered in the decision to increase CPAP in pediatric and adult patients. Specific guidelines for pediatric and adult CPAP titrations are depicted in **Figs 1** and **2**, respectively, and in **Box 1**.

GUIDELINES FOR BILEVEL POSITIVE AIRWAY PRESSURE TITRATION

In general, BPAP is not more effective than CPAP, and the following guidelines should not be construed to imply otherwise (**Figs 4** and **5**). A patient may be tried on BPAP for intolerance of high pressures on CPAP and if there are continued obstructive respiratory events at 15 cm H$_2$O of CPAP in the course of

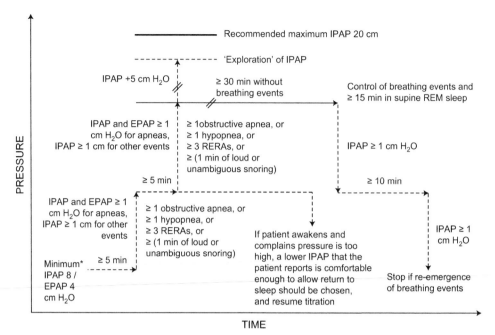

Fig. 4. Bilevel positive airway pressure (BPAP) titration algorithm for patients younger than 12 years during full- or split-night titration studies. Note, upward titration of inspiratory positive airway pressure (IPAP) and expiratory positive airway pressure (EPAP) greater than or equal to 1 cm H_2O for apneas and IPAP greater than or equal to 1 cm for other events over at least 5-minute periods is continued until at least 30 minutes without breathing events are achieved. A decrease in IPAP or setting BPAP in spontaneous-timed mode with backup rate may be helpful if treatment-emergent central apneas are observed. A higher starting IPAP and EPAP may be selected for patients who have an elevated BMI and for retitration studies (*). When transitioning from CPAP to BPAP, the minimum starting EPAP should be set at 4 cm H_2O or the CPAP level at which obstructive apneas were eliminated. An optimal minimum IPAP–EPAP differential is 4 cm H_2O, and an optimal maximum IPAP–EPAP differential is 10 cm H_2O. (*From* Kushida CA, Chediak A, Berry R, et al. Clinical guidelines for the manual titration of positive airway pressure in patients with obstructive sleep apnea. J Clin Sleep Med 2008;4:157–71; with permission.)

a CPAP titration. Efforts should be made to explore the cause of CPAP intolerance and to remedy the complaint before proceeding to BPAP titration. In full-night BPAP titration PSG and split-night PSG when BPAP is used in the titration arm of the study, BPAP should be increased until obstructive respiratory events are eliminated (apneas, hypopneas, RE-RAs, and snoring) or a recommended maximum IPAP is reached. The algorithm for split-night BPAP titration studies should be identical to that of full-night BPAP titration studies. Specific guidelines are listed in **Box 2**.

GUIDELINES FOR GRADING OF POSITIVE AIRWAY PRESSURE TITRATION STUDIES

The PAP settings prescribed following a titration study should reflect control of obstructive respiration by a low (preferably less than 5/h) RDI at the selected pressure, a minimum sea level oxyhemoglobin saturation (SaO_2) above 90% at the pressure, and with a leak within acceptable parameters at the pressure.

- An optimal titration is one that reduces RDI by less than 5 during at least 15 minutes of

sleep and includes sustained supine REM sleep at the selected pressure.
- A good titration is one that: Reduces RDI by no more than 10 or by 50% if the baseline RDI is less than 15/h and includes sustained supine REM sleep at the selected pressure.
- An adequate titration is one that does not reduce the overnight RDI by less than or equal to 10/h but does reduce the RDI by 75% from baseline. Additionally, the titration grading criteria for optimal or good are met with the exception that supine REM sleep did not occur at the selected pressure.
- An unacceptable titration is one that does not meet any of the previously described criteria for optimal, good, or acceptable titrations.

IDENTIFYING AND MANAGING UNINTENTIONAL MASK LEAKS DURING POSITIVE AIRWAY PRESSURE TITRATION STUDIES

PAP mask refit or readjustment should be performed whenever any significant unintentional leak is observed.

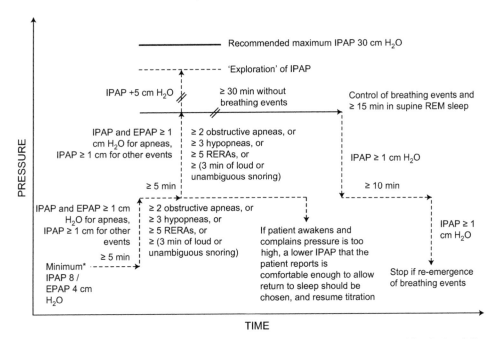

Fig. 5. Bilevel positive airway pressure (BPAP) titration algorithm for patients 12 years or older during full- or split-night titration studies. Note, upward titration of inspiratory positive airway pressure (IPAP) and expiratory positive airway pressure (EPAP) greater than or equal to 1 cm H_2O for apneas and IPAP greater than or equal to 1 cm for other events over at least 5-minute periods is continued until at least 30 minutes without breathing events are achieved. A decrease in IPAP or setting BPAP in spontaneous-timed mode with backup rate may be helpful if treatment-emergent central apneas are observed. A higher starting IPAP and EPAP may be selected for patients who have an elevated body mass index and for retitration studies (*). When transitioning from continuous positive airway pressure (CPAP) to BPAP, the minimum starting EPAP should be set at 4 cm H_2O or the CPAP level at which obstructive apneas were eliminated. An optimal minimum IPAP–EPAP differential is 4 cm H_2O, and an optimal maximum IPAP–EPAP differential is 10 cm H_2O. (*From* Kushida CA, Chediak A, Berry R, et al. Clinical guidelines for the manual titration of positive airway pressure in patients with obstructive sleep apnea. J Clin Sleep Med 2008;4:157–71; with permission.)

PAP mask air leakage can occur in several forms. The mask leak that washes out CO_2 and prevents rebreathing can be termed intentional leak, with the amount of intentional leak dependent on the interface used and the output pressure from the PAP device. Air unintentionally escaping by means of the mouth is called mouth leak, while air that escapes between the mask and the contact on the face or nose can be termed mask leak. A combination of intentional and unintentional leak can be termed total leak, and it is this latter value that most commercially available laboratory titration devices output to either a stand-alone monitor or plot directly on to the polygraph recording. Unintentional mask leak should be minimized by mask refit or readjustment, while unintentional mouth leak may be addressed by adding a chin strap to reduce mouth opening or by switching to a full-face/oronasal mask.[28,29]

The definition of a clinically significant leak during the course of PAP titration is difficult to define. A leak substantially higher than that

recorded at a given pressure from a well-fitted mask in general may be considered unacceptable. The acceptable leak depends on the interface and the applied pressure. The notion that unintentional leak always will exceed intentional leak can be used for laboratories to derive a range of acceptable total leak for a specific PAP mask and pressure. **Table 1** shows the expected intentional leak of selected interfaces at a fixed pressure. The reader is encouraged to contact the individual PAP interface manufacturer to ascertain the intentional leak for other or new interfaces, the latter as they reach the marketplace. Laboratories are encouraged to use the manufacturer-specific leak–pressure relationship for a given interface and clinical judgment to develop laboratory-specific guidelines of acceptable total leak.

POSITIONAL AND SLEEP STAGE FACTORS

As defined earlier, for an optimal PAP titration, the patient should be recorded in supine REM sleep for at least 15 minutes at the designated optimal

Box 2
Specific bilevel positive airway pressure filtration guidelines

In pediatric and adult patients, the recommended minimum starting IPAP and EPAP should be 8 cm H_2O and 4 cm H_2O, respectively. A priori determination of IPAP and EPAP cannot be supported by evidence. Nonetheless, a higher starting IPAP or EPAP is sensible in retitration studies, in those who have very high BMI, and in cases where patients experience air hunger on lower doses of IPAP or EPAP during the pretitration acclimation to BPAP.

The maximum IPAP should be 20 cm H_2O for patients younger than 12 years.

The maximum IPAP should be 30 cm H_2O for patients 12 years of age or older.

The minimum IPAP–EPAP differential should be 4 cm H_2O

The maximum IPAP–EPAP differential should be 10 cm H_2O.

IPAP or EPAP (based on the type of obstructive respiratory event) should be increased by at least 1 cm H_2O apiece with an interval no shorter than 5 minutes, with the goal of eliminating obstructive respiratory events.

Obstructive apnea

In patients younger than 12 years, increase IPAP and EPAP if at least one obstructive apnea is observed.

In patients 12 years of age or older, increase IPAP and EPAP if at least two obstructive apneas are observed.

Obstructive hypopnea

In patients younger than 12 years, increase IPAP if at least one hypopnea is observed.

In patients 12 years of age or older, increase IPAP if at least three hypopneas are observed.

RERA events

In patients younger than 12 years, increase IPAP if at least three RERAs are observed.

In patients 12 years of age or older, increase IPAP if at least five RERAs are observed.

Loud or unambiguous snoring

In patients younger than 12 years, one may increase IPAP if at least 1 minute of loud or unambiguous snoring is observed.

In patients 12 years of age or older, one may increase IPAP if at least 3 minutes of loud or unambiguous snoring are observed.

As described in the guidelines for CPAP titration, exploration of IPAP above the pressure at which control of abnormalities in respiratory parameters is achieved should not exceed 5 cm H_2O.

Exploiting hysteresis during BPAP titration has not been reported. Therefore, specific guidelines for up–down and up–down–up BPAP titration strategies are not offered.

Complaints of excess pressure during the course of BPAP titration may be addressed by resuming the BPAP titration at an IPAP or EPAP pressure at or just below that which the patient reported as uncomfortable.

If central apneas emerge in the course of BPAP titration, a decrease in IPAP or setting BPAP in spontaneous-timed (ST) mode with backup rate may be helpful.

pressure. If the patient is in REM sleep but not in the supine position while at the designated optimal pressure, the patient may be awakened and instructed to lie in the supine position.

Optimal CPAP in the supine position may exceed optimal CPAP while sleeping in the lateral position by 2 cm. This relationship is applicable in REM and non-REM (NREM) sleep, in obese and nonobese subjects and in those younger and older than 60 years.[30] Because treatment-emergent central sleep apnea is more likely to occur in NREM sleep, it is also important to evaluate patients at the designated optimal pressure during NREM sleep.[31–34] Because sleep efficiency is the sole independent PSG parameter that predicts PAP adherence, the decision to awaken the

Table 1
Intentional leak at various pressures (cm H_2O) for selected positive airway pressure interfaces

(a) Intentional leak of selected ResMed interfaces (L/min)[a]

Pressure	Extranasal			Intranasal			Mirage Full-Face/Oronasal	
	Mirage Micro	Mirage Activa	Ultra Mirage II	Swift LT	Swift II	Liberty	Quattro	Ultra
4	19.2	19.2	18.3	20.3	20.3	22.1	22.1	22.1
6	23.7	23.7	24.1	25.2	25.2	27.6	27.6	27.6
8	27.7	27.7	29.4	29.4	29.4	32.3	32.3	32.3
10	31.2	31.2	34.3	33.2	33.2	36.6	36.6	36.6
12	34.4	34.4	38.4	36.7	36.7	40.5	40.5	40.5
14	37.4	37.4	42.6	39.9	39.9	43.5	43.5	43.5
16	40.2	40.2	46.3	42.9	42.9	47.8	47.8	47.8
18	42.8	42.8	49.9	45.8	45.8	51.1	51.1	51.1
20	45.4	45.4	53.1	48.6	48.6	54.3	54.3	54.3

(b) Intentional leak of selected Respironics interfaces (L/min)[b]

Pressure	Extranasal					Intranasal	Full-Face/Oronasal	
	ComfortGel	ComfortSelect	ComfortClassic	Profile Lite	Simplicity	OptiLife	ComfortFull 2	ComfortGel Full[c]
5	17.9	17.9	17.9	17.9	15.6	16.1	18.6	17
10	25.5	25.5	25.5	25.5	22.4	23.1	27.5	26
15	31.4	31.4	31.4	31.4	27.5	28.7	34.2	33
20	36.7	36.7	36.7	36.7	31.9	33.7	39.7	40
25	41.1	41.1	41.1	41.1	35.7	37.9	44.2	45
30	45	45	45	45	39.2	41.7	48.4	50

[a] From http://www.resmed.com/en-us/assets/documents/product/102648-pressure-vs-flow-mask-flow-generator-settings-usa-eng.pdf.
[b] From http://sleepapnea.respironics.com/PDF/LeakRate.pdf.
[c] From ComfortGel (Murrysville, Pennsylvania) FULL instructions for use.

patient to sample supine REM must be considered in the light of potentially altering the value of sleep efficiency as a predictor of long-term PAP use.

SUMMARY

PAP therapy continues to be the most widely prescribed treatment for adult OSA, and PAP increasingly is offered to pediatric patients who have OSA. The current standard of practice involves performing attended PSG for the manual titration of PAP therapy. This article set out to provide a practical framework by which to manually titrate PAP therapy (CPAP and BPAP) during a laboratory PSG. Most of the recommendations and guidelines within this treatment on PAP titration have been derived by consensus with reliance on the relatively sparse available evidence for scientific review. The interested reader is referred to the AASM Positive Airway Pressure Titration Task Force publication[1] for details regarding the evidence-based and consensus findings behind the recommended approach for the manual titration of PAP during attended in-laboratory PSG.

REFERENCES

1. Juhasz J. The fine art of CPAP titration—will it ever become obsolete? Sleep Breath 2007;11:65–7.
2. Stepanski EJ. The need for a standardized CPAP titration protocol and follow-up procedures. J Clin Sleep Med 2005;1:311.
3. Stepanski EJ, Dull R, Basner RC. CPAP titration protocols among accredited sleep disorders centers. J Sleep Res 1996;25:374.
4. Mokhlesi B, Tulaimat A. Recent advances in obesity hypoventilation syndrome. Chest 2007;132:1322–6.
5. Weist GH, Fuchs FS, Harsch IA, et al. Reproducibility of a standardized titration procedure for the initiation of continuous positive airway pressure therapy in patients with obstructive sleep apnoea. Respiration 2001;68:145–50.
6. Berthon-Jones M, Lawrence S, Sullivan CE, et al. Nasal continuous positive airway pressure treatment: current realities and future. Sleep 1996; 19(Suppl 9):S131–5.
7. Kushida CA, Chediak AD, Berry RB, et al. Clinical guidelines for the manual titration of positive airway pressure in patients with obstructive sleep apnea. J Clin Sleep Med 2008;4:157–71.
8. Sullivan CE, Issa FG, Berthon-Jones M, et al. Home treatment of obstructive sleep apnoea with continuous positive airway pressure applied to a nosemask. Bull Eur Physiopathol Respir 1984;20:49–54.
9. Sforza E, Krieger J, Bacon W, et al. Determinates up effective continuous positive airway pressure in obstructive sleep apnea. Role of respiratory effort. Am J Respir Crit Care Med 1995;151:1852–6.
10. Nino-Murcia G, McCann CC, Bliwise DL, et al. Compliance and side effects in sleep apnea patients treated with nasal continuous positive airway pressure. West J Med 1989;150:165–9.
11. Miljeteig H, Hoffstein V. Determinants of continuous positive airway pressure level for treatment of obstructive sleep apnea. Am Rev Respir Dis 1993;147:1526–30.
12. Pevernagie DA, Shepherd JW Jr. Relations between sleep stage, posture and effective nasal CPAP levels in OSA. Sleep 1992;5:162–7.
13. Hoffstein V, Mateika S. Predicting nasal continuous positive airway pressure. Am J Respir Crit Care Med 1994;150:486–8.
14. Rowley JA, Tarbichi AG, Badr MS. The use of a predicted CPAP equation improves CPAP titration success. Sleep Breath 2005;9:26–32.
15. Gokcebay N, Hirshkowitz M. Optimal CPAP: titration versus. formula. Sleep 1997;20:237–8.
16. Slifer KJ, Kruglak D, Benore E, et al. Behavioral training for increasing preschool children's adherence with positive airway pressure: a preliminary study. Behav Sleep Med 2007;5:147–75.
17. Sleep-related breathing disorders in adults: recommendations for syndrome definition and measurement techniques and clinical research. The report of an American Academy of Sleep Medicine Task Force. Sleep 1999;22:667–89.
18. Iber C, et al. The AASM manual for the scoring of sleep and associated events: rules, terminology and technical specifications. 2. Westchester (NY): American Academy of Sleep Medicine; 2007.
19. Montgomery-Downs HE, O'Brien LM, Gulliver TE, et al. Polysomnographic characteristics in normal preschool and early school-aged children. Pediatrics 2006;117:741–53.
20. Silva RS, Truksinas V, de Mello-Fujita L, et al. An orientation session improves objective sleep quality and mask acceptance during positive airway pressure titration. Sleep Breath 2008;12:85–9.
21. Krakow B, Ulibarri V, Melendrez D, et al. A daytime, abbreviated cardiorespiratory sleep study (CPT 95807-52) to acclimate insomnia patients with sleep disordered breathing to positive airway pressure (PAP-NAP). J Clin Sleep Med 2008;4:212–22.
22. Marcus CL, Ward SL, Mallory GB, et al. Use of nasal continuous positive airway pressure as treatment of childhood obstructive sleep apnea. J Pediatr 1995; 127:88–94.
23. Rains JC. Treatment of obstructive sleep apnea in pediatric patients. Behavioral intervention for compliance with nasal continuous positive airway pressure. Clin Pediatr (Phila) 1995;35:535–41.
24. Montserrat JM, et al. Time-course of stepwise CPAP titration. Behavior of respiratory and neurological variables. Am J Respir Crit Care Med 1995;152:1854–9.

25. Guilleminault C, Stoohs R, Clerk A, et al. A cause of excessive daytime sleepiness. The upper airways resistance syndrome. Chest 1993;104:781–7.

26. Condos R, Norman RG, Krishnasamy I, et al. Flow limitation as a noninvasive assessment of residual upper-airway resistance during continuous positive airway pressure therapy of obstructive sleep apnea. Am J Respir Crit Care Med 1994;150:475–80.

27. Bureau MP, Series F. Comparison of two in-laboratory titration methods to determine effective pressure levels in patients with obstructive sleep apnoea. Thorax 2000;55:741–5.

28. Schwartz AR, Kacmarek RM, Hess DR. Factors affecting oxygen delivery with bilevel positive airway pressure. Respir Care 2004;49:270–5.

29. Berry RB. Medical therapy. In: Johnson JT, Gluckman JL, Sanders MH, editors. Obstructive sleep apnea. London: Martin Dunniz; 2002. p. 89–118.

30. Oksenberg A, Silverberg DS, Arons E, et al. The sleep supine position has a major effect on optimal nasal continuous positive airway pressure: relationship with rapid eye movements and non-rapid eye movements sleep, body mass index, respiratory disturbance index, and age. Chest 1999;116:1000–6.

31. Gilmartin GS, Daly RW, Thomas RJ. Recognition and management of complex sleep-disordered breathing. Curr Opin Pulm Med 2005;11:485–93.

32. Hoheisel GB, Teschler H. Clinical parameters for the prescription of minimally effective CPAP for the treatment of obstructive sleep apnea. Am J Respir Crit Care Med 1994;149:A496.

33. Goodwin JL, Kaemingk KL, Fregosi RF, et al. Clinical outcomes associated with sleep-disordered breathing in Caucasian and Hispanic children—the Tucson Children's Assessment of Sleep Apnea study (TuCASA). Sleep 2003;26:587–91.

34. Montserrat JM, Alarcon A, Lloberes P, et al. Adequacy of prescribing nasal continuous positive airway pressure therapy for sleep apnoea/hypopnoea syndrome on the basis of nighttime respiratory recording variables. Thorax 1995;50:967–71.

The Future of Sleep and Circadian Testing

David P. White, MD[a,b,*]

KEYWORDS

- Sleep • Diagnostic • Circadian • Future • Therapy

In looking back over the last 20 to 30 years, there has been very little actual progress in sleep testing, while circadian monitoring has not evolved into the clinical arena at all. That is not to say that the number of sleep laboratories/centers has not multiplied many fold over the last 25 years. That is certainly the case. Other than transitioning from paper recordings to digital ones, however, the standard polysomnogram (PSG) has remained very much the same over this span of years both in terms of the signals recorded and the methods used to score such records. Why so little progress has been made is arguable. At least part of the problem, however, likely has been that standard polysomnography has increasingly been used and well-reimbursed, leaving little motivation to change the status quo. This does not seem to be the case any longer, with several forces pushing for new methodologies that, in the end, will benefit both patients and sleep physicians. I will speculate here as to where these changes will take sleep physicians.

There is not space in this article to even attempt to cover all of the changes in sleep/circadian testing that will evolve in the years ahead. This is particularly the case as relates to specific sleep disorders. Thus examples will be given using a single sleep disorder or a single method of testing that could then be extrapolated to other disease processes or approaches to evaluation. Thus no attempt will be made to be exhaustive or comprehensive.

TESTING IN THE SLEEP LABORATORY
Sleep Disorders

Current polysomnographic testing in the sleep laboratory generally has yielded diagnostic information and has addressed a relatively limited number of disorders, with most such testing being conducted to diagnose obstructive sleep apnea (OSA). This testing also is used for initiating therapy (continuous positive airway pressure titration) and occasionally to assess therapeutic efficacy (eg, success of upper airway surgery). Standard polysomnography, however, is not used realistically to predict outcomes, as current measures of sleep fragmentation and disruption do not predict sleepiness or performance with any degree of accuracy.[1,2] Thus the sleep measures resulting from the standard PSG are not used commonly either diagnostically or therapeutically.

In the future, this must change. By the use of shorter-duration epochs, computer assessments of electroencephalogram (EEG) frequency, amplitude, and pattern, and both linear and nonlinear dynamic approaches, it seems feasible that more viable measures of sleep continuity and sleep disruption will emerge. These measures then can be used to assess the impact of a sleep disorder, such as periodic limb movement disorder, on sleep quality or the efficacy of a therapy, such as a hypnotic, on improving sleep. It would be presumptuous to try to outline the methods that will be used to accomplish such quantification of sleep in this article. Without marked improvement in the current measures, however, home diagnostics will become the dominant method by which all sleep disorders are diagnosed and followed, with little real use for direct measures of sleep. If such methodologies are developed, however, it seems likely that:

- A broader range of sleep disorders and totally new disease processes can be identified and diagnosed in the sleep laboratory.

[a] Division of Sleep Medicine, Department of Medicine, Brigham and Women's Hospital, 221 Longwood Ave, Boston, MA, USA
[b] Philips Respironics, 1505 Commonwealth Avenue, Suite # 420, Boston, MA 02135, USA
* Philips Respironics, 1505 Commonwealth Avenue, Suite # 420, Boston, MA 02135.
E-mail address: dpwhite@partners.org

Sleep Med Clin 4 (2009) 455–463
doi:10.1016/j.jsmc.2009.04.009

- The effects of a given sleep disorder on sleepiness and performance during wakefulness can be predicted based on the sleep study.
- Follow-up to assess the resolution of an abnormal sleep process or disruptor of sleep will be possible.

Phenotyping in the Sleep Laboratory

Although diagnosing a sleep disorder may be sufficiently straight-forward that it can be accomplished routinely in the home with relatively few signals, more complex testing in the laboratory may yield valuable additional information that allows for a more sophisticated or individualized approach to therapy. OSA will be used as the example. There are likely four or five anatomic/physiologic traits in a given individual that predict whether that person will have or develop OSA.[3] These traits likely vary substantially from one patient to the next, meaning that patients may have sleep apnea for quite different reasons. These traits likely include:

- pharyngeal anatomy (Pcrit, critical closing pressure, **Fig. 1**)
- pharyngeal muscle responsiveness during sleep and the ability of these muscles to dilate the airway
- the arousal threshold to a respiratory stimulus
- loop gain, a measure of respiratory control stability (**Fig. 2**).

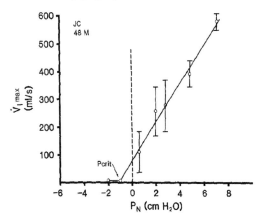

Fig. 1. Maximal airflow (Vimax) versus nasal pressure (Pn) is shown for a representative obstructive sleep apnea (OSA) patient. The figure demonstrates a Pcrit of -1.2 cm H_2O (defined by the nasal pressure at which airflow ceases). Vimax during tidal breathing at atmospheric Pn is shown by the level of flow at the intercept with the vertical dashed line. Each point represents the mean + SD for breaths sampled at each level of Pn shown. (*From* Gleadhill IC, Schwartz AR, Schubert N, et al. Upper airway collapsibility in snorers and in patients with obstructive hypopnea and apnea. Am Rev Res Dis 1991;143(6):1301; with permission. Copyright © 1991 American Thoracic Society.)

When one combines: (1) a carefully controlled nasal airway pressure device with the ability to generate both positive and negative airway pressure, (2) a smart data acquisition system with well-defined algorithms, and (3) real-time automated sleep staging, it seems probable that each of these traits could be defined accurately in a single night in a patient who has OSA. Doing so would be valuable only if these measures predicted responses to certain forms of therapy or other outcomes of the disorder. Individualization of therapy for OSA based on these traits seems quite possible in the relatively near future, however. An easy example would be loop gain. If loop gain is quite high (very unstable ventilatory control) and is the principle cause of the apnea, reducing loop gain could be accomplished with oxygen administration[4] at night or daily acetazolamide. Either could be tolerated better or more easily than many of the currently available therapies.

These same principles may apply to other sleep disorders also. If insomnia could be phenotyped more accurately allowing for quantitative assessment of hyperarousal, circadian phase, anxiety, or comorbidities, the entire approach to therapy might change, allowing for more focused strategies, be they behavioral or pharmacologic.

This concept likely applies to primary hypersomnia and central sleep apnea among others.

Assessing Psychiatric/Neurological Disease by Monitoring Brain Activity During Sleep

Although virtually all testing currently conducted in the sleep laboratory addresses sleep itself or disorders of sleep, recent work by Tononi[5,6] and his investigative team suggests that sleep may provide an opportunity to examine brain function that is impossible during wakefulness. Using 256 lead EEG and sophisticated signal processing, they have made a number of novel observations. First,[5] they observed that learning is a very focal neurological process that can be monitored during sleep on the night after the learning task. Following a rotation motor learning task with simultaneous positron emission tomography (PET) imaging, the subjects slept with the 256 lead EEG monitoring configuration. The principle observation was increased slow wave activity over the cortical site demonstrated by PET to be involved in the learning process. There was a direct correlation between the increase in slow wave activity and the improvement in the motor task the next day. Tononi interprets the slow wave activity to represent synaptic decompression, which is, he believes, one of the fundamental functions of sleep. On a more practical level, however, a fundamental brain function,

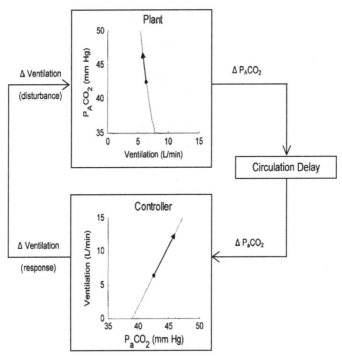

Fig. 2. Demonstrated is the respiratory control loop, the gain of which is referred to as loop gain. The main components are the plant gain (change in PCO_2 per unit change in ventilation, Ve), the controller gain (change in ventilation for each unit change in arterial PCO_2), and the circulatory delay (time for blood to move from the lung to the chemoreceptors [central and peripheral]). Thus a respiratory disturbance will be translated into a respiratory response based on the gain of the loop.

learning or memory consolidation, could be monitored during sleep.

The second observation using this technique[6] has even more obvious clinical relevance and addresses the disorder schizophrenia. Currently the diagnosis of schizophrenia is made largely based on clinical criteria without an effective objective test. Using the high-resolution 256 lead EEG approach, Tononi and his colleagues examined brain activity during sleep in a group of treated schizophrenics and compared the results with those obtained in healthy controls and subjects with a history of depression. The results showed a significant reduction in centroparietal EEG power from 13.75 to 15.0 Hz in the schizophrenic patients when compared to both control groups (**Fig. 3**). They also observed a significant reduction in sleep spindle number, amplitude, and duration in the schizophrenia patients in the same anatomic location when compared with the healthy and depressed controls. No difference in either variable was found between the healthy controls and the depressed subjects. Finally, they found that integrated spindle activity provided a greater than 90% ability to separate the schizophrenia patients from both control groups. This would suggest that this approach may be a sensitive and specific

method by which to diagnose schizophrenia. A more recent study[7] assessed the evoked response in the EEG (again using the 256 lead approach) to transcranial magnetic stimulation (TMS) in schizophrenic patients versus healthy controls. As is the previous study, clear differences between groups were evident, particularly in the frontal cortex in the first 100 milliseconds after stimulation. This again suggests the utility of such testing in the schizophrenic population.

Whether this 256 lead EEG approach or others similar to it can be used during sleep to diagnose other psychiatric or neurological disorders is unclear. As stated by Tononi, however, "spontaneous brain rhythms during sleep reflect brain function unconfounded by attention and motivation." Thus it seems likely that this methodology could evolve into a standard clinical tool with the test administered in the sleep laboratory, while the results address disorders not classically thought of as relating to sleep.

IMAGING IN SLEEP MEDICINE

Predicting the role imaging will take in future sleep testing is difficult, but several possibilities seem reasonable. As functional imaging (eg, PET, fMRI,

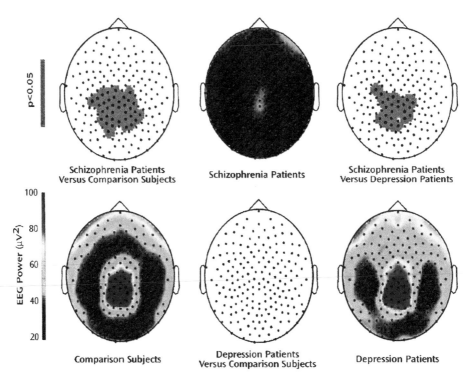

Fig. 3. White plots: topographical distribution of the electrodes showing significant power reduction (*gray*) at 13.75 to 15.00 Hz in schizophrenia versus comparison and schizophrenia versus depressed but not depressed versus comparison subjects. Color plots: topographical distribution of mean electroencephalogram (EEG) power at 13.75 to 15.00 Hz during the first non-rapid eye movement sleep episode in schizophrenia (N = 18), comparison (N = 17), and depressed (N = 15) subjects. Values (*color bar*) were plotted at the corresponding electrode position (*dots*) on the planar projection of the scalp surface. The schizophrenia subjects had significantly reduced power in the areas shown, while the other groups (comparison and depressed) did not differ from each other. (*From* Ferrarelli F, Huber R, Peterson MJ, et al. Reduced sleep spindle activity in schizophrenia patients. Am J Psychiatry 2007;164(3):487; with permission.)

single photon emission computed tomography) evolves into improved spatial and temporal resolution, the ability to use these methodologies to precisely evaluate brain activity awake and asleep in patients with a variety of sleep disorders will increase.[8] An obvious example would be insomnia. Functional imaging could be used to:

- aid differential diagnosis as different patterns of brain activation may characterize insomnia secondary to hyperarousal[9] versus depression[10] or other causes,
- assess treatment response by demonstrating changes in regional brain activity awake or asleep in response to a given intervention,
- select the best pharmacologic agent based on the individual's focus of abnormal brain activity and how this activity is affected by specific drugs.

Thus patients who have insomnia may undergo such imaging as the first step in their evaluation for diagnostic and therapeutic reasons. The other

obvious area for future imaging would be the pharyngeal airway in patients who have OSA. To date, such imaging has been helpful scientifically, but has provided little guidance clinically in managing individual patients.[11] The problems have been that the images are largely static, cannot reasonably be gathered during sleep, and are quite expensive. Dynamic MRI of the pharyngeal airway during sleep, however, could provide highly useful information regarding site of collapse, extent of collapse (length of collapsing airway segment), and possibly even localized tissue movement/deformation. These results could be used to guide surgery, surgical implants, and possibly other device-related therapies. As MRI and other dynamic imaging approaches continue to improve, such testing seems possible.

Whether imaging will have a role in diagnosing or managing disorders such as narcolepsy,[12] idiopathic hypersomnia, or movement disorders during sleep[13] is less clear. As the neurobiology of these disorders becomes understood better, however, a role for functional imaging may emerge.

CIRCADIAN TESTING

Circadian biology, although quite advanced at the basic science and physiologic level,[14] has not found its way into clinical practice in a meaningful way. The main cause for this probably relates, at least in part, to the fact that there is no readily available test to define circadian phase. Thus, the only way to identify a circadian abnormality is from the history obtained from the patient. This probably works reasonably well for overt circadian disorders, but many more subtle abnormalities likely are missed. Also, the primary method by which circadian phase can be manipulated or corrected is light,[15] which is cumbersome to administer. In addition, without clear information on circadian phase, when light should be administered to a given patient is largely guesswork.

This speaks to the imperative to develop a clinical test for circadian phase.

In the research setting, circadian phase is delineated most commonly using the dim light melatonin onset (DLMO) (**Fig. 4**).[16] This generally involves measuring plasma or salivary melatonin levels every 30 to 60 minutes with the subject lying in dim light or wearing goggles to block light exposure in the relevant wave lengths. As salivary levels are as useful as plasma, there would seem to be no particular reason why a kit could not be developed that would allow for multiple, timed saliva collections that could be sent to a laboratory for subsequent analysis. Whether this evaluation could be accomplished best and most reliably in the sleep laboratory or the home is probably arguable. The rapid evolution of such testing, however, would seem to be an imperative in this field. Once

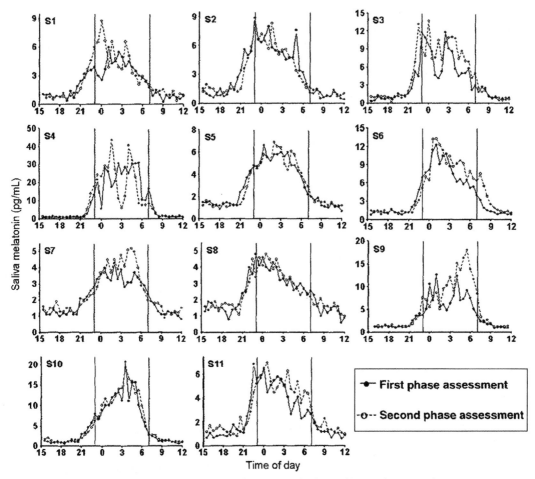

Fig. 4. Salivary melatonin profiles are shown for 11 subjects. In each, the profile was determined on two occasions separated by 1 week. The two vertical lines represent scheduled, weekday bedtime (23:00 hours) and wake time (07:00 hours). As can be seen, the determinations were quite consistent over time. (*From* Revell VL, Kim H, Tseng CY, et al. Circadian phase determined from melatonin profiles is reproducible after 1 week in subjects who sleep later on weekends. J Pineal Res 2005;39:198; with permission.)

such objective testing becomes available, its use in insomnia patients in whom the cause is not completely clear and in patients who have a suspected circadian rhythm disorder both to confirm the diagnosis and to guide the timing of light exposure would seem to be initial logical uses for such an evaluation. Others likely would evolve quickly. Finally, once the circadian phase is known, continuous monitoring of both actigraphy and light exposure likely would allow for the longitudinal monitoring of sleep and circadian phase, which could be quite useful in shift workers, some patients who have insomnia, and individuals who have frequent travel across multiple time zones.

Clinical testing of the circadian period, although not as urgent as circadian phase, probably will also evolve without great difficulty and likely will provide useful clinical information. Knowledge of the circadian period could explain circadian preference and, in some cases, the cause of a circadian rhythm abnormality. Such information likely would have therapeutic implications also. Determining the circadian period in a given individual in a research laboratory is a long and laborious process and does not lend itself to clinical utilization.[17] Individual circadian period, however, may be determined from dermal fibroblasts using a lentivirally delivered reporter system.[18] The amplitude of the circadian system and its ability to be phase-shifted or entrained to environmental signals also may be assessed in these cells. As a result, a wealth of clinically useful information could be derived from these cell cultures. If a sleep physician knew the circadian phase, period, amplitude, and susceptibility to phase shifting in a patient with a possible circadian rhythm abnormality, the ability to manage that patient would be improved immensely. Thus, several forms of circadian testing are likely the most near-term and clinically useful new evaluations for the clinical sleep field.

SLEEP DEPRIVATION AND PERFORMANCE

Acute sleep deprivation and chronic sleep deprivation have become increasingly common everywhere and have the potential to not only affect the health[19] and performance[20] of the afflicted individual, but also the safety of the sleep-deprived person and those around him or her. The safety issue surrounding this rapidly evolving problem could be addressed, at least in part, by two forms of testing:

- Fitness to perform (ie monitoring variables that influence sleep/circadian-based performance prior to a job [work shift] during which vigilance is required)

- A continuous measure of sleepiness or drowsiness

Fitness to perform monitoring ideally would include measures of previous sleep duration (over several nights), time since last sleep (to control for sleep inertia and the duration of the current period of wakefulness), and circadian phase. Most of this information could be obtained from an actigraph worn continuously in combination with one determination of the DLMO, as circadian phase is likely to be stable. Algorithms then could be generated to analyze this information and predict the level of performance or potential for a sleepiness-related error. There is obviously considerable individual variability in nightly sleep need, impact of sleep deprivation on performance, and sleep inertia. If properly calibrated, however, fairly simple devices could provide very useful information regarding an individual's ability to perform well in a job requiring sustained attention for a relatively long period of time. Such testing could be accomplished in the very near future.

A continuous measure of sleepiness also would have great value in any job requiring sustained vigilance or outside the workplace while driving. Several such devices have been developed over the years with quite variable success. An example of such a device would be infrared reflectance oculography, which provides a continuous measure of eye lid motion/position from an infra red sensor attached to a pair of glasses, combined with an algorithm that predicts sleepiness based on eyelid closure and reopening times/variability.[21] Although certainly not perfect, this particular device has a reasonable ability to detect sleepiness before frank sleep onset and could be programmed to intervene or alert the individual to prevent an accident or injury. This type of testing would have wide applicability in many settings in which sustained vigilance is required.

Programs and devices designed to monitor/document sleep loss and quantify sleepiness as described previously, would be best organized, distributed, and interpreted by sleep physicians who understand the strengths and weaknesses of the techniques and can guide their use into appropriate channels. As we become an increasingly 24-hour society, the need for such techniques is likely to be substantial.

SLEEP TESTING/SCREENING IN THE HOME

In the years ahead, there is likely to be substantial sleep testing, monitoring, and screening done in the home with several examples having been described already. Home testing not only allows for this assessment in a more natural sleep environment, but in many cases makes it possible to monitor the individual over several nights, which is likely to provide more complete and representative information. Such testing likely would fall into several categories, which will be discussed in the following sections.

Diagnostic Testing

There is already a great deal of sleep apnea diagnostic testing being conducted in the home, with most devices utilized in this role simply recording standard respiratory signals with or without some measure of sleep.[22] This practice is likely to increase and rapidly become the standard method by which disorders of breathing during sleep are diagnosed. This may be accomplished with sensors attached to the subject as is now generally the case, or by the use of specialized materials placed on the surface of the bed that can detect movement, respiration, and heart rate.[23] Video recording also may have a role in the future. Circadian sleep disorders likely will be diagnosed with actigraphs or easily utilized monitors of sleep/wake, with such testing again being conducted primarily in the home.[24] This may require assessment of the DLMO, for which samples also could be obtained easily in the home setting. These approaches also apply to insomnia. Combined, time-synched, multinight recordings of EEG and video from the bedroom at home could be quite useful in diagnosing parasomnias, movement disorders, and seizures. Thus, most sleep and circadian disorders likely will be diagnosed more conveniently and effectively in the home setting.

Sleep Monitoring

In some disorders, with insomnia being an obvious example, monitoring of sleep over a longer period of time (weeks to months) can yield useful diagnostic information or actively assess ongoing therapy. This can be accomplished at this time with actigraphs from which several weeks of sleep/wake information can be obtained easily.[25] In time, more complete sleep monitoring with full sleep staging likely will be possible with easily utilized dry electrodes.[26] Thus, on a nightly basis, a physician could follow the sleep of his or her patient, making interventions as required. Such monitoring devices likely will move into the consumer market, such that people can follow their own sleep duration and quality, adjusting their habits and lifestyles as needed to improve their sleep and subsequently their quality of life. As a result, chronic, home-based sleep monitoring likely will become quite common in the future and will require either individual or algorithmic guidance from the sleep physician.

Screening for Sleep Disorders

Active screening for sleep disorders likely will not come into general practice until there is clear evidence that the disorder, if untreated, leads to adverse health consequences, and there are acceptable, effective therapies available. The only sleep disorder that could fill both of these criteria in the near future would be sleep apnea. If current and future studies demonstrate an indisputable association between sleep apnea and adverse cardiovascular outcomes,[27] then home-based screening likely would evolve rapidly. Such screening could be home-based monitoring using only a few signals or utilize a biomarker if such a test can be developed. Screening for other sleep disorders seems unlikely in the near future.

GENETIC TESTING

How genetic testing will be used for diagnosing and managing sleep disorders is controversial. There are several possibilities, however:

- Genetic predisposition to disease is a well-established phenomenon and has been demonstrated in people who have narcolepsy and restless leg syndrome (RLS).[28] Genes predisposing to parasomnias like sleep paralysis, sleep walking, or the disorder Klein Levin syndrome seem probable based on existing family studies. Genetic causes for circadian rhythm abnormalities have been demonstrated in a few families.[29] Whether these genetic associations are strong enough to have meaningful diagnostic utility is unclear at this time.
- Understanding the pathophysiology of various disease processes (like OSA) likely will result from genetic approaches such as genome-wide association studies.[30] Such testing therefore may be able to distinguish the different routes by which an individual develops sleep apnea, allowing for different therapeutic approaches based on the phenotypic information.
- The susceptibility to the complications of sleep disorders also may depend highly on individual genetics. An example would be the cardiovascular complications of OSA. As the risk for cardiovascular disease in general is known to have a genetic basis, who develops these complications in OSA is likely genetic also. Thus, an asymptomatic OSA patient who has a high genetic

risk for cardiovascular disease might receive therapy when this would not be the case otherwise.

- Individual susceptibility to important decrements in performance from sleep deprivation may vary substantially based on genetics.[31] Thus, genetic testing could be used to select individuals for jobs during which vigilance is required yet adequate sleep may not always be possible.

Thus, genetic testing in sleep medicine may become quite common, as will be the case in most areas of medicine.

SUMMARY

Although sleep testing has been somewhat limited, with a focus on one procedure (PSG) with circadian testing being virtually nonexistent, the future possibilities seem promising and exciting. Clinically available methods to define circadian phase and period stand to remarkably improve sleep physicians' ability to care for patients who have circadian abnormalities and to lead to a substantially better understanding of these disorders. Improved techniques to measure and quantify sleep itself will allow for more meaningful assessment of sleep disruption, and lead to both the recognition of new disorders and better predictions of the outcomes of these disorders. Sleep also may provide a window on the brain, allowing for understanding of certain diseases not possible from recordings made during wakefulness. Genetic testing and imaging, now actively used clinically in many fields, need to evolve in the sleep arena to provide improved insights into both disease pathophysiology and hopefully new therapies. Thus, there is potential for remarkable advances if sleep physicians can both recognize these possibilities and not remain mired in the past.

REFERENCES

1. Roehrs T, Zorick F, Wittig R, et al. Predictors of objective level of daytime sleepiness in patients with sleep-related breathing disorders. Chest 1989; 95(6):1202–6.
2. Bennett LS, Langford BA, Stradling JR, et al. Sleep fragmentation indices as predictors of daytime sleepiness and nCPAP response in obstructive sleep apnea. Am J Respir Crit Care Med 1998; 158(3):778–86.
3. White DP. Pathogenesis of obstructive and central sleep apnea. Am J Respir Crit Care Med 2005; 172(11):1363–70.
4. Wellman A, Malhotra A, Jordan AS, et al. Effect of oxygen in obstructive sleep apnea: role of loop gain. Respir Physiol Neurobiol 2008;162(2):144–51.
5. Huber R, Ghilardi MF, Massimini M, et al. Local sleep and learning. Nature 2004;430(6995):78–81.
6. Ferrarelli F, Huber R, Peterson MJ, et al. Reduced sleep spindle activity in schizophrenia patients. Am J Psychiatry 2007;164(3):483–92.
7. Ferrarelli F, Massimini M, Peterson MJ, et al. Reduced evoked gamma oscillations in the frontal cortex in schizophrenia patients: a TMS/EEG study. Am J Psychiatry 2008;165(8):996–1005.
8. Desseilles M, Dang-Vu T, Schabus M, et al. Neuroimaging insights into the pathophysiology of sleep disorders. Sleep 2008;31(6):777–94.
9. Nofzinger EA, Buysse DJ, Germain A, et al. Functional neuroimaging evidence for hyperarousal in insomnia. Am J Psychiatry 2004;161(11):2126–8.
10. Milak MS, Parsey RV, Keilp J, et al. Neuroanatomic correlates of psychopathologic components of major depressive disorder. Arch Gen Psychiatry 2005;62(4):397–408.
11. Schwab RJ, Pasirstein M, Pierson R, et al. Identification of upper airway anatomic risk factors for obstructive sleep apnea with volumetric magnetic resonance imaging. Am J Respir Crit Care Med 2003;168(5):522–30.
12. Draganski B, Geisler P, Hajak G, et al. Hypothalamic gray matter changes in narcoleptic patients. Nat Med 2002;8(11):1186–8.
13. Michaud M, Soucy JP, Chabli A, et al. SPECT imaging of striatal pre- and postsynaptic dopaminergic status in restless legs syndrome with periodic leg movements in sleep. J Neurol 2002;249(2):164–70.
14. Czeisler CA, Gooley JJ. Sleep and circadian rhythms in humans. Cold Spring Harb Symp Quant Biol 2007;72:579–97.
15. Duffy JF, Wright KP Jr. Entrainment of the human circadian system by light. J Biol Rhythms 2005; 20(4):326–38.
16. Lewy AJ. The dim light melatonin onset, melatonin assays, and biological rhythm research in humans. Biol Signals Recept 1999;8:79–83.
17. Czeisler CA, Duffy JF, Shanahan TL, et al. Stability, precision, and near-24-hour period of the human circadian pacemaker. Science 1999;284(5423): 2177–81.
18. Brown SA, Kunz D, Dumas A, et al. Molecular insights into human daily behavior. Proc Natl Acad Sci U S A 2008;105(5):1602–7.
19. Knutson KL, Spiegel K, Penev P, et al. The metabolic consequences of sleep deprivation. Sleep Med Rev 2007;11(3):163–78.
20. Czeisler CA. Sleep deficit: the performance killer. A conversation with Harvard Medical School Professor Charles A. Czeisler. Harv Bus Rev 2006;84(10):53–9, 148.

21. Michael N, Johns M, Owen C, et al. Effects of caffeine on alertness as measured by infrared reflectance oculography. Psychopharmacology (Berl) 2008;200(2):255–60.

22. Collop NA, Anderson WM, Boehlecke B, et al. Clinical guidelines for the use of unattended portable monitors in the diagnosis of obstructive sleep apnea in adult patients. Portable Monitoring Task Force of the American Academy of Sleep Medicine. J Clin Sleep Med 2007;3(7):737–47.

23. Polo O, Brissaud L, Sales B, et al. The validity of the static charge sensitive bed in detecting obstructive sleep apnoeas. Eur Respir J 1988;1(4):330–6.

24. Morgenthaler TI, Lee-Chiong T, Alessi C, et al. Practice parameters for the clinical evaluation and treatment of circadian rhythm sleep disorders. An American Academy of Sleep Medicine report. Sleep 2007;30(11):1445–59.

25. Morgenthaler T, Alessi C, Friedman L, et al. Practice parameters for the use of actigraphy in the assessment of sleep and sleep disorders: an update for 2007. Sleep 2007;30(4):519–29.

26. Wright K, Johnstone J, Febregas S, et al. Evaluation of a portable dry sensor based on autonomatic sleep monitoring system. Sleep 2008;31:A337.

27. Marin JM, Carrizo SJ, Vicente E, et al. Long-term cardiovascular outcomes in men with obstructive sleep apnoea–hypopnoea with or without treatment with continuous positive airway pressure: an observational study. Lancet 2005;365(9464): 1046–53.

28. Schormair B, Kemlink D, Roeske D, et al. PTPRD (protein tyrosine phosphatase receptor type delta) is associated with restless legs syndrome. Nat Genet 2008;40(8):946–8.

29. Toh KL, Jones CR, He Y, et al. An hPer2 phosphorylation site mutation in familial advanced sleep phase syndrome. Science 2001;291(5506):1040–3.

30. Palmer LJ, Buxbaum SG, Larkin E, et al. A whole-genome scan for obstructive sleep apnea and obesity. Am J Hum Genet 2003;72(2):340–50.

31. Viola AU, Archer SN, James LM, et al. PER3 polymorphism predicts sleep structure and waking performance. Curr Biol 2007;17(7):613–8.

Index

Note: Page numbers of article titles are in **boldface** type.

A

Actigraphy, in diagnosis of nocturnal movements, 362

Action potential, of a neuron, 324

Airflow measurement, in diagnosis of
  sleep-disordered breathing, 353–354
    nasal pressure cannula, 354
    pneumotachograph, 354
    thermal technology, 353–354
  in polysomnography, 337

Airflow monitoring, in pediatric polysomnography, 399

Ambulatory polysomnography, pediatric, 398

Amplifiers, differential, and associated filters, 328–331

Anxiety disorders, and treatments for, polysomnographic features of, 412–413

Apnea. *See* Sleep apnea.

Architecture, sleep, drug effects on, 410–411
  in pediatric polysomnography scoring, 402–404

Arousals, confusional, nocturnal movement in, 365
  in pediatric polysomnography scoring, 404

Arterial blood gas, measurement of gas exchange with, 356

Artifacts, on polysomnography, **423–436**
  identifying, 423–424
  nonphysiologic, 424–426
    at 60Hz, 424
    channel blocking, 426
    electrode popping, 424–425
    electromagnetic interference, 424
    equipment malfunction, 426
    implanted medical device, 426
    moisture artifact, 425–426
  optimizing analysis, 434–436
    channel inversion, 435
    electrode selector feature, 434
    filters and sensitivity, 434
    montage display, 435
  physiologic, 426–433
    electrocardiogram artifact, 429–430
    eye movement artifact, 431
    movement intrusion, 428–429
    muscle intrusion, 426–428
    sweat sway, 431–433
  troubleshooting, 433–434

B

Balloons, esophageal pressure measurement of respiratory effort with, 355

Benign epilepsy of childhood, with centrotemporal spikes, nocturnal movement in, 367–368

Benign sleep myoclonus of infancy, nocturnal movement in, 369

Bilevel positive airway pressure, manual titration of, in patients with obstructive sleep apnea, **445–455**

Bipotentials, recording of, 325–326

Body position, in pediatric polysomnography, 402

Brain activity, history of physiologic recordings of, 313
  laboratory assessment of psychiatric/neurologic disease by monitoring during sleep, future of, 458–459

Breathing disorders, sleep-related, nocturnal movement in, 370

Bruxism, sleep-related, diagnostic features, 364
  polysomnographic findings, 364

C

Capnometry, in pediatric polysomnography, 401–402

Carbon dioxide, gas exchange measurement, 356
  arterial blood gas, 356
  end tidal, 356
  transcutaneous, 356

Cardiac monitoring, during sleep, **373–384**
  clinical scenarios, 377–380
    Cheyne-Stokes breathing, 378–380
    obstructive sleep apnea, 377–378
    risk of sudden cardiac death, 377
  normal cardiac rhythm changes during sleep, 374–377
  standardized methods, 380–381
    data acquisition and display, 380–381
    reporting cardiac activity, 381
    scoring of cardiac events, 381

Cardiac rhythm evaluation, during sleep, by electrocardiography, 338–339

Cardiovascular disease, and treatments for, polysomnographic features of, 415–416

Central apnea, pediatric, polysomnography for, 395–396

Central hypoventilation syndrome, pediatric, polysomnography for, 395–396

sleep.theclinics.com

Channel blocking, artifacts on polysomnography due to, 426

Channel inversion, avoiding polysomnography artifacts with, 435

Cheyne-Stokes breathing, cardiac monitoring during polysomnography in patients with, 378–380

Choking, sleep-related abnormal, 371

Circadian testing, future of, 461–462

Confusional arousals, nocturnal movement in, 365

Continuous positive airway pressure, manual titration of, in patients with obstructive sleep apnea, **445–455**
    pediatric ventilator titration studies, 397

D

Daytime sleepiness, excessive, pediatric, polysomnography for, 397–398

Death, sudden cardiac, risk of, cardiac monitoring during polysomnography, 377

Dementia, and treatments for, polysomnographic features of, 415

Diaphragmatic electromyography, measurement of respiratory effort with, 355–356

Differential amplifiers, and associated filters, 328–331

Differential diagnosis, of nocturnal movements, 362

Drugs, pharmaceutical, effects on sleep architecture, 410–411
    sleep-related movement disorders related to, 364

E

Eating disorder, sleep-related, nocturnal movement in, 366

Effort, respiratory, measurement of, in diagnosis of sleep-disordered breathing, 354–356
    diaphragmatic EMG, 355–356
    esophageal pressure measurement, 355
    piezoelectric sensors, 355
    respiratory inductance plethysmography, 355

Electrocardiography (ECG, EKG), advanced signal processing in, 357
    artifacts on, 429–430
    cardiac rhythm evaluation by, 338–339
    of sleep, 327–328

Electrode popping, artifacts on polysomnography due to, 424–425

Electrode selector feature, avoiding polysomnography artifacts with, 434

Electrodes, in polysomnography, **333–341**
    airflow measurement, 337
    cardiac rhythm evaluation, 338–339
    electro-oculography, 335–336
    electroencephalogram and the 10-20 electrode system, 333–335
    electromyogram, 336–337

other monitoring devices, 339–340

oxygen saturation, 339

respiratory effort measurement, 337–338

sleep system modifications, 340

Electroencephalography (EEG), 10-20 electrode system and, 333–335
    monitoring in pediatric polysomnography, 399
    of sleep, 326–327

Electromagnetic interference, artifacts on polysomnography due to, 424

Electromyography (EMG), diaphragmatic, measurement of respiratory effort with, 355–356
    electrodes for, 336–337
    of sleep, 327–328

Electro-oculography (EOG), electrodes for, 335–336
    of sleep, 327–328

End tidal carbon dioxide, measurement of gas exchange with, 356

Epilepsy, nocturnal movements in, 366–368
    benign, of childhood, 367–368
    early or late onset occipital, 368
    juvenile myoclonic, 368
    nocturnal frontal lobe, 367
    sleep-related, 366–367

Esophageal pH, in pediatric polysomnography, 402

Esophageal pressure measurement, in measurement of respiratory effort, 355

Excessive daytime sleepiness, pediatric, polysomnography for, 397–398
    testing for, **385–393**
        alternative tests of sleepiness, 392
        clinical history, 385–386
        maintenance of wakefulness test, 390–391
        multiple sleep latency test, 386–390
        polysomnography, 386
        potential applications of tests, 391–392

Eye movement, artifact on polysomnography due to, 430

F

Filters, avoiding polysomnography artifacts with, 434
    differential amplifiers and, 328–331

Fluid-filled catheters, esophageal pressure measurement of respiratory effort, 355

Foot tremor, hypnagogic, and alternating leg muscle activation during sleep, 369

Fragmentary myoclonus, excessive, 370

Future, of sleep testing, **457–465**
    circadian testing, 461–462
    genetic testing, 463–464
    imaging in, 459–460
    in the home, 462–463
        diagnostic testing, 463
        screening for sleep disorders, 463
        sleep monitoring, 463

in the sleep laboratory, 457–459
    assessing psychiatric/neurological disease, 458–459
    phenotyping, 458
    sleep disorders, 457–458
sleep deprivation and performance, 462

G

Gas exchange measurement, in diagnosis of sleep-disordered breathing, 356
    carbon dioxide, 356
        arterial blood gas, 356
        end tidal, 356
        transcutaneous, 356
    oxygen, 356
        arterial blood gas, 356
        pulse oximetry, 356
        transcutaneous oximetry, 356
Gastrointestinal disease, and treatments for, polysomnographic features of, 416
Genetic testing, for sleep disorders, future of, 463–464

H

History, clinical, in diagnosis of nocturnal movements, 361
    of polysomnography, **313–321**
        from recording to scoring sleep, 316
            development of new scoring manual, 316
            Rechtschaffen and Kales Manual, 316
        of sleep staging, 343–344
        parallel growth of field of sleep technology, 318–319
        recording sleep, 313–315
            physiologic recordings of brain, 313
            physiologic recordings of sleep, 313–315
        role in development of sleep medicine, 316–318
            barriers to use of, 318
            growth of clinical application, 318
            narcolepsy, 316–317
            sleep apnea, 317–318
            Stanford Narcolepsy Clinic, 317
Home, sleep testing in, future of, 462–463
    diagnostic testing, 463
    screening for sleep disorders, 463
    sleep monitoring, 463
Hypnagogic foot tremor, and alternating leg muscle activation during sleep, 369

I

Imaging, in sleep medicine, future of, 459–461
Implanted medical devices, artifacts on polysomnography due to, 426

Infancy. *See also* Pediatrics.
    benign sleep myoclonus of, nocturnal movement in, 369
Ion channels, of the neuron, 324

J

Juvenile myoclonic epilepsy, nocturnal movement in, 368

L

Laboratory, sleep, creating a child-friendly, 398–399
    future of testing in, 457–459
        assessing psychiatric/neurological disease, 458–459
        phenotyping, 458
        sleep disorders, 457–458
Landau-Kleffner syndrome, nocturnal movement in, 368
Laryngospasm, sleep-related abnormal, 371
Leg cramps, sleep-related, diagnostic features, 363
    polysomnographic findings, 363
Leg muscle activation, alternating, during sleep, hypnagogic foot tremor and, 369
Lung disease, chronic pediatric, polysomnography for, 396

M

Maintenance of wakefulness test, for excessive daytime sleepiness, 390–391
    case study, 391
    potential applications of, 391–392
Malfunction, equipment, artifacts on polysomnography due to, 426
Medical devices, implanted, artifacts on polysomnography due to, 426
Medical disorders, and treatments for, polysomnographic features of, 415–417
    cardiovascular disease, 415–416
    common medications, 416–417
    gastrointestinal disorders, 416
    renal disease, 416
    rheumatologic illness, 416
    sleep-related movement disorders related to, 364
Medications, effects on sleep architecture, 410–411
Millar catheters, esophageal pressure measurement of respiratory effort, 355
Moisture, artifacts on polysomnography due to, 425–426
Monitoring. *See also* Polysomnography.
    cardiac, **373–384**
    portable, **437–444**
        considerations for usage, 441–443

Monitoring (*continued*)
 diagnostic accuracy, 438–441
 outcome studies using, 441
 timeline of, 437–438
 sleep, in the home, future of, 463
Montage display, avoiding polysomnography
 artifacts with, 435–436
Mood disorders, and treatments for,
 polysomnographic features of, 411–412
Movement artifact, on polysomnography, 428–429
Movements, body, in sleep staging, 349–350
 nocturnal, differentiation of, **361–372**
 approaching the diagnosis of, 361–362
 actigraphy and polysomnography, 362
 clinical history, 361
 physical examination, 361–362
 constructing a differential diagnosis, 362
 important diagnostic features and criteria,
 362–364
 drugs and substances, 364
 medical conditions, 364
 sleep-related movement disorders,
 362–364
 miscellaneous symptoms and conditions,
 368–371
 benign sleep myoclonus of infancy, 369
 excessive fragmentary myoclonus, 370
 hypnagogic foot tremor and alternating leg
 muscle activation during sleep, 369
 propriospinal myoclonus at sleep onset,
 369–370
 sleep starts, 368–369
 sleep-related abnormal swallowing, 371
 sleep-related breathing disorders, 370
 sleep disorders, 365–368
 neurologic disorders, 366–368
 parasomnias, 365–366
Multiple sleep latency test, for excessive daytime
 sleepiness, 386–390
 case study, 389–390
 potential applications of, 391–392
Muscle intrusion, artifacts on polysomnography due
 to, 426–428
Myoclonus, benign sleep, of infancy, nocturnal
 movement in, 369
 excessive fragmentary, 370
 propriospinal, at sleep onset, 369–370

N

Narcolepsy, history of polysomnography in,
 316–317
 Stanford Narcolepsy Clinic, 317
Nasal pressure cannula, airflow measurement using,
 354
Neurodegenerative disorders, and treatments for,
 polysomnographic features of, 415

Neurologic disorders, and treatments for,
 polysomnographic features of, 414–415
 dementias and other neurodegenerative
 disorders, 415
 Parkinson's disease, 414–415
 seizure disorders, 414
 nocturnal movements in, 366–368
 benign epilepsy of childhood, 367–368
 continuous spike waves during non-rapid eye
 movement sleep, 368
 early or late onset occipital epilepsy, 368
 juvenile myoclonic epilepsy, 368
 Landau-Kleffner syndrome, 368
 nocturnal frontal lobe epilepsy, 367
 sleep-related epilepsies, 366–367
Neurological disease, laboratory assessment by
 monitoring brain activity during sleep, future of,
 458–459
Neuromuscular disorders, pediatric,
 polysomnography for, 396
Neuron, physical and electrical properties, 323–325
Neurotransmitters, 325
Nightmare disorder, nocturnal movement in, 366
Nocturnal frontal lobe epilepsy, nocturnal movement
 in, 367
Nocturnal movements. *See* Movements, nocturnal.
Non-rapid eye movement sleep, continuous spike
 waves during, nocturnal movement in, 368
 in sleep staging, 346–348
 stage N1 sleep, 346
 stage N2 sleep, 346–348
 stage N3 sleep, 348

O

Obstructive sleep apnea, cardiac monitoring during
 polysomnography in patients with, 377–378
 manual titration of positive airway pressure in,
 445–455
 bilevel positive airway pressure titration
 guidelines, 449–450
 continuous positive airway pressure titration
 guidelines, 449
 general recommendations for, 447–449
 guidelines for grading of positive airway
 pressure titration studies, 450
 identifying and managing unintentional mask
 leaks, 450–451
 positional and sleep stage factors, 451–454
 pediatric, polysomnography for, 395
 portable monitoring for, 437–443
Occipital epilepsy, early of late onset, nocturnal
 movement in, 368
Onset, of sleep, problem of, in sleep staging, 346
Oxford Sleep Resistance Test, 392
Oximetry, in pediatric polysomnography, 399

Oxygen, gas exchange measurement, 356
    arterial blood gas, 356
    pulse oximetry, 356
    transcutaneous oximetry, 356

P

Parasomnias, nocturnal movements in, 365–366
    confusional arousals, 365
    nightmare disorder, 366
    rapid eye movement sleep behavior disorder, 365–366
    sleep terrors, 365
    sleep-related eating disorder, 366
    sleepwalking, 365
    pediatric, polysomnography for, 397
Parkinson's disease, and treatments for, polysomnographic features of, 414–415
Pediatrics, benign epilepsy of childhood with centrotemporal spikes, nocturnal movement in, 367–368
    benign sleep myoclonus of infancy, nocturnal movement in, 369
    juvenile myoclonic epilepsy, nocturnal movement in, 368
    polysomnography, **395–408**
        clinical implications of scoring, 406–407
        creating a child-friendly laboratory, 398–399
        indications for, 395–398
            ambulatory and unattended polysomnography, 398
            central apnea, periodic breathing, and central hypoventilation syndromes, 395–396
            chronic lung disease, 396
            continuous positive airway pressure ventilator titration studies, 397
            excessive daytime sleepiness, 397–398
            neuromuscular disorders, 396
            obstructive sleep apnea syndrome, 395
            parasomnias, 397
            restless legs syndrome and periodic limb movement disorder, 397
            tracheostomy decannulation, 397
        reproducibility of results, 406
        scoring, 402–405
            arousals, 404
            respiratory, 404–405
            sleep architecture, 402–404
        techniques, 399–402
            airflow monitoring, 399
            body position, 402
            capnometry, 401–402
            EEG monitoring, 399
            esophageal pH, 402
            oximetry, 399

            respiratory effort, 402
            videotaping, 402
        sleep staging considerations in, 350
Performance, sleep deprivation and, future of testing for, 462
Periodic breathing, pediatric, polysomnography for, 395–396
Periodic limb movement disorder, diagnostic features, 362–363
    pediatric, polysomnography for, 397
    polysomnographic findings, 363
Peripheral arterial tonometry, assessment of, in sleep-disordered breathing, 357–358
Phenotyping, in the sleep laboratory, future of, 458
Physical examination, in diagnosis of nocturnal movements, 361–372
Piezoelectric sensors, in measurement of respiratory effort, 355
Plethysmography, respiratory inductance, in measurement of respiratory effort, 355
Pneumotachograph, airflow measurement using, 354
Polysomnography, artifacts, **423–436**
    identifying, 423–424
    nonphysiologic, 424–426
    optimizing analysis, 434–436
    physiologic, 426–433
    troubleshooting, 433–434
    cardiac monitoring during sleep, **373–384**
        clinical scenarios, 377–380
        normal cardiac rhythm changes during sleep, 374–377
        standardized methods, 380–381
    electrodes, recording systems, and specifications for, **333–341**
        airflow measurement, 337
        cardiac rhythm evaluation, 338–339
        electro-oculography, 335–336
        electroencephalogram and the 10-20 electrode system, 333–335
        electromyogram, 336–337
        other monitoring devices, 339–340
        oxygen saturation, 339
        respiratory effort measurement, 337–338
        sleep system modifications, 340
    features of medical and psychiatric disorders and their treatments on, **409–421**
        drug effects on sleep architecture, 410–411
        medical disorders, 415–417
        neurologic disorders, 414–415
        psychiatric disorders, 411–414
    for excessive daytime sleepiness, **385–393**
        alternative tests of sleepiness, 392
        clinical history, 385–386
        maintenance of wakefulness test, 390–391
        multiple sleep latency test, 386–390
        potential applications of tests, 391–392
    future of sleep testing, **457–465**

Polysomnography (*continued*)
    circadian testing, 461–462
    genetic testing, 463–464
    imaging in, 459–460
    in the home, 462–463
    in the sleep laboratory, 457–459
    sleep deprivation and performance, 462
    generating a signal, **323–331**
        differential amplifier and associated filters,
            328–331
        electroencephalography of sleep, 326–327
        electromyogram, electrooculogrm, and EKG of
            sleep, 327–328
        neuron, physical and electrical properties of,
            323–325
        recording bipotentials, 325–326
    history of, **313–321**
        from recording to scoring sleep, 316
        parallel growth of field of sleep technology,
            318–319
        recording sleep, 313–315
        role in development of sleep medicine,
            316–318
            barriers to use of, 318
            growth of clinical application, 318
            narcolepsy, 316–317
            sleep apnea, 317–318
            Stanford Narcolepsy Clinic, 317
    manual titration of positive airway pressure in
        obstructive sleep apnea, **445–455**
        bilevel positive airway pressure titration
            guidelines, 449–450
        continuous positive airway pressure titration
            guidelines, 449
        general recommendations for, 447–449
        guidelines for grading of positive airway
            pressure titration studies, 450
        identifying and managing unintentional mask
            leaks, 450–451
        positional and sleep stage factors, 451–454
    nocturnal movements, differentiation of, **361–372**
        approaching the diagnosis of, 361–362
        constructing a differential diagnosis, 362
        important diagnostic features and criteria,
            362–364
            drugs and substances, 364
            medical conditions, 364
            sleep-related movement disorders,
                362–364
        miscellaneous symptoms and conditions,
            368–371
            benign sleep myoclonus of infancy, 369
            excessive fragmentary myoclonus, 370
            hypnagogic foot tremor and alternating leg
                muscle activation during sleep, 369
            propriospinal myoclonus at sleep onset,
                369–370

        sleep starts, 368–369
        sleep-related abnormal swallowing, 371
        sleep-related breathing disorders, 370
    sleep disorders, 365–368
        neurologic disorders, 366–368
        parasomnias, 365–366
    pediatric, **395–408**
        clinical implications of scoring, 406–407
        creating a child-friendly laboratory, 398–399
        indications for, 395–398
        reproducibility of results, 406
        scoring, 402–405
        techniques, 399–402
    portable monitoring, **437–444**
        considerations for usage, 441–443
        diagnostic accuracy, 438–441
        outcome studies using, 441
        timeline of, 437–438
    respiratory monitoring, **353–360**
        airflow measurement, 353–354
        definitions, 358–359
        effort measurement, 354–356
        gas exchange measurement, 356
        new applications of old technology, 357
        new technology, 357–358
    staging sleep, **343–352**
        derivations and montages, 344–345
        future trends, 350
        historic survey, 343–344
        major body movements, 349–350
        pediatric considerations, 350
        terminology and scoring principles, 345–349
            non-rapid eye movement sleep, 346–348
            rapid eye movement sleep, 348–349
            wakefulness, 345–346
Polyvinyl fluoride film airflow sensors, 354
Portable monitoring, for polysomnography, **437–444**
    considerations for usage, 441–443
    diagnostic accuracy, 438–441
    outcome studies using, 441
    timeline of, 437–438
Position, body, in pediatric polysomnography, 402
Positive airway pressure, manual titration of, in
    obstructive sleep apnea, **445–455**
    bilevel positive airway pressure titration
        guidelines, 449–450
    continuous positive airway pressure titration
        guidelines, 449
    general recommendations for, 447–449
    guidelines for grading of positive airway
        pressure titration studies, 450
    identifying and managing unintentional mask
        leaks, 450–451
    positional and sleep stage factors, 451–454
Propriospinal myoclonus, at sleep onset, 369–370
Psychiatric disorders, and treatments for,
    polysomnographic features of, 411–414

anxiety disorders, 412–413
   mood disorders, 411–412
   psychotic disorders, 413–414
  laboratory assessment by monitoring brain activity
   during sleep, future of, 458–459
Psychotic disorders, and treatments for,
  polysomnographic features of, 413–414
Pulse oximetry, advanced signal processing in, 357
  measurement of gas exchange with, 356
Pulse transit time, assessment of, in sleep-disordered
  breathing, 357
Pupillometry, 392

R

Rapid eye movement sleep, in sleep staging,
  348–349
Rapid eye movement sleep behavior disorder,
  nocturnal movement in, 365–366
Rechtschaffen and Kales Manual, 316
Recording systems, for sleep. See
  Polysomnography.
Renal disease, and treatments for, polysomnographic
  features of, 416
Reproducibility, of pediatric polysomnography
  results, 406
Respiratory effort, in pediatric polysomnography, 402
  measurement in polysomnography, 337–338
Respiratory inductance plethysmography, in
  measurement of respiratory effort, 355
Respiratory monitoring, in diagnosis of
  sleep-disordered breathing, **353–360**
   airflow measurement, 353–354
    nasal pressure cannula, 354
    pneumotachograph, 354
    thermal technology, 353–354
   definitions, 358–359
   effort measurement, 354–356
    diaphragmatic EMG, 355–356
    esophageal pressure measurement, 355
    piezoelectric sensors, 355
    respiratory inductance plethysmography,
     355
   gas exchange measurement, 356
    carbon dioxide, 356
    oxygen, 356
   new applications of old technology, 357
    advanced signal processing of ECG, 357
    advanced signal processing of pulse
     oximetry, 357
   new technology, 357–358
    peripheral arterial tonometry, 357–358
    pulse transit time, 357
Respiratory scoring, in pediatric polysomnography,
  404–405
Restless legs syndrome, pediatric, polysomnography
  for, 397

Rheumatologic illness, and treatments for,
  polysomnographic features of, 416
Rhythmic movement disorders, sleep-related,
  diagnostic features, 364
  polysomnographic features, 364

S

Scoring, polysomnography, pediatric, 402–405
  clinical implications of, 406–407
  See also Staging.
Screening, for sleep disorders, in the home, 463
Seizure disorders, and treatments for,
  polysomnographic features of, 414
Sleep, onset of, problem in sleep staging, 346
  recording of. See Polysomnography.
  staging, **343–352**
   derivations and montages, 344–345
   historic survey, 343–344
   major body movements, 349–350
   terminology and scoring principles, 345–349
    non-rapid eye movement sleep, 346–348
    rapid eye movement sleep, 348–349
    wakefulness, 345–346
Sleep apnea, cardiac monitoring during
  polysomnography in patients with obstructive,
  377–378
  central, pediatric, polysomnography for, 395–396
  history of polysomnography in, 317–318
  manual titration of positive airway pressure in
   patients with obstructive, **445–455**
  obstructive, portable monitoring for, 437–443
  pediatric obstructive, polysomnography for, 395
Sleep architecture, drug effects on, 410–411
  in pediatric polysomnography scoring, 402–404
Sleep deprivation, performance and, future of testing
  for, 462
Sleep disorders, nocturnal movements in, 365–368
   neurologic disorders, 366–368
    benign epilepsy of childhood, 367–368
    continuous spike waves during non-rapid
     eye movement sleep, 368
    early or late onset occipital epilepsy, 368
    juvenile myoclonic epilepsy, 368
    Landau-Kleffner syndrome, 368
    nocturnal frontal lobe epilepsy, 367
    sleep-related epilepsies, 366–367
   parasomnias, 365–366
    confusional arousals, 365
    nightmare disorder, 366
    rapid eye movement sleep behavior
     disorder, 365–366
    sleep terrors, 365
    sleep-related eating disorder, 366
    sleepwalking, 365
  screening for, in the home, 463
  testing in the sleep laboratory, future of, 457–458

Sleep medicine, role of polysomnography in development of, 316–318

Sleep monitoring, in the home, future of, 463

Sleep starts, nocturnal movement in, 368–369

Sleep technology, field of, history of growth of, 318–319

Sleep terrors, nocturnal movement in, 365

Sleep-disordered breathing, portable monitoring for, 437–443
respiratory monitoring in diagnosis of, **353–360**

Sleep-related breathing disorders, manual titration of positive airway pressure in patients with, **445–455**

Sleep-related epilepsies, nocturnal movement in, 366–367

Sleep-related movement disorders, important diagnostic features, 362–364
bruxism, 364
leg cramps, 363
periodic limb movement disorder, 362–363
rhythmic movement disorder, 364

Sleepiness, excessive daytime, pediatric, polysomnography for, 397–398

Sleepiness, excessive daytime, testing for, **385–393**
alternative tests of sleepiness, 392
clinical history, 385–386
maintenance of wakefulness test, 390–391
multiple sleep latency test, 386–390
polysomnography, 386
potential applications of tests, 391–392

Sleepwalking, 365

Staging, sleep, **343–352**
derivations and montages, 344–345
historic survey, 343–344
major body movements, 349–350
terminology and scoring principles, 345–349
non-rapid eye movement sleep, 346–348
rapid eye movement sleep, 348–349
wakefulness, 345–346

Stanford Narcolepsy Clinic, history of, 317

Starts, sleep, nocturnal movement in, 368–369

Stimulants, sleep-related movement disorders related to, 364

Sudden cardiac death, risk of, cardiac monitoring during polysomnography, 377

Swallowing, sleep-related abnormal, 371

Sweat sway, artifact on polysomnography due to, 430–433

T

Techniques, polysomnographic, for pediatric patients, 399–402

Terrors, sleep, nocturnal movement in, 365

Thermal technology, in measurement of airflow, 353–354
polyvinyl fluoride film airflow sensors, 354

Tonometry, peripheral arterial, assessment of, in sleep-disordered breathing, 357–358

Tracheostomy decannulation, pediatric, polysomnography for, 397

Transcutaneous carbon dioxide, measurement of gas exchange with, 356

Transcutaneous oximetry, measurement of gas exchange with, 356

Troubleshooting, artifacts and, on polysomnography, **423–436**

U

Unattended polysomnography, pediatric, 398

V

Videotaping, in pediatric polysomnography, 402

W

Wakefulness, in sleep staging, 345–346
criteria for, 345–346
problem of sleep onset, 346

Moving?

Make sure your subscription moves with you!

To notify us of your new address, find your **Clinics Account Number** (located on your mailing label above your name), and contact customer service at:

Email: journalscustomerservice-usa@elsevier.com

800-654-2452 (subscribers in the U.S. & Canada)
314-447-8871 (subscribers outside of the U.S. & Canada)

Fax number: 314-447-8029

Elsevier Health Sciences Division
Subscription Customer Service
3251 Riverport Lane
Maryland Heights, MO 63043

*To ensure uninterrupted delivery of your subscription, please notify us at least 4 weeks in advance of move.